I0894736

Integrating Oral and General Health Epidemiology Through Data Science and AI:

EpiDentomics

Muhammad Farooq Umer
Department of Preventive Dental Sciences, College of Dentistry, King Faisal University, Hofuf, Saudi Arabia

IGI Global
Scientific Publishing
Publishing Tomorrow's Research Today

Vice President of Editorial	Melissa Wagner
Director of Acquisitions	Mikaela Felty
Director of Book Development	Jocelynn Hessler
Production Manager	Mike Brehm
Cover Design	Jose Rosado

Published in the United States of America by
IGI Global Scientific Publishing
701 East Chocolate Avenue
Hershey, PA, 17033, USA
Tel: 717-533-8845 | Fax: 717-533-7115
Website: https://www.igi-global.com E-mail: cust@igi-global.com

Library of Congress Cataloging-in-Publication Data

Names: Umer, Muhammad Farooq, 1979- editor
Title: Integrating oral and general health epidemiology through data science and AI : epiDentomics / edited by Muhammad Farooq Umer.
Other titles: EpiDentomics
Description: Hershey, PA : IGI Global Scientific Publishing, [2027] | Includes bibliographical references and index. | Summary: "This book integrates oral and general health epidemiology through the transformative lens of data science, artificial intelligence, and digital health analytics. This book introduces a unified paradigm-EpiDentomics-that conceptualizes oral health as an integral part of systemic well-being, moving beyond the traditional siloed approaches in epidemiological research. Combining population-based methodologies with machine learning, predictive modeling, and digital surveillance, EpiDentomics demonstrates how oral-systemic interconnections can guide precision prevention, policymaking, and global health strategies"-- Provided by publisher.
Identifiers: LCCN 2026015572 (print) | LCCN 2026015573 (ebook) | ISBN 9798337384023 h/c | ISBN 9798337384030 s/c | ISBN 9798337384047 ebook
Subjects: LCSH: Teeth--Diseases--Epidemiology | Epidemiology--Data processing | Dentistry--Data processing | Dental public health | Artificial intelligence--Medical applications
Classification: LCC RK305 .I568 2026 (print) | LCC RK305 (ebook)
LC record available at https://lccn.loc.gov/2026015572
LC ebook record available at https://lccn.loc.gov/2026015573

British Cataloguing in Publication Data
A Cataloguing in Publication record for this book is available from the British Library.

This book is lovingly dedicated to my family, whose unwavering love, encouragement, and sacrifices have been the foundation of every milestone in my academic and professional journey.

To my beloved parents, my cherished wife, my three wonderful children, and my dear siblings—thank you for your constant support, patience, and faith in me. Your strength, kindness, and inspiration have sustained me throughout this journey and continue to motivate me in the pursuit of knowledge and service.

This work is a tribute to all of you, with my deepest love, gratitude, and respect.

Table of Contents

Detailed Table of Contents

EpiDentomics is an emerging interdisciplinary field that integrates epidemiology, dentistry, and multi-omics to provide a more comprehensive understanding of oral diseases. Unlike traditional approaches that focus on isolated risk factors, this framework considers the interaction between genetic, microbial, environmental, and behavioral determinants. Recent advances in high-throughput technologies and data analytics have enabled the exploration of complex biological mechanisms and their population-level implications. This chapter outlines the foundations, evolution, and core components of EpiDentomics, highlighting its role in disease prediction, risk assessment, and precision oral healthcare. It also discusses current challenges, including data integration, ethical considerations, and the translation of research findings into clinical and public health practice. Overall, EpiDentomics represents a promising shift toward more integrated and personalized approaches in oral health research and care.

Epidemiological principles provide the foundation for understanding, preventing, and controlling diseases across populations, including the growing burden of oral conditions and their links with systemic health. This chapter presents a comprehensive overview of core epidemiological concepts applied to both oral and general health, emphasizing their relevance in contemporary public health practice. Key measures of disease frequency and association, such as incidence, prevalence, risk ratios, and population-attributable fractions, are discussed alongside their interpretation for clinical and policy decision-making. The chapter further explores confounding, bias, and effect modification, highlighting strategies to ensure valid and reliable inference. Disease causation is framed through multicausal models, including the web of causation and social determinants of health, integrating behavioral and environmental influences across the life course. Together, these principles support evidence-informed interventions, implementation strategies, and health policy development globally.

Muhammad Farooq Umer, Department of Preventive Dental Sciences, College of Dentistry, King Faisal University, Hofuf, Saudi Arabia

The global burden of oral and systemic diseases shows a major public health challenge, presenting intricate connections between social, biological, and environmental factors. Over recent years, epidemiological transitions have led to a change from communicable to non-communicable diseases, with oral conditions, for instance, dental caries, periodontal disease, and oral cancers remaining highly prevalent globally. They are deeply connected with systemic diseases, which include diabetes mellitus, cardiovascular illnesses, and respiratory infections, reflecting a reciprocal relationship that worsens the global burden of disease. Currently, trends reveal that there continue to be inconsistencies in the distribution of disease, which are generally affecting underdeveloped nations and marginalized communities. Inadequate healthcare facilities, socio-economic differences, insufficient knowledge regarding health issues, and imbalance in resource distribution cause these disparities.

Muhammad Mohsin Javaid, School of Dentistry, Shaheed Zulfiqar Ali Bhutto Medical University, Islamabad, Pakistan & School of Public Health, Health Services Academy Islamabad, Pakistan
Hasan Mujtaba, School of Dentistry, Shaheed Zulfiqar Ali Bhutto Medical University, Islamabad, Pakistan
Najam Ul Hassan, School of Dentistry, Shaheed Zulfiqar Ali Bhutto Medical University, Islamabad, Pakistan
Muhammad Shoaib, Multan Medical and Dental College, Ibne Sina Hospital, Multan, Pakistan
Shahzad Ahmad, The University of Buckingham, Buckingham, UK

The shared risk factor approach (SRFA) provides a comprehensive framework that can effectively manage the growing global burden of oral and systemic diseases using a common modifiable risk factors approach. Oral health and major non-

This chapter explores digital Public Health Campaigns, social media epidemiology and nudging for oral and systemic health promotion and also demonstrates the rise of "digital persuasion ecosystems", public health environments driven by social media data, real-time surveillance, AI-enabled communication, and behavioural science models. As global health systems move toward precision public health and data-informed decision-making, digital campaigns have grown more impactful, reshaping how health education is created, delivered, and consumed. Within the broader EpiDentomics framework, digital public health becomes a central pillar for preventing both oral diseases and systemic conditions connected to oral health.

This chapter examines the bidirectional relationship between oral hygiene and mental health through a comprehensive review of current evidence on psychodental interactions. It synthesizes epidemiological findings, biological mechanisms, behavioural pathways, psychosocial consequences, and shared social determinants linking oral health and psychological wellbeing. This chapter further discusses the influence of mental illness on oral hygiene behaviours, identifies vulnerable populations, and explores emerging innovations, including digital health and integrated models of care. An Integrated Psychodental Framework is proposed to illustrate the multidirectional pathways connecting oral hygiene, biological mediators, mental health outcomes, and broader social determinants. This chapter highlights the importance of interdisciplinary collaboration and holistic healthcare approaches to improve oral health, mental wellbeing, and future research in psychodentistry.

R. Alfiya Roofi, Department of Microbiology, Sacred Heart College, Tirupattur, India
B. Lokeshwari, Department of Microbiology, Sacred Heart College, Tirupattur, India
P. Saranraj, Department of Microbiology, Sacred Heart College, Tirupattur, India
A. Mubarak Ali, Department of Microbiology, Sacred Heart College, Tirupattur, India
S. Mayilazhagan, Department of Microbiology, Sacred Heart College, Tirupattur, India

Oral mucositis (OM) is a pain and suffering condition associated with cancer treatment, negatively affecting the patient's quality of life and treatment outcomes. The oral cavity houses the second largest community of microbes in the human body, and the perturbation of this microbiome has been shown to be associated with many systemic diseases, including cardiovascular, diabetes, and inflammatory diseases. Studies of transcriptome and proteome of Candida albicans infection have identified immune responses in hosts and strategies used by fungi to escape, offering targets for potential therapies. Although there have been remarkable developments in the field, there are still challenges such as cost, lack of standardization, and need for validation studies.

Artificial intelligence (AI) is rapidly transforming oral healthcare by enabling the integration of diverse oral biomarkers with systemic health information for more accurate, preventive, and personalized clinical decision-making. This chapter explores the potential applications of machine learning, deep learning, natural language processing and predictive analytics in analyzing multimodal data, such as dental radiographs, intraoral images, electronic health records, salivary protein profiles, oral microbiome, genomic data, outputs from wearable sensors, and patient-reported data. Standardized collection of data, clear model development, prospective multicenter validation, data sharing systems, and ongoing professional supervision are needed to overcome these barriers. AI offers a promising pathway toward predictive, preventive, personalized, and participatory healthcare, while strengthening the role of oral health as an essential component of whole-body medicine.

Studies on oral health at the population level are changing through artificial intelligence and data science. This chapter argues that integrating dental imaging data, electronic health records, and systemic outcome registries creates new opportunities for epidemiological research through the EpiDentomics framework. These advances move beyond minor adjustments to current survey techniques and may lead to a structural shift in the measurement, tracking, and correlation of oral

Preface

INTRODUCTION

The convergence of oral health, systemic medicine, epidemiology, artificial intelligence (AI), and data science is reshaping the future of population health research. Historically, oral health has remained largely separated from mainstream epidemiological investigations despite overwhelming evidence demonstrating its intimate relationship with chronic systemic diseases, including diabetes mellitus, cardiovascular disease, respiratory disorders, neurodegenerative conditions, and adverse pregnancy outcomes. Simultaneously, advances in genomics, microbiome science, digital health technologies, electronic health records, wearable sensors, and machine learning have created unprecedented opportunities to study health as an interconnected biological and societal phenomenon.

This book, Integrating Oral and General Health Epidemiology Through Data Science and AI: EpiDentomics, introduces EpiDentomicsas an emerging interdisciplinary paradigm that integrates oral health epidemiology, systemic disease epidemiology, multi-omics, digital technologies, and artificial intelligence into a unified scientific framework. Rather than treating oral diseases as isolated clinical entities, EpiDentomics recognizes them as integral components of whole-body health influenced by complex interactions among biological, behavioral, environmental, social, and technological determinants.

To our knowledge, this is the first edited volume dedicated exclusively to integrating oral epidemiology, systemic health, artificial intelligence, and data science within a unified conceptual framework.

The objective of this volume is to provide researchers, clinicians, epidemiologists, public health professionals, educators, policymakers, and data scientists with a comprehensive understanding of how contemporary epidemiology is evolving through digital innovation and interdisciplinary collaboration. The chapters examine both theoretical foundations and practical applications, covering epidemiological methods, global disease burden, shared risk factor approaches, digital epidemiology, AI-enabled surveillance, biomarker integration, imaging analytics, omics sciences, behavioral sciences, health communication, and precision population health.

A distinguishing feature of this book is its emphasis on integrating diverse sources of health information, including clinical records, dental imaging, omics data, microbiome profiles, wearable technologies, environmental exposures, and real-time digital surveillance, through advanced computational methods. Artificial intelligence serves not merely as an analytical tool but as an enabling technology capable of transforming disease prediction, personalized prevention, healthcare delivery, and public health decision-making.

Beyond technological advances, the contributors emphasize critical issues surrounding ethics, data governance, interoperability, equity, explainable AI, and global health policy. The vision of EpiDentomics extends beyond improving diagnostic accuracy; it seeks to establish a comprehensive ecosystem in which oral and systemic health are monitored, understood, and managed through integrated data infrastructures that support evidence-based interventions across clinical and population settings.

This volume brings together contributions from internationally recognized researchers representing multiple disciplines and geographical regions. Their collective expertise reflects the global nature of contemporary health challenges and the necessity of collaborative, multidisciplinary solutions. We hope this work serves as both a foundational reference and an inspiration for future research, innovation, and policy development that bridges dentistry, medicine, epidemiology, computer science, and public health.

As healthcare increasingly moves toward predictive, preventive, personalized, and participatory models, EpiDentomics offers a timely and forward-looking framework for understanding health across the oral–systemic continuum. It is my sincere hope that this book will stimulate new collaborations, encourage interdisciplinary thinking, and contribute to advancing integrated population health for future generations.

The successful completion of this volume reflects the dedication and expertise of the contributing authors, whose scholarly efforts have made this interdisciplinary work possible. I sincerely thank each contributor for sharing their knowledge and commitment to advancing oral and systemic health research. I am also grateful to the editorial team at IGI Global Scientific Publishing for their guidance and support throughout the development of this book.

CHAPTER OVERVIEW

This book is organized into thirteen interconnected chapters that progressively build the conceptual, methodological, technological, and clinical foundations of EpiDentomics.

Chapter 1 introduces the foundations of EpiDentomics by tracing its evolution from traditional oral epidemiology toward an integrated framework combining epidemiology, dentistry, multi-omics, and data science. The chapter establishes the conceptual basis for precision oral healthcare while discussing opportunities and challenges associated with data integration and translational research.

Chapter 2 reviews the core principles of epidemiology relevant to oral and systemic health. Fundamental concepts including disease frequency, measures of association, causal inference, confounding, bias, effect modification, and social determinants of health are presented as essential tools for evidence-based clinical and public health decision-making.

Chapter 3 examines the global burden of oral and systemic diseases, emphasizing epidemiological transitions, health inequalities, and socioeconomic disparities that shape disease distribution worldwide. The chapter highlights the interconnected nature of oral diseases and chronic non-communicable diseases while discussing implications for global health policy.

Chapter 4 explores the Shared Risk Factor Approach (SRFA), demonstrating how common behavioral and environmental determinants simultaneously influence oral diseases and major systemic conditions. Particular emphasis is placed on the periodontal–cardiovascular–diabetes triad and the development of integrated policy frameworks that promote health equity and resource optimization.

Chapter 5 investigates the digital transformation of epidemiology through big data, cloud computing, Internet of Things technologies, and real-time surveillance systems. The chapter illustrates how digital infrastructures facilitate integrated oral-systemic epidemiological research while addressing privacy, ethics, interoperability, and emerging computational approaches such as federated learning.

Chapter 6 presents the EpiDentomic paradigm as a novel epidemiological model situated at the oral–systemic–digital interface. Integrating systems epidemiology, artificial intelligence, and global health policy, the chapter proposes an Oral Systemic Digital Epidemiology Nexus that links biological, behavioral, environmental, and digital determinants across multiple levels of healthcare.

Chapter 7 introduces the concept of a Global EpiDentomic Observatory, describing how AI-driven surveillance, predictive analytics, and international collaboration can transform epidemiological research while simultaneously promoting educational innovation through data-driven learning environments and knowledge exchange.

Chapter 8 focuses on digital health communication, behavioral science, and technology-enabled nudging strategies within the EpiDentomics framework. The chapter examines how artificial intelligence, social media analytics, and precision public health campaigns can enhance oral-systemic disease prevention, health promotion, and population engagement.

Chapter 9 explores the bidirectional relationship between oral hygiene and mental health through the emerging field of psychodental epidemiology. An integrated framework is presented to explain the biological, behavioral, psychosocial, and social determinants that connect oral conditions with psychological well-being and overall quality of life.

Chapter 10 examines integrative multi-omics approaches for understanding oral-systemic health relationships. Drawing upon genomics, transcriptomics, proteomics, metabolomics, and microbiome research, the chapter discusses how molecular epidemiology contributes to biomarker discovery, disease mechanisms, and precision medicine while identifying current methodological challenges.

Chapter 11 investigates the integration of oral biomarkers with systemic health data using artificial intelligence. Machine learning applications involving dental imaging, salivary diagnostics, microbiome profiling, electronic health records, wearable technologies, and predictive analytics are presented as important components of personalized healthcare and precision epidemiology.

Chapter 12 reviews the expanding role of artificial intelligence in dental radiographic and clinical epidemiology. Deep learning, cone-beam computed tomography (CBCT), cephalometric analysis, explainable AI, and image-based diagnostics are examined for their contributions to large-scale epidemiological studies and improved understanding of oral-systemic disease relationships.

Chapter 13 concludes the volume by exploring AI-driven epidemiology in endodontic and restorative diseases. The chapter demonstrates how predictive modeling, radiographic analytics, and electronic health record integration strengthen our understanding of oral infections and their associations with cardiovascular disease, diabetes, inflammatory disorders, and other systemic health outcomes, illustrating the practical application of the EpiDentomics framework in precision healthcare.

CONCLUSION

Collectively, these chapters establish EpiDentomics as a transformative interdisciplinary field that unites epidemiology, dentistry, artificial intelligence, omics sciences, and digital health technologies. Together they provide a comprehensive roadmap for future research, clinical innovation, public health practice, and policy development aimed at advancing integrated oral and systemic health worldwide.

Acknowledgment

Funding Statement The Deanship of Scientific Research, Vice Presidency supported this Book for Graduate Studies and Scientific Research, King Faisal University, Saudi Arabia. [Project Number: KFU264122].

Chapter 1
Introduction to EpiDentomics:
Foundations, Evolution, and Conceptual Framework

Amany Osama Kassem
http://orcid.org/0009-0001-2968-5336
Riyadh Elm University, Saudi Arabia

Shumaila Zofeen
http://orcid.org/0000-0003-3190-7548
Xi'an Jiaotong University, China

ABSTRACT

EpiDentomics is an emerging interdisciplinary field that integrates epidemiology, dentistry, and multi-omics to provide a more comprehensive understanding of oral diseases. Unlike traditional approaches that focus on isolated risk factors, this framework considers the interaction between genetic, microbial, environmental, and behavioral determinants. Recent advances in high-throughput technologies and data analytics have enabled the exploration of complex biological mechanisms and their population-level implications. This chapter outlines the foundations, evolution, and core components of EpiDentomics, highlighting its role in disease prediction, risk assessment, and precision oral healthcare. It also discusses current challenges, including data integration, ethical considerations, and the translation of research findings into clinical and public health practice. Overall, EpiDentomics represents a promising shift toward more integrated and personalized approaches in oral health research and care.

DOI: 10.4018/979-8-3373-8402-3.ch001

1. INTRODUCTION

Oral health plays an integral role in overall well-being. Poor oral health negatively influences chewing, speech, and socialization; therefore, it affects one's quality of life (Petersen, 2003). Despite the development of effective measures for disease prevention and treatment, oral diseases, including tooth decay, periodontal conditions, and oral cancer, continue to prevail worldwide (Peres et al., 2019). These diseases pose both health and economic risks (Peres et al., 2019). Most oral diseases are preventable, yet they are associated with multiple biological, behavioral, environmental, and social determinants (Peres et al., 2019).

Conventional epidemiological studies are commonly used to investigate the transmission and causation of oral diseases in populations. Such research draws attention to modifiable risk factors, such as poor oral hygiene, unhealthy dietary habits, tobacco consumption, and poverty. Epidemiology can facilitate disease prevention and control in public health (Friis & Sellers, 2021). However, the identification of specific biological determinants of oral diseases remains beyond the scope of epidemiology due to the individual differences in the disease mechanisms (Divaris, 2016).

With recent rapid advancements in biomedical science, innovative approaches to investigating diseases were needed. Multi-omics science encompasses genomics, epigenomics, transcriptomics, proteomics, and microbiomics (Hasin et al., 2017). The use of high-throughput technologies allows researchers to study biological systems in detail at the molecular level, thereby increasing understanding of disease processes (Hasin et al., 2017). Investigations of oral health conditions via multi-omics helped to reveal the interaction between the host and its microbiome, immune system regulation, and molecular mechanisms underlying the initiation, progression, and treatment of diseases, such as cavities and periodontitis (Kilian et al., 2016). The oral cavity is the habitat of a highly diverse range of microorganisms that function as a bridge between the body and the external environment (Kilian et al., 2016).

These significant developments fostered the emergence of EpiDentomics as an interdisciplinary scientific methodology for advancing knowledge about oral diseases and related clinical practices (Kau et al., 2011). EpiDentomics represents a novel way to explore oral diseases by integrating epidemiology and multi-omics (Divaris et al., 2017).

The advent of EpiDentomics aligns with the recent changes in modern healthcare toward precision medicine that aims to prevent, diagnose, and treat individuals in accordance with their biological uniqueness and environmental characteristics (Collins & Varmus, 2015). In turn, the transition to precision oral health care strives to advance risk assessment, early diagnosis, and targeted interventions (Giannobile & Lang, 2016).

From the perspective of population health, EpiDentomics contributes to the identification of factors associated with oral disease risk and the development of preventive strategies informed by scientific evidence (Peres et al., 2019). Furthermore, it improves our understanding of oral health disparities (Friis & Sellers, 2021). Nevertheless, the adoption of the new paradigm faces various methodological and practical barriers, including data integration and ethics (Manolio et al., 2015).

2. FOUNDATIONS OF EPIDENTOMICS

This study aims to review the concept of EpiDentomics which is an interdisciplinary field that combines elements of epidemiology, dentistry, and omics sciences to understand oral diseases comprehensively. Traditionally, oral health research has involved epidemiology and dentistry but not their combination with omics sciences (Petersen, 2003; Peres et al., 2019; Hasin et al., 2017). As a result, understanding the interaction of genetic, microbial, environmental, and behavioral risk factors in oral disease pathogenesis was not well understood. In addition, EpiDentomics is part of the current shift to precision medicine (Collins & Varmus, 2015).

As mentioned earlier, EpiDentomics uses epidemiology which is a scientific discipline that focuses on studying the occurrence and determinants of diseases in populations (Rothman et al., 2008). Historically, epidemiology has been critical in the identification of risk factors associated with oral diseases, including diet, smoking, and social environment (Peres et al., 2019). Various epidemiological designs, such as cross-sectional and cohort studies, have enhanced our knowledge about the global patterns of oral diseases (Petersen & Baez, 2013). Nevertheless, it is unable to explain the biology of those associations (Wild, 2005).

In contrast, dentistry is an academic discipline that involves diagnosis, prevention, and management of oral diseases (Fejerskov & Kidd, 2008). Clinicians play a crucial role in elucidating the course of a disease and its response to treatment (Newman et al., 2019). Also, the practice of dentistry generates valuable patient data that can be used for further analysis. Nonetheless, traditional dentistry emphasizes treatment and does not consider omic information.

Genomics, proteomics, metabolomics, and microbiomics are parts of omics sciences that constitute another pillar of EpiDentomics (Hasin et al., 2017). The former allows determining susceptibility to disease because of specific mutations (Vieira, 2012). In addition, omics science recognizes the importance of the oral microbiome in the formation of certain conditions like caries and periodontal disease (Kilian et al., 2016; Dewhirst et al., 2010). Finally, proteomics and metabolomics help to uncover the underlying molecular mechanisms (Nicholson et al., 2012). At the same time, omics data must be placed into appropriate context (Ginsburg & Willard, 2009).

Integration of the discussed disciplines is vital since oral diseases depend on various biological, behavioral, and environmental factors whose relationship is intricate. In turn, traditional approaches examine those determinants individually which limits the depth of the understanding of oral diseases (Wild, 2005). EpiDentomics can combine different data sets and link molecular aspects with trends in populations (Khoury et al., 2013). As a consequence, such research improves the ability to predict risk, detect early signs, and deliver appropriate intervention (Ashley, 2016).

Also, conventional studies suffer from such problems as use of self-reported data, focusing on separate risk factors, and failure to validate findings biologically (Ioannidis, 2005). On one hand, epidemiological research can be subject to bias and confounding. On the other hand, clinical investigations often lack generalizability. Besides, omics research produces complicated results requiring careful consideration (Hasin et al., 2017). These facts indicate the need for integration in studying oral diseases (Khoury et al., 2013).

The interdisciplinary nature of EpiDentomics helps to adopt a systems perspective for understanding oral diseases. Such perspective facilitates the development of precision dentistry when treatments are customized based on patients' biological features (Divaris, 2016). For example, integration of genomic and microbiome data can increase the accuracy of detecting individuals at high risk of developing periodontal disease (Kilian et al., 2016). In turn, EpiDentomics has great public health significance due to disease surveillance and informing policymakers about evidence-based practices (Petersen & Baez, 2013). It can enable the discovery of biomarkers for disease diagnosis and evaluation of interventions (Ashley, 2016). In such a way, it offers an all-inclusive approach to oral diseases (Watt et al., 2019).

To sum up, EpiDentomics uses epidemiology, dentistry, and omics sciences to avoid weaknesses of other research paradigms and develop a holistic view of oral diseases (Peres et al., 2019).

3. EVOLUTION OF EPIDENTOMICS

The evolution of EpiDentomics can be seen as one of the paradigm shifts in the history of research in oral health that moved it from the traditional descriptive epidemiology toward integrative and more biologically informed paradigms. The early period in oral epidemiology involved studying the distribution and determinants of oral diseases through clinical indicators (e.g., DMFT and periodontal measures) and observational designs (Petersen, 2003; Peres et al., 2019). Those methods made it possible to determine key risk factors for oral diseases, such as dietary habits, oral hygiene, smoking, and socio-economic inequalities, and identify them as a significant global public health problem (Peres et al., 2019; Watt et al., 2019). However, the aforementioned paradigm is limited due to the reliance on clinical and self-reported measures, bias and confounding, and lack of consideration for risk factors as part of a system (Ioannidis, 2005; Rothman et al., 2008). Besides, it cannot account for the biological mechanisms involved in disease development and progression, thus failing to explain individual variations in vulnerability and outcome (Wild, 2012).

The subsequent stage of oral health investigation included molecular biology. With this technique, it was possible to study genetic, cellular, and biochemical pathways associated with the development of various diseases (Collins & Varmus, 2015). Applying molecular biology techniques for studying oral diseases helped understand how a particular genetic profile of an individual could predispose one to the development of diseases such as dental caries and periodontitis, enhanced knowledge regarding inflammation mechanisms and defense reactions, as well as elucidated the ways pathogens and hosts interacted (Vieira, 2012; Kinane et al., 2017). However, molecular biological studies were usually conducted without reference to population-based approaches, which negatively affected their applicability within public health (Wild, 2012).

Next, multi-omics techniques emerged. Multi-omics refers to the ability to conduct a multi-scale analysis of biological systems, including genomics, transcriptomics, proteomics, metabolomics, and microbiomics (Hasin et al., 2017). They are used to map complex biological networks and mechanisms related to diseases. Multi-omics has significantly contributed to the investigation of the oral microbiome in relation to dental caries, periodontitis, and oral cancers (Kilian et al., 2016; Dewhirst et al., 2010). For instance, microbiome research indicated that dysbiosis was responsible for the majority of cases of oral diseases, but not individual pathogens, which made the problem much more complicated (Dewhirst et al., 2010). Moreover, metabolomics and proteomics have helped identify biomarkers for the diagnosis and monitoring the progression of diseases (Nicholson & Lindon, 2008). As omics data is typically massive, it should be analyzed and interpreted in combination with additional information, for example, clinical data (Hasin et al., 2017; Ginsburg & Willard, 2009).

All of the aforementioned advancements made a significant contribution to the development of precision dentistry. It represents an approach that aims at preventing, diagnosing, and treating oral diseases on a case-by-case basis based on individual genetic and non-genetic factors (Divaris, 2016; Schork, 2015). Unlike the earlier adopted generalized approaches implying uniform treatment, precision dentistry implies targeted strategies taking into account individual risk profiles, dysbiosis, and lifestyle-related variables. It is expected to result in the improvement of prediction capacity, earlier identification of potential problems, and, ultimately, better clinical outcomes. Precision dentistry requires the integration of data of different types, which is why an interdisciplinary framework such as EpiDentomics is necessary.

EpiDentomics refers to an innovative cross-disciplinary paradigm that unites the concepts of epidemiology, clinical dentistry, and omics sciences (Peres et al., 2019; Hasin et al., 2017). It makes it possible to gain new insights about the nature and progression of diseases by correlating population-based patterns with molecular mechanisms (Peres et al., 2019; Hasin et al., 2017). It allows detecting high-risk subjects, developing personalized preventive programs, and assessing the effectiveness of interventions at various levels (Khoury et al., 2016). EpiDentomics complements the objectives of precision medicine and public health, whose goal is to combine the data of the individual and population levels (Ashley, 2016).

The transition to EpiDentomics demonstrates the complexity of oral diseases, which develops due to a complicated interaction of biological, environmental, behavioral, and social factors (Watt et al., 2019). Traditional unidimensional models focusing on individual risk factors fail to provide sufficient assistance in solving this problem, which is why advanced integrated and systems-based models are necessary (Wild, 2012). The adoption of EpiDentomics is required to solve the existing problems through modern technology and data diversity.

The process of EpiDentomics development can be described as the progressive shift from traditional descriptive epidemiology towards molecular studies, and, finally, to the integrated and targeted approaches of recent years. This strategy leverages the benefits provided by molecular biology and multi-omics, while eliminating the weaknesses. The emergence of the interdisciplinary paradigm under consideration represents another stage in this transition.

4. CORE COMPONENTS OF EPIDENTOMICS

EpiDentomics involves several connected components, making it possible to investigate diseases through a multidimensional lens. In contrast to conventional approaches, the present methodology combines biological, environmental, behavioral, and computational aspects within one framework. This characteristic reflects the nature of the problems studied since oral diseases arise as a result of a complex interaction of several factors (Peres et al., 2019; Watt et al., 2019; Hasin et al., 2017). Such an integrative perspective leads to novel discoveries.

4.1 Genomics

Genomics constitutes the first component of EpiDentomics and involves the study of genetic differences. Modern technologies, especially genome-wide association studies (GWAS), have identified a great number of loci associated with periodontal disease, dental caries, and oral cancer (Vieira, 2012; Shaffer et al., 2011). These variations affect a wide range of processes, such as immunity, inflammation, and enamel production (Kinane et al., 2017). Genomics also helps understand the connections between genetic variations, environmental factors, and the microbial ecosystem. There may be certain genetic profiles that predispose patients to heightened inflammatory responses when they are in contact with certain microbial communities or exposed to environmental risks (e.g., smoking) (Kinane et al., 2017).

Another important application of the genomic component in EpiDentomics is related to the creation of predictive models of diseases. With such an approach, one can detect people who belong to high-risk groups and implement preventive measures in relation to them. However, genetic predisposition cannot be considered independently, which is why it should be combined with other components.

4.2 Epigenomics

Epigenomics represents another component of EpiDentomics that examines changes in gene expression without altering the DNA sequence. These changes are called modifications, and they can be associated with DNA methylation, histone modifications, etc. Moreover, they are dynamic, which means that they can be influenced by external environmental and behavioral factors (Bird, 2007). Thus, epigenomics can serve as a bridge between exogenous and endogenous variables in a disease process.

Oral diseases have long been linked to epigenetic changes in some cases. For instance, epigenetics plays an important role in the pathogenesis of periodontal disorders, cancer, and inflammatory conditions (Zhang et al., 2013). Changes in the methylation pattern of immune-related genes might impact the response of the organism to microbial colonization of the mouth. Therefore, epigenetic changes can be understood as cumulative exposures, which is why they should be viewed from the perspective of the life course.

Another characteristic of epigenetic changes is their reversible nature. This fact suggests that there might be ways of reversing these changes by regulating gene expression. The information obtained through this component of EpiDentomics might be useful when creating targeted interventions for prevention and therapy.

4.3 Oral Microbiome

Oral microbiome is the third component of EpiDentomics that deals with the microorganisms present in the oral cavity. With the help of next-generation sequencing techniques, it became clear that oral microbiomes are very complex communities (Kilian et al., 2016; Dewhirst et al., 2010). Instead of being caused by a single pathogen, dental caries and periodontitis are the results of dysbiosis or an imbalance in the microbiome (Hajishengallis, 2015).

Interaction between the microbiome and the organism is also bi-directional, meaning that both parties can affect each other. Host's genotype, immune system, and lifestyle affect the oral microbiome, which responds to these changes in certain ways. For instance, it can change the level of immune response and health of tissues in the mouth (Kilian et al., 2016). On the other hand, environment and behavior shape the microbiome, which affects oral diseases directly.

Apart from the structural diversity of the oral microbiome, there is also its functionality that can be important when considering the causes of disease onset. For instance, acid-producing bacteria cause enamel demineralization, while inflammatory communities affect periodontal tissues (Hajishengallis, 2015). This information is helpful when creating targeted interventions, such as probiotics and microbiome regulation therapy.

4.4 Environmental and Behavioral Determinants

The fourth component of EpiDentomics is concerned with the environmental and behavioral factors that significantly affect the occurrence of oral diseases. They include diet, smoking and alcohol consumption, oral hygiene practices, education, socioeconomic status, etc. (Peres et al., 2019; Watt, 2012). As in the case with genomics and microbiome, such factors work at the personal and population levels. Moreover, they affect other components, contributing to disparities in diseases.

The idea of exposome can serve as a framework for incorporating environmental factors into the research conducted in the field of EpiDentomics (Wild, 2012). Exposome refers to all kinds of factors, both internal and external, that accumulate throughout one's life. With this concept in mind, it becomes easier to investigate and control the effects of such variables.

Behavioral factors are important because they regulate oral health through the interaction with the microbiome. For example, poor oral hygiene is likely to cause higher microbial load in the mouth, while certain diets alter the microbial composition and responses of the organism (Watt, 2012). Moreover, sociodemographic and educational characteristics influence people's access to care.

4.5 Data Science and Bioinformatics

Data science and bioinformatics are enabling components of EpiDentomics that are needed for analysis and management of large datasets. Technological advancements in molecular biology resulted in a flood of high-dimensional omics data that requires effective analysis and interpretation (Hasin et al., 2017). Thus, data science and bioinformatics become extremely important in this context.

Thus, with the help of bioinformatics, one can unite various datasets to analyze how different factors are related to each other. Scientists can create predictive models that explain how the disease will unfold or demonstrate the relationship between specific elements. Moreover, machine learning and artificial intelligence can also be implemented into this process. Predictive diseases, biomarker discoveries, and optimization can be done using these tools (Libbrecht & Noble, 2015).

In addition to this, data science and bioinformatics might be useful for putting EpiDentomics into practice in a clinical setting. Through the combination of electronic databases, epidemiological and omics data, one will be able to make relevant and valuable conclusions on treatment and prevention of oral disorders. Such a part might be helpful for the implementation of precision medicine.

5. CONCEPTUAL FRAMEWORK OF EPIDENTOMICS

Unlike traditional approaches that pay attention either to one risk factor or single pathways, EpiDentomics perceives oral diseases as the outcome of dynamic interactions of several elements at different levels. As a consequence, EpiDentomics provides an example of how the systems-based approach to health sciences may look like by acknowledging the existence of multifactorial, complex molecular, individual, and social mechanisms behind oral disorders (Peres et al., 2019; Hasin et al., 2017; Ginsburg & Willard, 2009). With its holistic approach to the matter, it becomes possible to better comprehend the onset and evolution of oral diseases. Moreover, EpiDentomics might give us opportunities to develop precise medicine hypotheses.

First of all, biological components of EpiDentomics consist of the study of genomics, epigenomics, immunobiology, and oral microbiome. Together, these factors define the predisposition to the disease and responses of an organism to both environment and behavior. Genetic polymorphisms can influence immune reactions, inflammation, and tissue susceptibility, thus increasing predisposition to the particular disease and influencing disease development (Vieira, 2012). Epigenomics affects gene expression in response to environmental and behavioral impacts, providing a dynamic link between environment and biologic outcomes (Bird, 2007). Finally, the adaptive and interactive character of the oral microbiomes helps either maintain health or trigger diseases through dysbiosis (Kilian et al., 2016).

Secondly, we need to consider a wide range of environmental factors that impact oral health at different stages of people's life course. In addition to actual exposures to physical stressors, it is important to take into consideration such determinants of oral disorders as diet, pollution, presence of fluoridated water, dental care accessibility, and others (Watt et al., 2019). In light of the presented understanding, environmental factors should be considered within the concept of exposome.

In turn, behaviors of individuals mediate the relationships between environmental and biological factors. Thus, the quality of people's oral hygiene, eating habits, smoking, and drinking behaviors, as well as access to and consumption of dental services, have profound implications for their oral health status (Watt et al., 2019; Fisher-Owens et al., 2007). These behaviors depend on personal knowledge and socioeconomic circumstances.

On the highest level, the EpiDentomics framework is complemented by information obtained from population-based data and epidemiology. Namely, it contributes vital insight into the prevalence, distribution, determinants, and patterns of incidence of oral diseases in specific populations, allowing to identify inequalities and disparities (Petersen & Baez, 2013). By combining the evidence from molecular and population-level studies, this model builds a link between lab-based and applied aspects of research.

The key feature of the EpiDentomics model is its systems-based character, implying the presence of dynamic connections between all elements of the framework. The interactions are characterized by numerous feedback loops and, therefore, do not operate in a linear fashion (Bird, 2007).

It should be noted that one of the key enabling factors facilitating the implementation of EpiDentomics is data science and bioinformatics – areas dedicated to integration and analysis of big datasets (Hasin et al., 2017). Indeed, advances in biotechnologies generated massive amounts of high-dimensional data necessitating special approaches for their proper processing (Hasin et al., 2017). In addition, machine learning and artificial intelligence open up opportunities for constructing predictive models and discovering new biomarkers for disease (Topol, 2019).

From the conceptual point of view, the structure of EpiDentomics can be presented in the form of a multi-layered network illustrating interactions between biological systems, environmental exposures, behavioral factors, and population-level determinants within a dynamic systems-based approach (Figure 1).

Figure 1. EpiDentomics conceptual framework showing key determinant interactions.

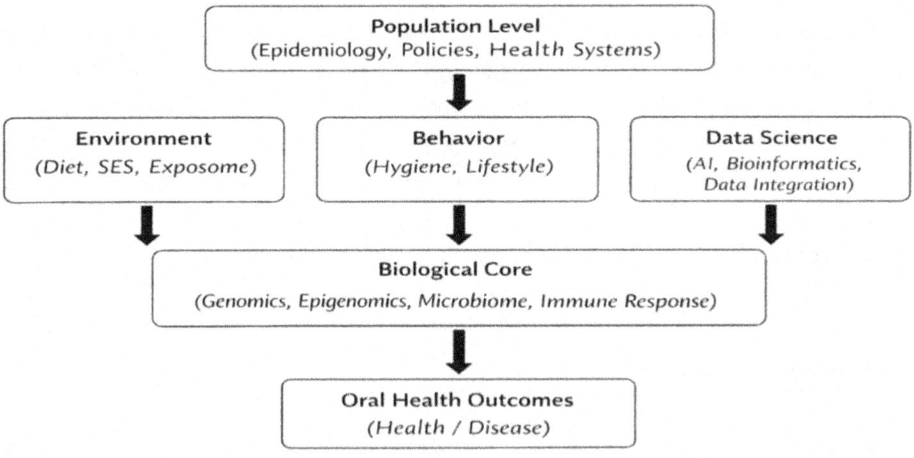

This framework consists of several interacting levels:

- **Core Biological Layer:** Genomics, epigenomics, microbiome, immune responses
- **Intermediate Layer:** Behavioral factors and environmental exposures (lifestyle, diet, tobacco use, healthcare access)
- **Population Layer:** Epidemiological patterns, health systems, social determinants, and policies
- **Integrative Layer:** Data science, bioinformatics, artificial intelligence

These layers are continuously interacting through rapid feedback loops. For instance, health information can be used to inform evidence-based public health interventions, which impact behaviors and exposures, which in turn impact biology and health outcomes. This iterative approach allows for improvement of knowledge and optimization of oral health policies.

The EpiDentomics approach is compatible with the concepts of precision dentistry and precision public health, whereby individualized care is provided in accordance with the patients' risk profiles while considering broader population-level factors (Khoury et al., 2016). It further facilitates a life-course perspective on oral health, recognizing that experiences and exposures throughout life stages can influence health outcomes over time.

6. APPLICATIONS OF EPIDENTOMICS

Integration of epidemiology, dentistry, and multi-omics is capable of revolutionizing oral healthcare services by merging evidence-based science and practice with genomics, proteomics, transcriptomics, epigenomics, metagenomics, and metabolomics into viable applications. Integration of diverse types of data would allow for transitioning from reactive approaches to proactive, personalized, and predictive oral healthcare provision. The applications of EpiDentomics include disease prediction and assessment, patient-specific healthcare service delivery, public health, and scientific innovations.

6.1 Disease Prediction

An important application of EpiDentomics is disease prediction. Traditional disease prediction typically utilizes a limited number of parameters related to clinical manifestations and behavioral risk factors (Featherstone, 2003; Selwitz et al., 2007). Inclusion of biological and microbial factors as well as environmental and behavioral determinants enhances the accuracy of prediction.

Genomic information can contribute to disease prediction, specifically with regard to dental caries and periodontal diseases due to their impact on immune system function and tissue integrity (Vieira, 2012). Microbiome analysis provides indicators of early-stage dysbiosis. Epigenetic biomarkers are valuable for the prediction of inflammation and subsequent disease progression (Kilian et al., 2016; Hajishengallis, 2012).

Machine learning and artificial intelligence provide the opportunity to investigate more complex interactions of different factors contributing to the prediction of disease, thus allowing for the improvement of predictions and real-time risk assessment (Libbrecht & Noble, 2015; Topol, 2019).

6.2 Risk Assessment

Risk assessment is an essential aspect of preventive dentistry, and the inclusion of omics and other data sources makes this process more accurate and multidimensional. Traditionally, risk assessment is conducted based on only a few parameters such as previous disease experience or oral hygiene practices (Featherstone, 2003).

Through EpiDentomics, one will have the possibility of analyzing different biological, microbial, environmental, and behavioral aspects that are responsible for individual risk of developing certain diseases. This means that those who have high-risk microbiomes and are genetically predisposed to dental caries, but do not experience any issues, are classified into the high-risk category (Kilian et al., 2016).

At the same time, risk assessment becomes more dynamic since all of the data can be analyzed and evaluated regularly, allowing for the identification of any changes in the condition that should lead to personalized preventive measures (Tellez et al., 2013).

6.3 Precision Oral Healthcare

Precision oral healthcare is a very revolutionary application of EpiDentomics. In this case, there is a transition from the generalized “one-size-fits-all” approach to individualization of care according to the patient's profile (Divaris, 2016).

The use of genetic, microbiome, and other types of data will facilitate the creation of personalized prevention and treatment plan for the patient. For example, when a person is at the risk of having periodontal disease due to his/her genetics, he/she needs more regular checks and additional intervention measures (Vieira, 2012). Another example involves the utilization of microbiome data in order to prescribe the appropriate antimicrobial therapy and normalize the microbial balance (Hajishengallis, 2012).

Biomarkers revealed through omics can be used for early diagnosis and disease progression monitoring. This will ensure more precise treatment and improve patient satisfaction and outcomes.

6.4 Public Health Planning

There are many opportunities for public health planning in EpiDentomics because of the possibility to analyze data of various types. The combination of epidemiology with the identification of biological, microbial, and environmental determinants gives a better understanding of the distribution and causes of diseases among population (Peres et al., 2019; Watt, 2012).

For example, by integrating epidemiological data and environmental factors, the development of preventive programs in particular communities can be considered (Watt, 2012). EpiDentomics can facilitate precision public health, which means that the interventions will be developed specifically for particular groups of people rather than implemented uniformly. Moreover, big data will provide opportunities for real-time surveillance and monitoring of disease trends and program outcomes (Bibault et al., 2016).

6.5 Research and Innovation

EpiDentomics has great potential for driving innovations in science as it facilitates the integration of different types of data and promotes interdisciplinary collaboration (Hasin et al., 2017; Ashley, 2016). Omics allows identifying new biomarkers, discovering the targets for the intervention, and predicting disease progression. As a result, research will become more effective, as the discoveries can easily be translated to practice, which will lead to the emergence of innovative solutions and approaches in the field (Patel et al., 2018). All in all, there are many promising applications of EpiDentomics that can transform oral healthcare positively. A summary of these applications is presented in Table 1.

Table 1. Applications of EpiDentomics in oral healthcare and public health:

Application Area	Description	Example in Practice
Disease Prediction	Uses genomic, microbiome, and behavioral data to detect disease early	Identifying high-risk caries patients using microbiome analysis
Risk Assessment	Integrates multiple determinants to stratify patient risk	Classifying patients into risk categories
Precision Oral Healthcare	Provides personalized prevention and treatment strategies	Tailoring recall intervals and therapies
Public Health Planning	Supports targeted interventions and policy development	Designing community-based programs
Research and Innovation	Enables biomarker discovery and new therapies	Developing salivary diagnostics

7. CHALLENGES AND LIMITATIONS

Despite its immense promise to revolutionize oral healthcare, EpiDentomics is also associated with several challenges and limitations. As an integrative and data-driven approach, Data integration and complexity are critical for the successful development and implementation of the field of EpiDentomics, as it heavily relies on combining various types of data from biology, clinics, and public health. Such data integration poses particular challenges for EpiDentomics.

7.1 Data Integration and Complexity

One of the major obstacles lies in the significant diversity of the available data types. For instance, EpiDentomics deals with data of biological, clinical, epidemiological, behavioral, environmental, genetic, and other omics nature (Ginsburg &

Willard, 2009; Misra et al., 2019). Each of these datasets has a high level of complexity and heterogeneity, requiring particular technical approaches.

Namely, genomic and other omics data are highly complex and require high-tech computational tools, while epidemiological data are structured differently and come from a population sample (Kilian et al., 2016). Moreover, there are particular challenges related to missing data, differences between studies, and a lack of standardization that have adverse effects on the quality, accuracy, and reproducibility of data (Ioannidis, 2005). In order to overcome the identified constraints, special bioinformatic and machine learning techniques are required, although they can be a source of new challenges associated with validation of such information (Libbrecht & Noble, 2015).

7.2 Ethical and Privacy Issues

The problem of ethics arises in the case of EpiDentomics due to a high degree of sensitivity of the collected information. There are strict requirements regarding the protection of genomic and other health-related data to ensure security and avoid abuse (McGuire et al., 2008).

There is a need for obtaining informed consent of patients for reuse and transferring their data from one institution to another. Patients must know the purpose of analyzing, storing, and protecting their data (McGuire et al., 2008; Shabani et al., 2016). Otherwise, there is a risk of biases, leading to discrimination and misinterpretation of biomarkers and their importance in disease development (Obermeyer et al., 2019). Thus, ethical policies and steps should be undertaken to facilitate the utilization of EpiDentomics.

7.3 Cost and Accessibility

Another limitation is associated with high costs and low accessibility of the necessary technology, as EpiDentomics requires advanced approaches including genotyping, other omics, and microbial analysis that require significant financial investments and are commonly available in developed regions only (Ginsburg & Willard, 2009; Goodwin et al., 2016).

Moreover, in many developing countries, such technologies remain unaffordable due to a lack of funds, which exacerbates global inequalities within health care. Consequently, there is a need to develop cost-reducing strategies and improve infrastructure and health professionals' competence.

7.4 Translation to Clinical Practice

Another constraint concerns difficulties in translation of results into regular clinical practice. Numerous studies reveal significant insights concerning biological and molecular mechanisms of oral disease pathogenesis, yet implementation of such discoveries is a complicated task (Divaris, 2016).

It becomes particularly difficult for healthcare professionals to interpret the obtained omic data in the context of providing medical assistance. Furthermore, there is a lack of relevant guidelines and practical tools for translating such results into routine practices (Divaris, 2016; Collins & Varmus, 2015).

Some predictive models and biomarkers require further testing in clinical settings before they can be applied to practice. Besides, limited time and insufficiently organized workflow are among the constraints preventing implementation of EpiDentomics.

There is a need to develop clinical guidelines, decision support systems, and training for health workers. Overcoming these limitations will help to achieve successful implementation of EpiDentomics in clinical and public health fields (Figure 2)

Figure 2. Key challenges and limitations of EpiDentomics.

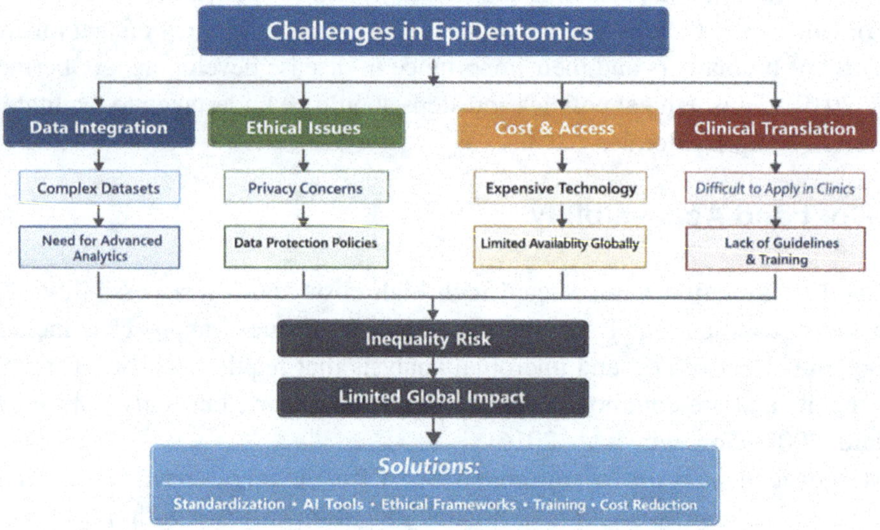

8. FUTURE DIRECTIONS

Consequently, the future development of EpiDentomics is expected to involve applications of artificial intelligence, big data, and precision medicine for transforming oral health care from reactive approaches to proactive and personalized preventive strategies (Hasin et al., 2017; Nicholson & Lindon, 2008; Peres et al., 2019). Furthermore, future work on EpiDentomics can contribute to improving population health and eliminating disparities in global oral health.

8.1 Artificial Intelligence in Dentistry

Artificial intelligence (AI) will have a crucial role in EpiDentomics through machine learning and deep learning methods. AI technologies will facilitate data analysis of complex big data sets, such as genome, microbiome, environmental, and behavioral data, that can predict disease occurrence and evaluate risk (Libbrecht & Noble, 2015; Topol, 2019).

Currently, AI technology has a variety of applications in dentistry, such as diagnostics, image analysis, prediction, and decision-making. AI can analyze the data from different sources, such as patient history, images, and test results, to estimate the risk of tooth decay, periodontal diseases, or oral cancers (Esteva et al., 2019).

In the future, more sophisticated methods of deep learning and neural network modelling can increase the transparency and reliability of the predictions made by clinicians (Topol, 2019; Obermeyer et al., 2019). Such advancements will help clinicians make informed decisions, work more effectively, and avoid diagnostic errors.

8.2 Big Data and Data Integration

Big data can serve as an excellent basis for developing EpiDentomics because electronic health records, genetic databases, microbiome data, and epidemiological research allow investigating relations between various oral health factors (Hasin et al., 2017; Bibault et al., 2016).

Future research needs to address data integration issues since effective data analysis of multi-omics data and clinical records will require harmonizing formats, procedures, and methods and applying advanced data-processing capabilities (Misra et al., 2019).

Cloud computing and data-sharing systems will also play a significant role in facilitating cooperation between researchers and organizations. Real-time data analysis will help to monitor disease progression and effects of various preventive measures (Bates et al., 2014).

8.3 Personalized Prevention and Precision Care

Personalized prevention and precision care are promising developments in EpiDentomics. Using biological, environmental, and behavioral data can help to personalize prevention strategies based on individual risk profile (Divaris, 2016).

Such an approach allows identifying patients with high risk early and applying targeted preventive measures. For instance, analyzing microbiome data will allow choosing appropriate probiotic and antimicrobial treatment based on genetic predisposition to gum disease and tooth decay (Kilian et al., 2016).

Furthermore, precision oral healthcare will also influence therapy options since biological characteristics will be considered during treatment planning. Advanced omics-based biomarkers, such as saliva tests, can facilitate the detection of diseases and monitoring the process of treatment (Zhang et al., 2012). In other words, EpiDentomics aligns with principles of precision medicine (Divaris, 2016; Ginsburg & Willard, 2009).

8.4 Global Health Impact

Applications of EpiDentomics can have an immense impact on global oral health by contributing to equalizing health care distribution around the world. Currently, oral diseases are a prevalent issue in the field of global health, especially in LMICs with no proper infrastructure for delivering health care services (Peres et al., 2019).

Thus, EpiDentomics can contribute to the development of preventive public health policies that would account for oral disease distribution across countries. This would contribute to developing and implementing precision public health strategies aimed at addressing specific needs of each community (Khoury et al., 2016).

Furthermore, further work needs to facilitate wider application of EpiDentomics solutions globally. It will be vital to develop skills in underserved populations and promote international cooperation and data sharing (Ginsburg & Willard, 2009). In addition, mobile health and telemedicine will help deliver personalized oral health services in underserved areas.

8.5 Emerging Technologies and Interdisciplinary Innovation

New emerging technologies will have an impact on further development of EpiDentomics. Advances in omics technologies, such as single-cell sequencing, metagenomics, and metabolomics, will allow gaining more insight into the pathogenesis of oral diseases (Hasin et al., 2017; Ashley, 2016).

Digital health technologies, such as wearable devices and apps, will allow continuous monitoring of behaviors and environment. This will facilitate acquiring real-time data and using it to design personalized intervention strategies (Bates et al., 2014).

Collaboration in the fields of dentistry, genomics, data sciences, and public health can foster innovation and accelerate translating research into practice. In summary, further developments in EpiDentomics are expected to involve advanced technologies, data-driven approaches, and personalized health services. AI, big data, and precision medicine will help overcome the existing limitations and advance EpiDentomics even further.

9. CONCLUSION

The presented concept represents a revolutionary advancement in the field of oral health research and practice. The current chapter discussed fundamental aspects of the new paradigm, including its theoretical background, core components, and basic framework. The transition from traditional approaches to oral epidemiology to a systemic vision makes it evident that understanding of oral diseases necessitates accounting for multiple dimensions.

EpiDentomics can establish links between molecular mechanisms of disease development and population trends. Incorporating biological data with data related to environment and behaviors will enable gaining a deeper understanding of the pathogenesis of oral diseases. EpiDentomics can also be applied to disease prediction, risk assessment, and evidence-based intervention design.

Application of EpiDentomics in clinical settings and public health demonstrates promising results in promoting better oral health among individuals and communities. However, there are some obstacles to further success, such as data integration challenges, ethical concerns, financial barriers, and difficulties in the implementation of advances. Further research and collaboration are crucial for overcoming these limitations.

AI, big data, and precision medicine are expected to facilitate further developments of EpiDentomics. These technologies will help deliver personalized, effective, and data-driven care in dentistry. EpiDentomics will also contribute to global health care improvement in terms of equalizing access to oral health care services in underserved regions.

Figure 3 illustrates the main concepts of the EpiDentomics framework that combines multi-omics and epidemiology in order to predict disease, assess risk, deliver precision oral care, and improve population health. Future work will involve validating predictive models, facilitating data integration, and translating scientific innovations into clinical practice. Collaboration between researchers, practitioners, and policymakers will be crucial for success.

Figure 3. EpiDentomics framework integrating multi-omics and epidemiological data for precision oral health.

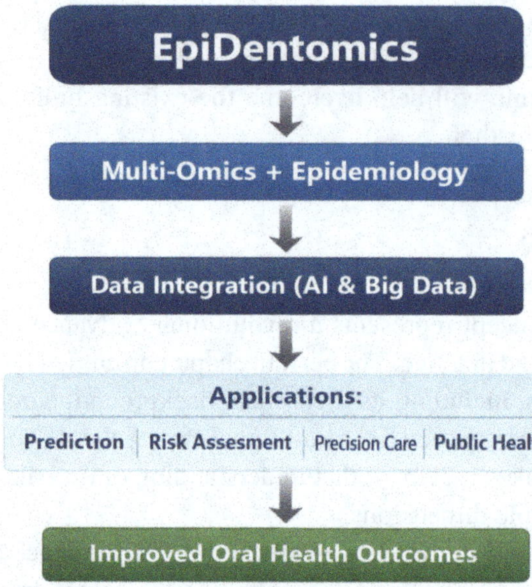

REFERENCES

Ashley, E. A. (2016). Towards precision medicine. *Nature Reviews. Genetics*, *17*(9), 507–522. DOI: 10.1038/nrg.2016.86 PMID: 27528417

Bates, D. W., Saria, S., Ohno-Machado, L., Shah, A., & Escobar, G. (2014). Big data in health care: Using analytics to identify and manage high-risk and high-cost patients. *Health Affairs (Project Hope)*, *33*(7), 1123–1131. DOI: 10.1377/hlthaff.2014.0041 PMID: 25006137

Bibault, J.-E., Giraud, P., & Burgun, A. (2016). Big data and machine learning in radiation oncology: State of the art and future prospects. *Cancer Letters*, *382*(1), 110–117. DOI: 10.1016/j.canlet.2016.05.033 PMID: 27241666

Bird, A. (2007). Perceptions of epigenetics. *Nature*, *447*(7143), 396–398. DOI: 10.1038/nature05913 PMID: 17522671

Collins, F. S., & Varmus, H. (2015). A new initiative on precision medicine. *The New England Journal of Medicine*, *372*(9), 793–795. DOI: 10.1056/NEJMp1500523 PMID: 25635347

Dewhirst, F. E., Chen, T., Izard, J., Paster, B. J., Tanner, A. C. R., Yu, W.-H., Lakshmanan, A., & Wade, W. G. (2010). The human oral microbiome. *Journal of Bacteriology*, *192*(19), 5002–5017. DOI: 10.1128/JB.00542-10 PMID: 20656903

Divaris, K. (2016). Precision dentistry: Moving toward personalized oral health care. *Journal of Dental Research*, *95*(9), 965–970.

Divaris, K., Lee, J. Y., Baker, A. D., & Vann, W. F.Jr. (2017). Precision oral health in the era of omics and systems biology. *Journal of Dental Research*, *96*(5), 487–493. PMID: 28425840

Esteva, A., Robicquet, A., Ramsundar, B., Kuleshov, V., DePristo, M., Chou, K., Cui, C., Corrado, G., Thrun, S., & Dean, J. (2019). A guide to deep learning in healthcare. *Nature Medicine*, *25*(1), 24–29. DOI: 10.1038/s41591-018-0316-z PMID: 30617335

Featherstone, J. D. B. (2003). The caries balance: Contributing factors and early detection. *Journal of the California Dental Association*, *31*(2), 129–133. DOI: 10.1080/19424396.2003.12224144 PMID: 12636316

Fejerskov, O., & Kidd, E. (Eds.). (2008). *Dental caries: The disease and its clinical management* (2nd ed.). Blackwell Munksgaard.

Fisher-Owens, S. A., Gansky, S. A., Platt, L. J., Weintraub, J. A., Soobader, M.-J., Bramlett, M. D., & Newacheck, P. W. (2007). Influences on children's oral health: A conceptual model. *Pediatrics*, *120*(3), e510–e520. DOI: 10.1542/peds.2006-3084 PMID: 17766495

Friis, R. H., & Sellers, T. A. (2021). *Epidemiology for public health practice* (6th ed.). Jones & Bartlett Learning.

Giannobile, W. V., & Lang, N. P. (2016). Are dental implants a panacea or should we better strive to save teeth? *Journal of Dental Research*, *95*(1), 5–6. DOI: 10.1177/0022034515618942 PMID: 26701917

Ginsburg, G. S., & Willard, H. F. (2009). Genomic and personalized medicine: Foundations and applications. *Translational Research : The Journal of Laboratory and Clinical Medicine*, *154*(6), 277–287. DOI: 10.1016/j.trsl.2009.09.005 PMID: 19931193

Goodwin, S., McPherson, J. D., & McCombie, W. R. (2016). Coming of age: Ten years of next-generation sequencing technologies. *Nature Reviews. Genetics*, *17*(6), 333–351. DOI: 10.1038/nrg.2016.49 PMID: 27184599

Hajishengallis, G. (2015). Periodontitis: From microbial immune subversion to systemic inflammation. *Nature Reviews. Immunology*, *15*(1), 30–44. DOI: 10.1038/nri3785 PMID: 25534621

Hasin, Y., Seldin, M., & Lusis, A. (2017). Multi-omics approaches to disease. *Genome Biology*, *18*(1), 83. DOI: 10.1186/s13059-017-1215-1 PMID: 28476144

Ioannidis, J. P. A. (2005). Why most published research findings are false. *PLoS Medicine*, *2*(8), e124. DOI: 10.1371/journal.pmed.0020124 PMID: 16060722

Kau, A. L., Ahern, P. P., Griffin, N. W., Goodman, A. L., & Gordon, J. I. (2011). Human nutrition, the gut microbiome and the immune system. *Nature*, *474*(7351), 327–336. DOI: 10.1038/nature10213 PMID: 21677749

Khoury, M. J., Iademarco, M. F., & Riley, W. T. (2016). Precision public health for the era of precision medicine. *American Journal of Preventive Medicine*, *50*(3), 398–401. DOI: 10.1016/j.amepre.2015.08.031 PMID: 26547538

Kilian, M., Chapple, I. L. C., Hannig, M., Marsh, P. D., Meuric, V., Pedersen, A. M. L., Tonetti, M. S., Wade, W. G., & Zaura, E. (2016). The oral microbiome—An update for oral healthcare professionals. *British Dental Journal*, *221*(10), 657–666. DOI: 10.1038/sj.bdj.2016.865 PMID: 27857087

Kinane, D. F., Stathopoulou, P. G., & Papapanou, P. N. (2017). Periodontal diseases. *Nature Reviews. Disease Primers*, *3*(1), 17038. DOI: 10.1038/nrdp.2017.38 PMID: 28805207

Libbrecht, M. W., & Noble, W. S. (2015). Machine learning applications in genetics and genomics. *Nature Reviews. Genetics*, *16*(6), 321–332. DOI: 10.1038/nrg3920 PMID: 25948244

Manolio, T. A., Abramowicz, M., Al-Mulla, F., Anderson, W., Balling, R., Berger, A. C., Bleyl, S., Chakravarti, A., Chantratita, W., Chisholm, R. L., Dissanayake, V. H. W., Dunn, M., Dzau, V. J., Han, B.-G., Hubbard, T., Kolbe, A., Korf, B., Kubo, M., Lasko, P., & Ginsburg, G. S. (2015). Global implementation of genomic medicine: We are not alone. *Science Translational Medicine*, *7*(290), 290ps13. DOI: 10.1126/scitranslmed.aab0194 PMID: 26041702

McGuire, A. L., Caulfield, T., & Cho, M. K. (2008). Research ethics and the challenge of whole-genome sequencing. *Nature Reviews. Genetics*, *9*(2), 152–156. DOI: 10.1038/nrg2302 PMID: 18087293

Newman, M. G., Takei, H. H., Klokkevold, P. R., & Carranza, F. A. (Eds.). (2019). *Newman and Carranza's clinical periodontology* (13th ed.). Elsevier.

Nicholson, J. K., & Lindon, J. C. (2008). Systems biology: Metabonomics. *Nature*, *455*(7216), 1054–1056. DOI: 10.1038/4551054a PMID: 18948945

Obermeyer, Z., Powers, B., Vogeli, C., & Mullainathan, S. (2019). Dissecting racial bias in an algorithm used to manage the health of populations. *Science*, *366*(6464), 447–453. DOI: 10.1126/science.aax2342 PMID: 31649194

Peres, M. A., Macpherson, L. M. D., Weyant, R. J., Daly, B., Venturelli, R., Mathur, M. R., Listl, S., Celeste, R. K., Guarnizo-Herreño, C. C., Kearns, C., Benzian, H., Allison, P., & Watt, R. G. (2019). Oral diseases: A global public health challenge. *Lancet*, *394*(10194), 249–260. DOI: 10.1016/S0140-6736(19)31146-8 PMID: 31327369

Petersen, P. E. (2003). The World Oral Health Report 2003: Continuous improvement of oral health in the 21st century—The approach of the WHO Global Oral Health Programme. *Community Dentistry and Oral Epidemiology*, *31*(s1, Suppl. 1), 3–23. DOI: 10.1046/j..2003.com122.x PMID: 15015736

Petersen, P. E., & Baez, R. J. (2013). *Oral health surveys: Basic methods* (5th ed.). World Health Organization.

Rothman, K. J., Greenland, S., & Lash, T. L. (2008). *Modern epidemiology* (3rd ed.). Lippincott Williams & Wilkins.

Selwitz, R. H., Ismail, A. I., & Pitts, N. B. (2007). Dental caries. *Lancet*, *369*(9555), 51–59. DOI: 10.1016/S0140-6736(07)60031-2 PMID: 17208642

Shaffer, J. R., Wang, X., Feingold, E., Lee, M., Begum, F., Weeks, D. E., Cuenco, K. T., Barmada, M. M., Wendell, S. K., Crosslin, D. R., Laurie, C. C., Doheny, K. F., Pugh, E. W., Zhang, Q., Feenstra, B., Geller, F., Boyd, H. A., Zhang, H., Melbye, M., & Marazita, M. L. (2011). Genome-wide association scan for childhood caries implicates novel genes. *Journal of Dental Research*, *90*(12), 1457–1462. DOI: 10.1177/0022034511422910 PMID: 21940522

Topol, E. J. (2019). High-performance medicine: The convergence of human and artificial intelligence. *Nature Medicine*, *25*(1), 44–56. DOI: 10.1038/s41591-018-0300-7 PMID: 30617339

Vieira, A. R. (2012). Genetics and dental caries: Prospects for the future. *Journal of Dental Research*, *91*(Suppl.), S23–S28.

Watt, R. G. (2012). Social determinants of oral health inequalities: Implications for action. *Community Dentistry and Oral Epidemiology*, *40*(s2, Suppl. 2), 44–48. DOI: 10.1111/j.1600-0528.2012.00719.x PMID: 22998304

Watt, R. G., Daly, B., Allison, P., Macpherson, L. M. D., Venturelli, R., Listl, S., Weyant, R. J., Mathur, M. R., Guarnizo-Herreño, C. C., Celeste, R. K., Peres, M. A., Kearns, C., & Benzian, H. (2019). Ending the neglect of global oral health: Time for radical action. *Lancet*, *394*(10194), 261–272. DOI: 10.1016/S0140-6736(19)31133-X PMID: 31327370

Wild, C. P. (2012). The exposome: From concept to utility. *International Journal of Epidemiology*, *41*(1), 24–32. DOI: 10.1093/ije/dyr236 PMID: 22296988

Zhang, A., Sun, H., & Wang, X. (2012). Metabolomics in biomarker discovery. *Mass Spectrometry Reviews*, *31*(2), 270–298.

Chapter 2
Epidemiological Principles in Oral and General Health

Muhammad Arshed
http://orcid.org/0009-0005-0683-9610
Baqai Medical University, Karachi, Pakistan & College of Public Health, Ziauddin University, Karachi, Pakistan

ABSTRACT

Epidemiological principles provide the foundation for understanding, preventing, and controlling diseases across populations, including the growing burden of oral conditions and their links with systemic health. This chapter presents a comprehensive overview of core epidemiological concepts applied to both oral and general health, emphasizing their relevance in contemporary public health practice. Key measures of disease frequency and association, such as incidence, prevalence, risk ratios, and population-attributable fractions, are discussed alongside their interpretation for clinical and policy decision-making. The chapter further explores confounding, bias, and effect modification, highlighting strategies to ensure valid and reliable inference. Disease causation is framed through multicausal models, including the web of causation and social determinants of health, integrating behavioral and environmental influences across the life course. Together, these principles support evidence-informed interventions, implementation strategies, and health policy development globally.

DOI: 10.4018/979-8-3373-8402-3.ch002

1. INTRODUCTION

1.1 Scope and Significance of Epidemiology in Oral and General Health

Epidemiology, defined as the study of the distribution and determinants of health-related states or events in specified populations and the application of this study to control health problems, is the underpinning of public health science (Ahlbom, 2021; Hajat, 2011; Thacker & Centers for Disease Control and Prevention, 2006). Epidemiology historically focused on infectious diseases, but has expanded to encompass chronic diseases, behaviors, environmental exposures, health systems, and other areas (Ahlbom, 2021; Hajat, 2011). Among these, oral health epidemiology has become a key yet under-integrated sub-discipline, despite the significant global burden of oral diseases including dental caries, periodontal disease, and oral cancers (Kassebaum et al., 2017; Petersen et al., 2005).

Oral diseases impact almost 3.5 billion people globally and are among the most common non-communicable diseases (NCDs), with shared risk factors with major systemic diseases, including cardiovascular diseases, diabetes, and cancers (Kassebaum et al., 2017; Petersen et al., 2005). These common risk factors, such as unhealthy diets and high intake of free sugars, smoking, alcohol, and poor oral hygiene practices, emphasize the need for a holistic epidemiological approach to oral and general health. The science of epidemiology offers the analytical framework for the measurement of disease burden, recognition of risk factors, assessment of interventions, and development of policy and strategies in both areas (Watt et al., 2019).

The importance of epidemiology in oral and general health goes beyond descriptive analysis to inferring causality and evaluating interventions. Using analytical study designs and sophisticated statistical techniques, epidemiology can identify associations and causal pathways between exposures and health outcomes. Epidemiological studies have shown associations of periodontal disease with poor systemic health outcomes, including diabetes and cardiovascular disease, but whether the latter are actually caused by periodontal disease is still under investigation (Tonetti et al., 2017). This knowledge is essential to inform the development of multimodal prevention strategies and health promotion programs that target multiple outcomes. Figure 1 illustrates an integrated oral and general health epidemiology framework. Figure 1 showing integrated oral and general health epidemiology framework.

Figure 1. Integrated oral and general health epidemiology framework

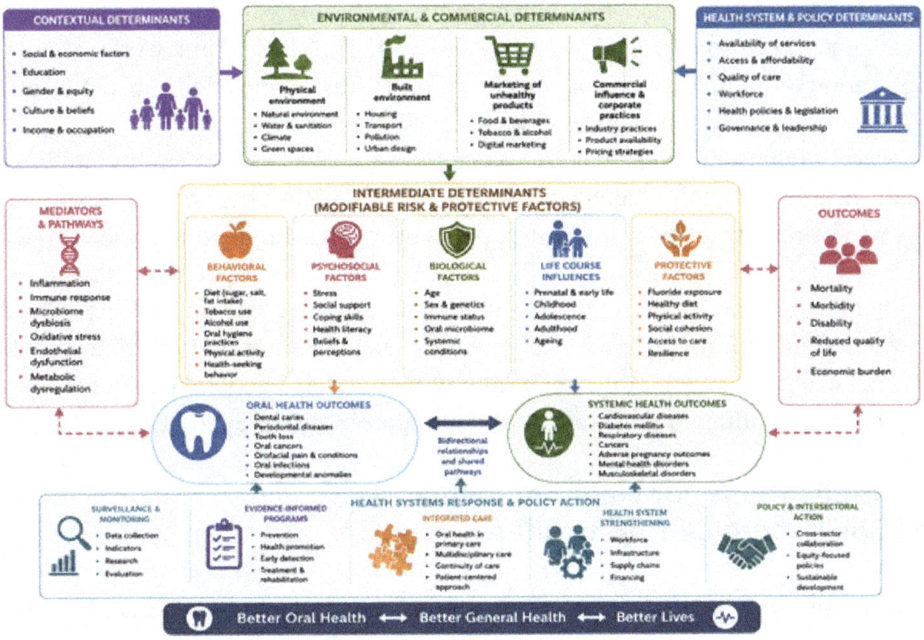

1.2 Epidemiology of Integrated Oral and Systemic Health

The historical distinction between oral health and systemic health has become blurred as evidence emerges of their interrelated nature. The idea of oral-systemic health integration acknowledges that the mouth is not a separate part of the body but an integral part of the whole and, therefore, is a reflection of general health(Hajat, 2011; Peres et al., 2019). Epidemiology offers a common denominator approach to examining these multifaceted relationships by exploring common risk factors, pathways and population health outcomes.

A key driver of integration between oral and general health epidemiology has been the common risk factor approach (CRFA). This approach underlines that multiple diseases can be prevented by targeting a few common risk factors, such as dietary factors, smoking, and oral hygiene (Hajat, 2011; Peres et al., 2019). Public health interventions that address these common factors can have a wide range of health benefits, improving efficiency and sustainability. For example, limiting sugar intake lowers the risk of dental caries, as well as obesity and type 2 diabetes (Moynihan & Kelly, 2014).

In terms of research methodology, the connection between oral and systemic health epidemiology requires cross-disciplinary research designs and analysis. Multilevel models, life-course epidemiology and systems epidemiology are increasingly being used to understand the inter-relationship between biological, behavioral, social and environmental factors in health (Diez Roux, 2012)). These frameworks allow the exploration of complex webs of causation, rather than simplified cause-and-effect relationships, in line with models like the web of causation.

Also, integration is critical for surveillance and systems. Traditionally, oral health data have been gathered independently from other health data, resulting in siloes information systems and lost opportunities for integrated analyses (Thacker & Centers for Disease Control and Prevention, 2006). Linking oral health measures to other health surveillance data can increase data quality, enable tracking of health disparities and inform policy making. For instance, adding oral health sections to national health surveys enables the evaluation of oral and general health conditions in parallel, providing opportunities for comparative and integrated analyses.

1.3 Implications for Data Science and AI (EpiDentomics Perspective)

Data science and artificial intelligence (AI) have revolutionized epidemiology through the ability to analyses large and complex data sets and provide real-time information about the epidemiology of diseases and their risk factors. This convergence, known as EpiDentomics, provides new avenues for improving research, monitoring and intervention in oral and public health (Beam & Kohane, 2018).

Data science refers to the use of methods including machine learning, data mining and predictive analytics, on a wide range of data sources, including electronic health records, mobile health apps, wearable and social media (Salathé et al., 2012; Topol, 2019). Such high-dimensional data enhance the effectiveness and timeliness of epidemiological studies. For instance, predictive models can help estimate who or which communities are at risk of developing dental caries or periodontal disease, to inform prevention and early intervention strategies.

The use of AI also supports precision public health via targeted interventions based on individual or population risk (Khoury et al., 2016). In the context of oral health, this could mean detecting vulnerable school communities or developing tailored strategies for behavioral change to enhance oral hygiene. Further, digital epidemiology enables real-time surveillance of health behaviors and health trends using alternative data sources, beyond traditional surveillance systems ((Salathé et al., 2012; Topol, 2019).

However, issues of data quality, privacy, bias and interpretability need to be solved to ensure the valid and ethical application of AI in epidemiology, (Salathé et al., 2012; Topol, 2019). Hence, epidemiologists need to embrace data science skills while maintaining their methodological rigor.

In summary, the convergence of epidemiology and data science with AI is revolutionizing oral and general health research, allowing more targeted, effective and fair public health strategies in the new era of EpiDentomics. EpiDentomics integrates epidemiology, oral health, and data science to improve population-level surveillance, risk assessment, and precision public health.

2. FOUNDATIONS OF EPIDEMIOLOGY IN ORAL AND GENERAL HEALTH

2.1. Definition, Aims, and Core Functions of Epidemiology

Epidemiology is the study of the distribution and determinants of health-related states or events in specified populations, and the application of this study to control health problems (Thiébaut & Thiessard, 2017). This encompasses the broad spectrum of epidemiology, including its application to not only infectious diseases but chronic diseases, injuries, behaviors and health. Epidemiology offers a rigorous scientific framework for understanding the distribution and determinants of disease, and guiding prevention efforts in oral and general health.

Epidemiology has a number of interrelated aims. The aims include describing the distribution of disease, identifying risk factors, understanding the natural history of disease, evaluating interventions and informing health policy and planning (Thacker & Centers for Disease Control and Prevention, 2006; Thiébaut & Thiessard, 2017). In dentistry, these are crucial for understanding the prevalence of oral diseases (dental caries, periodontal disease, tooth loss and oral cancer), and their association with systemic diseases (like diabetes and heart diseases).

These include surveillance, the identification of risk factors, evaluation of programs and the provision of evidence for policy (Thacker & Centers for Disease Control and Prevention, 2006; Thiébaut & Thiessard, 2017). While oral diseases are chronic, these are still important functions for identifying risk groups, tracking inequalities and evaluating interventions. Epidemiology therefore has a scientific and practical contribution to population health.

2.2. Distribution and Determinants of Disease

Epidemiology rests on the idea that disease occurs in patterns and is not random by person, place and time. Disease distribution is the frequency and pattern in populations, and is usually measured as incidence and prevalence and examined by demographic and geographic factors (Thiébaut & Thiessard, 2017). Patterns can help identify the at-risk population and guide hypotheses on risk factors.

Disease determinants are biological, behavioral, environmental and social factors that affect disease. Many determinants are common in oral and general health, such as consumption of sugars, use of tobacco and alcohol, poor oral hygiene and lack of health care (Watt et al., 2019). This concept of shared risk is fundamental to integrated epidemiology, which shows how multiple diseases can be caused by shared exposures.

Oral diseases are one of the world's most common diseases, and are closely linked to social inequalities (Peres et al., 2019). Their pattern of distribution is influenced by biological and social determinants including poverty, education and limited access to health care. Epidemiological studies, therefore, should not only focus on individual risk factors but also social and environmental factors that contribute to the risk of disease.

2.3. Population-based View of Oral and General Health

Epidemiology has a population perspective. Epidemiology takes a different approach to clinical medicine in that it looks at diseases from a population perspective. This is crucial because a large proportion of health gains are achieved through preventive population-based measures (Thacker & Centers for Disease Control and Prevention, 2006; Thiébaut & Thiessard, 2017).

In oral and general health, the population perspective explains the disproportionate burden of disease in certain disadvantaged groups. Dental caries and periodontal disease, for example, are affected by factors such as diet, socioeconomic status, education and health care (Peres et al., 2019; Thiébaut & Thiessard, 2017). As such, epidemiology can answer questions about inequalities, risk, and the effect of population-level interventions.

This view also underpins the common risk factor approach, which recognizes that improving shared determinants (such as sugar and smoking) can impact on both oral and general health. Epidemiology plays a key role in setting these priorities and assessing interventions to ensure their effectiveness and fairness.

2.4. Natural History of Disease and Disease Progression

The natural history of disease refers to the course of disease in the absence of intervention, from onset of disease to the outcome (Thacker & Centers for Disease Control and Prevention, 2006; Thiébaut & Thiessard, 2017). This term is important in epidemiology because it allows for the identification of points of intervention for prevention, early detection, and treatment.

Chronic diseases in the mouth, such as dental caries and periodontal disease, progress slowly. For dental caries, demineralization of enamel can progress to cavitation and tooth loss, while for periodontal disease, inflammation of the gums can lead to destruction of the connective tissue and tooth attachment. These can be interrupted through early intervention (Thiébaut & Thiessard, 2017).

The natural history of disease also forms the basis of the prevention levels: primary prevention prevents disease, secondary prevention focuses on early detection, and tertiary prevention reduces complications (Thacker & Centers for Disease Control and Prevention, 2006; Thiébaut & Thiessard, 2017). A life-course approach also highlights the importance of early exposures and cumulative risks for the development of disease. This means epidemiology aids in determining the timing and nature of interventions.

2.5. Epidemiological Triad and Multifactorial Disease

The epidemiological triad of agent, host and environment is a traditional explanation of disease (van Seventer & Hochberg, 2017). It shows disease results from the interactions between a number of factors, rather than a single factor, and it is helpful to conceptualize disease, especially infectious disease.

Yet, many oral and general diseases are complex. Dental caries, periodontal disease, diabetes, and cardiovascular diseases are multifactorial, involving interactions between biological, behavioral and environmental factors. Dental caries is affected by microorganisms, sugars consumed, oral hygiene, fluoride exposure, and time, and periodontal disease is the result of interactions between microorganisms, host response, and systemic factors (Peres et al., 2019).

Multifactorial approaches are important in contemporary epidemiology as they align with the real world. It fits with other models, including the web of causation and social determinants of health that acknowledge that diseases have common risk factors and tend to cluster in populations (Peres et al., 2019). Integrative epidemiological methods are therefore needed to tackle oral and general health problems.

3. EPIDEMIOLOGICAL TRANSITION AND ORAL-SYSTEMIC DISEASE PATTERNS

3.1 Transition From Infectious to Chronic Diseases

Epidemiological transition is the long-term shift in disease and mortality patterns from infectious diseases, malnutrition, and high maternal and infant mortality to chronic non-communicable diseases (NCDs), injuries and degenerative diseases. This shift has not been universally experienced; low- and middle-income countries are increasingly burdened with having a "double burden" of both infectious and chronic diseases. This transition is reflected in oral health. While acute oral infections remain, the burden of oral diseases globally is now dominated by chronic diseases such as dental caries, periodontal diseases, tooth loss, and oral cancers, which are influenced by long-term exposures, behaviors and social determinants, rather than a single cause (Peres et al., 2019).

This shift has implications for epidemiology. Chronic oral and systemic diseases typically have slow onset, modifiable risk factors, and require a prevention-focused and systems-oriented approach, rather than a cure-focused approach. Urbanization, dietary patterns, population ageing and exposure to commercial determinants (e.g. sugary foods, tobacco, alcohol), have played a role in shifting disease patterns in many countries. Therefore, oral epidemiology should now be increasingly considered in the broader context of NCD epidemiology and health-system change (Peres et al., 2019).

3.2 Burden of Oral Diseases

Oral diseases are one of the most prevalent health conditions and a significant global health burden. Untreated dental caries, severe periodontal (gum) diseases, edentulism (being toothless), and cancers of the lip and oral cavity are among the global burden of oral diseases. They result in pain, infections, difficulty chewing and communicating, decreased productivity at school and work, as well as lower quality of life. They also have significant social and economic impacts on individuals, families and health systems (Peres et al., 2019).

The burden of oral diseases is still high despite innovations in clinical dental practice and technologies for oral health. This ongoing burden is due to inadequate prevention and access to basic oral health care, lack of integration of oral health in the public health agenda, and social and economic inequalities. The prevention potential of most oral diseases, despite their high prevalence, suggests better epidemiology surveillance, risk factor modification and population prevention efforts are urgently needed (Peres et al., 2019; Watt et al., 2019).

3.3 Common Risk Factors for Oral Diseases

A major advance in epidemiology is to recognize the overlap of risk factors between oral diseases and NCDs. Excessive sugar consumption, smoking, excessive alcohol consumption, poor oral hygiene, low socioeconomic status, low health literacy and lack of access to preventive services are common risk factors for oral diseases but also for obesity, diabetes, heart disease, respiratory disease and a range of different cancers. This demonstrates that oral diseases should not be considered in isolation, but as part of a web of risk factors for chronic diseases (Peres et al., 2019; Watt et al., 2019).

For instance, high sugar dietary intake is a major risk factor for dental caries and also obesity and diabetes. Smoking is a risk factor for periodontal disease, tooth loss, oral cancer and many other diseases. These common risks make oral health conditions particularly pertinent in integrated health policy, as measures to address common risks have the potential to improve both oral and overall health. Thus, epidemiological assessment is critical to discover these associations and to measure their population impact (Peres et al., 2019; Watt et al., 2019).

3.4 Common Risk Factor Approach

The common risk factor approach is a leading public health strategy to tackle multiple diseases via common prevention measures. The approach seeks to address multiple diseases simultaneously, rather than developing separate, disease-specific programs, through the shared risk factors. Unhealthy diet, smoking, problematic alcohol use and poor social and environmental factors are common risk factors affecting oral and general health. This approach is particularly relevant in low-resource settings, where it is often more practical and cost-effective to offer integrated, holistic programs, rather than disease-specific ones (Peres et al., 2019; Watt et al., 2019).

Table 1 shows common risk factor approach has both scientific and practical merits. Scientifically, it is consistent with the fact that oral and non-communicable system diseases share common causes. Pragmatically, it guides integrated approaches like school health promotion, sugar reduction, tobacco control, promotion of improved hygiene, and integration of oral health into primary care and universal health coverage (Arshed, Kazi, Ashraf, et al., 2025). Epidemiology supports this approach by identifying the most important shared risks, tracking the burden of diseases, and assessing whether integrated interventions have beneficial effects on health outcomes across various aspects (Peres et al., 2019; Watt et al., 2019).

Table 1. Common risk factors linking oral and general health

Risk Factor	Oral Diseases	General Diseases
High sugar intake	Dental caries	Obesity, Diabetes
Tobacco	Periodontitis, Oral cancer	CVD, COPD, Cancer
Alcohol	Oral cancer	Liver disease, Cancer
Poor diet	Caries	NCDs
Low SES	All oral diseases	Most chronic diseases
Poor health literacy	Poor oral hygiene	Poor disease management

3.5 Health Inequalities in Oral and Overall Health

Diseases of the mouth, oral cavity and general health are not equally distributed within populations. There is a social gradient of disease with a greater burden in the poor and socially disadvantaged. People with poorer socioeconomic status (low income and education, limited access to health services, and exposure to unhealthy environments) have poorer oral and general health. Such disparities exist at a global level and within countries, communities and schools and households (Peres et al., 2019; Watt et al., 2019).

These inequities demonstrate that disease burden cannot be explained solely by genetic factors or individual behavior. It is also determined by broader factors such as the food system, accessibility to services, marketing practices, education, housing and the political climate. As such, oral epidemiology needs to take an equity lens. Knowing who is impacted, why the disease burden is concentrated in some groups, and how interventions may work across social groups, is vital to effective and equitable public health practice. Thus, epidemiological transition in oral and systemic health cannot be considered without regard to inequality, social determinants, and political and socioeconomic context of health (Peres et al., 2019; Watt et al., 2019).

4. STUDY DESIGNS IN ORAL AND GENERAL HEALTH EPIDEMIOLOGY

4.1 Descriptive Study Designs

Descriptive study designs are employed to describe the nature and distribution of diseases by person, place, and time. They are primarily used to estimate the burden of disease, identify risk groups, monitor trends, and suggest hypothesis for etiological research (Thiébaut & Thiessard, 2017). Descriptive epidemiology is crucial in oral and general health to describe the burden of dental diseases (dental caries, periodontal disease, tooth loss, oral cancer), and major non-communicable diseases (NCDs) (Peres et al., 2019; Watt et al., 2019).

Examples of descriptive designs include case reports, case series, ecological and cross-sectional studies. Case reports and case series describe rare or new conditions, diseases, or health problems. While they provide limited evidence for causality, they are helpful in detecting new relationships and generating hypotheses. Ecological studies examine group-level associations, such as regional sugar intakes and caries prevalence. They are valuable for hypothesis generation but are subject to ecological fallacy, where associations at the group level may not hold at the individual level (Hajat, 2011; Peres et al., 2019).

Cross-sectional designs are the most common in oral epidemiology. They measure exposure and outcome at one time and are well suited to estimating prevalence, determining treatment needs, and depicting population disparities (Hajat, 2011; Peres et al., 2019) . Cross-sectional designs are often implemented in national oral health surveys because they are efficient and appropriate for planning and surveillance. However, they measure exposure and outcome at the same time, so cannot provide information about temporal precedence and are thus limited in their ability to infer a causal relationship (Hajat, 2011; Peres et al., 2019). Contemporary cross-sectional studies continue to play an important role in estimating disease prevalence, evaluating health-related behaviours, and identifying associated factors to inform public health policy and intervention planning (Gillani et al., 2024; M et al., 2025).

4.2 Analytical Observational Study Designs

Analytical observational studies offer more than description, and investigate the association between exposure and outcome without artificially manipulating the exposure. The two most common designs are case-control and cohort studies, which have been extensively used in oral and health epidemiology (Hajat, 2011; Peres et al., 2019).

Case-control studies start with people who have the outcome and compare them to those who do not, and examine exposures retrospectively. They are particularly appropriate for rare diseases, those with long latency or outcomes that are difficult to assess. In dentistry, they are typically applied to study risk factors for oral cancer, severe periodontitis or rare diseases. They are efficient and cost-effective but can be prone to recall bias, selection bias and lack confirmation of the temporal relationship (Peres et al., 2019; Watt et al., 2019).

Cohort studies, on the other hand, start with the exposure and monitor the outcome, which may be retrospective or prospective. These can be prospective or retrospective and are ideal for studying incidence, progression, and temporal associations. In dentistry, cohort studies are used to study the progression of dental caries, the development of periodontal disease, life course inequalities, and the relationship between oral and general health. They allow for calculation of risk and determination of temporal relationships, but are often costly and time consuming (Peres et al., 2019; Watt et al., 2019).

Subtypes like nested case-control and case-cohort studies increase efficiency by involving a sample of participants from an existing cohort. They combine some of the key features of cohort designs and lower costs and complexity, particularly when there are limited data on exposure (Peres et al., 2019; Watt et al., 2019). Table 2 shows a comparison of epidemiological study designs in oral and general health.

Table 2. Comparison of epidemiological study designs in oral and general health

Study Design	Primary Purpose	Direction of Inquiry	Measure(s) Produced	Major Strengths	Major Limitations	Common Sources of Bias	Typical Oral & General Health Applications
Case Report / Case Series	Describe unusual or novel clinical conditions	No comparison group	Descriptive only	Identifies new diseases, adverse events, or rare conditions; generates hypotheses	Cannot establish causality or estimate frequency	Selection bias	Rare oral lesions, medication-related osteonecrosis, unusual oral manifestations of systemic diseases
Ecological Study	Compare disease patterns across populations or regions	Group-level comparisons	Correlation coefficients, ecological associations	Simple, inexpensive, useful for hypothesis generation and policy evaluation	Ecological fallacy; cannot infer individual-level associations	Ecological bias, confounding	Sugar availability vs. caries prevalence; fluoridation policies; regional oral cancer patterns
Cross-sectional Study	Estimate prevalence and identify associated factors	Exposure and outcome measured simultaneously	Prevalence, prevalence ratio, prevalence odds ratio	Rapid, cost-effective, suitable for surveillance and burden estimation	Cannot establish temporal sequence or causality	Selection bias, information bias	National oral health surveys, DMFT prevalence, periodontal disease burden, KAP studies
Case–Control Study	Identify factors associated with rare diseases	Outcome → previous exposure	Odds Ratio (OR)	Efficient for rare diseases and long latency periods; relatively inexpensive	Cannot directly estimate incidence or risk; recall of past exposure may be inaccurate	Recall bias, selection bias	Risk factors for oral cancer, cleft anomalies, severe periodontitis
Cohort Study (Prospective/ Retrospective)	Determine disease incidence and natural history	Exposure → outcome	Incidence, Risk Ratio (RR), Hazard Ratio (HR), Incidence Rate Ratio (IRR)	Establishes temporal relationship; evaluates multiple outcomes	Expensive, time-consuming, loss to follow-up	Attrition bias, confounding	Caries progression, periodontal disease incidence, oral-systemic disease associations
Randomized Controlled Trial (RCT)	Evaluate the efficacy of interventions under controlled conditions	Random allocation → outcome	Relative Risk, Risk Difference, Number Needed to Treat (NNT)	Highest internal validity; minimizes confounding; strongest evidence for causality	Expensive; strict eligibility may limit generalizability; ethical constraints	Performance bias, attrition bias (if poorly managed)	Fluoride therapies, oral hygiene interventions, behavioral interventions, and pharmacological trials

continued on following page

Table 2. Continued

Study Design	Primary Purpose	Direction of Inquiry	Measure(s) Produced	Major Strengths	Major Limitations	Common Sources of Bias	Typical Oral & General Health Applications
Cluster Randomized Trial (CRT)	Evaluate community or organizational interventions	Randomization of clusters (schools, clinics, communities) → outcome	RR, Mean Difference, ICC-adjusted estimates	Reduces contamination; ideal for public health and implementation research	Requires larger sample size; complex statistical analysis accounting for clustering	Recruitment bias, contamination between clusters	School oral health promotion, community fluoridation, mHealth implementation programs
Quasi-experimental Study	Evaluate interventions when randomization is infeasible	Before–after or non-randomized comparison	Mean Difference, OR, RR, Interrupted Time-Series estimates	Practical for health systems and policy evaluation; reflects real-world implementation	Lower internal validity; greater susceptibility to confounding	Selection bias, history bias, maturation bias	National oral health policies, service integration, and community prevention programs
Pragmatic Trial	Evaluate effectiveness under routine clinical or public health conditions	Real-world intervention → outcome	Effectiveness estimates, patient-centered outcomes	High external validity; informs policy and scale-up	Less control over intervention delivery; greater heterogeneity	Performance bias, implementation variability	School-based oral health programs, primary care integration, and digital health interventions
Hybrid Effectiveness–Implementation Trial	Simultaneously evaluate clinical effectiveness and implementation outcomes	Intervention → clinical and implementation outcomes	Clinical effect estimates plus implementation metrics (e.g., adoption, fidelity, reach)	Accelerates translation into routine practice; supports scale-up decisions	Methodologically complex; requires multidisciplinary expertise	Implementation bias, context-related variation	RE-AIM–based programs, implementation of preventive oral health interventions in schools and primary care
Mixed-Methods Study	Integrate quantitative outcomes with qualitative insights	Parallel or sequential quantitative and qualitative approaches	Quantitative estimates plus thematic findings	Explains not only whether an intervention works, but how and why; enhances contextual understanding	Requires expertise in multiple methodologies; resource-intensive	Researcher interpretation bias	Evaluation of acceptability, barriers, facilitators, stakeholder experiences, and implementation research

Abbreviations: DMFT = Decayed, Missing and Filled Teeth; HR = Hazard Ratio; ICC = Intracluster Correlation Coefficient; IRR = Incidence Rate Ratio; KAP = Knowledge, Attitudes and Practices; NNT = Number Needed to Treat; OR = Odds Ratio; RCT = Randomized Controlled Trial; RR = Risk Ratio.

4.3 Experimental and Quasi-Experimental Designs

Experimental designs include intervention assignments by the researcher. The randomized controlled trial (RCT) is the best method for assessing intervention effects because it reduces confounding and allows causal inference. In the fields of oral and general health, RCTs are commonly used to evaluate preventive, behavioral, and clinical interventions, including fluoride use, oral health education, dietary interventions, and smoking cessation interventions (Thacker & Centers for Disease Control and Prevention, 2006; Thiébaut & Thiessard, 2017).

In public health, cluster randomized trials (CRTs) are preferred to individual RCTs. These involve random assignment of groups, such as schools, clinics, or communities (Arshed, Mahmud, et al., 2025). They are useful for oral health promotion interventions, such as school toothbrushing and community fluoridation, where the intervention is applied at the group level. Cluster trials minimize contamination, but increase the sample size needed and require statistical techniques for clustered data (Thacker & Centers for Disease Control and Prevention, 2006; Thiébaut & Thiessard, 2017).

Quasi-experimental designs are applied when randomization is not possible or ethical. These include before-and-after, non-equivalent control group, interrupted time series, and natural experiments. They are particularly useful for public health policy and systems interventions. While they are more susceptible to bias than RCTs, good quasi-experimental studies can offer important evidence of effectiveness (Thacker & Centers for Disease Control and Prevention, 2006; Thiébaut & Thiessard, 2017). Evidence shows that experimental healthcare designs are feasible and acceptable in LMIC settings (Arshed, Mahmud, et al., 2025).

4.4 Mixed-Methods and Implementation-Oriented Designs

Contemporary epidemiology has been moving toward a recognition that, while it's important to know if an intervention works, it's also important to know how and why it works in the real world. As a result, there is increased application of mixed-methods and implementation-focused designs. Mixed-methods designs use both quantitative and qualitative data collection methods to integrate data on outcomes and context. For example, in oral health, clinical outcomes may be complemented by interviews, focus groups and observations to understand effectiveness, acceptability and contextual factors (Green et al., 2015).

Implementation-focused designs ephasize the delivery, uptake and sustainability of interventions. Hybrid effectiveness-implementation studies, pragmatic trials, and process evaluations embedded within trials address outcomes and processes of implementation. These study designs are crucial in oral health, as many interventions fail even when they are effective due to issues of feasibility, fidelity, acceptability or health system integration (Curran et al., 2012; Proctor et al., 2011).

Pragmatic trials are particularly important for informing policy. Pragmatic trials, as opposed to explanatory trials that take place in idealized conditions, assess interventions in real-world practice. They often involve diverse populations, flexible delivery of interventions, and relevant outcomes. So, they are very useful to examine scalability and health system impact, despite the lack of internal control (Zwarenstein et al., 2008).

In summary, there is no one best design. It is more a question of the research question, rarity of the outcome, ethical aspects, and causal inference. For oral and general health epidemiology, strong evidence is usually derived from the combination of various designs, from descriptive and observational through experimental and implementation research (Curran et al., 2012; Proctor et al., 2011). Frameworks such as RE-AIM and CFIR facilitate the translation of epidemiological evidence into sustainable public health practice by evaluating implementation, adoption, and long-term impact (Curran et al., 2012; Proctor et al., 2011). Figure 2 shows hierarchy of different epidemiological study designs.

Figure 2. Epidemiological study designs hierarchy

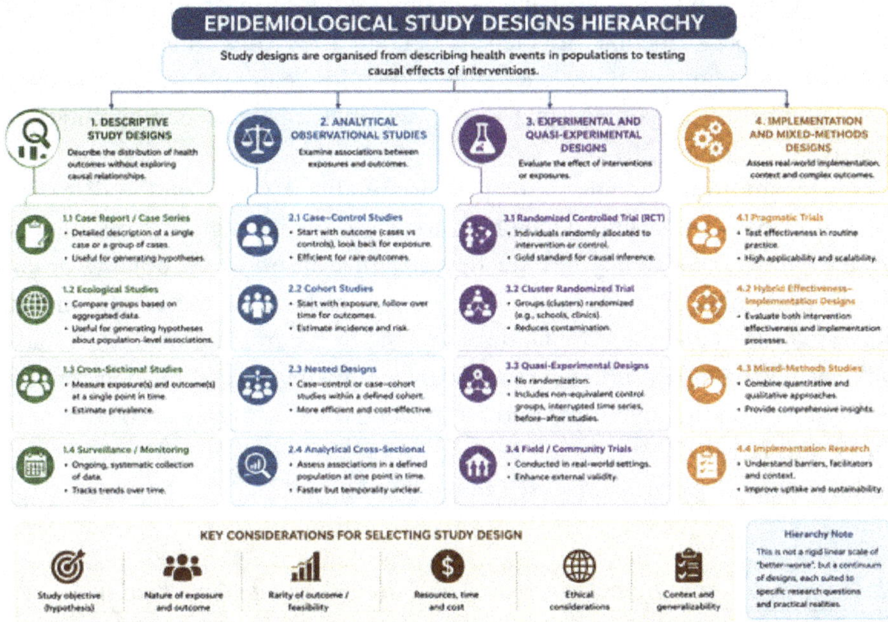

5. MEASURES OF DISEASE FREQUENCY, BURDEN, AND ASSOCIATION

5.1 Measures of Disease Frequency: Incidence and Prevalence

Disease frequency measures are key to epidemiology as they describe the frequency of health events in populations and enable comparisons between populations, geographic areas, and over time. The most common measures are incidence and prevalence. Incidence is the occurrence of a new disease within a defined population at risk during a time period, whereas prevalence is the number of all existing cases at a point in time or during a specified period, regardless of when they started (Thacker & Centers for Disease Control and Prevention, 2006; Thiébaut & Thiessard, 2017). They answer different questions and are not interchangeable. Incidence measures are more relevant when addressing questions of disease causality and risk, while prevalence measures are more relevant to estimating disease burden and health service requirements.

In oral and general health, incidence is particularly useful in research on the onset of new diseases, such as new caries, attachment loss, or oral cancer. It is particularly useful for studies of disease causation and prevention because it measures disease progression. By contrast, prevalence is commonly used in oral health surveys to assess the number of people affected by dental caries, gingivitis, edentulism, or unmet need for treatment. Prevalence is important for health planning as it captures the total number of people who may need preventive, restorative, rehabilitative, or supportive care (Hajat, 2011).

The decision to use incidence or prevalence also depends on the disease. Incidence may be low but prevalence high for diseases of long duration; incidence may be high and prevalence low for diseases that are resolved quickly or cause death. In oral epidemiology, this can be important because the conditions, such as untreated caries and periodontal disease, tend to accumulate with time, making prevalence particularly useful for monitoring and planning. But incidence remains vital for understanding dynamics and for preventive efforts (Hajat, 2011; Thiébaut & Thiessard, 2017).

Table 3 shows key measures used in epidemiology.

Table 3. Key epidemiological measures used in oral and general health

Measure	Definition	Primary Purpose	Typical Study Design	Example in Oral & General Health
Incidence	Number of new cases occurring in a population at risk over a specified period	Measure disease occurrence and risk	Cohort studies, RCTs	Incidence of new dental caries among schoolchildren
Prevalence	Total existing cases in a population at a specific point or period	Estimate disease burden and service needs	Cross-sectional studies	Prevalence of periodontitis or untreated dental caries
Mortality Rate	Frequency of deaths in a population during a specified period	Measure fatal disease burden	Cohort studies, surveillance	Mortality due to oral cancer

Measure	Definition	Primary Purpose	Typical Study Design	Example in Oral & General Health
DALYs	Years of life lost plus years lived with disability	Quantify overall population disease burden	Burden of disease studies	Burden of oral diseases globally
Risk Ratio (RR)	Ratio of disease risk in exposed versus unexposed groups	Compare disease risk between exposure groups	Cohort studies, RCTs	Risk of periodontal disease among smokers
Odds Ratio (OR)	Ratio of odds of exposure or disease between groups	Measure strength of association	Case–control studies, logistic regression	Association between tobacco use and oral cancer
Risk Difference (RD)	Difference in disease risk between exposed and unexposed groups	Measure absolute excess risk	Cohort studies, RCTs	Excess caries attributable to frequent sugar intake
Population Attributable Fraction (PAF)	Proportion of disease attributable to a specific exposure	Estimate potential disease prevention	Population-based studies	Percentage of oral cancer attributable to tobacco use

Abbreviations: DALYs = Disability-Adjusted Life Years; OR = Odds Ratio; PAF = Population Attributable Fraction; RD = Risk Difference; RR = Risk Ratio.

5.2 Measures of Morbidity, Mortality and Burden

Epidemiology also employs measures of morbidity, mortality and burden to quantify the impact of disease, in addition to frequency. Morbidity is a measure of illness or less-than-perfect health; mortality is a measure of death. Mortality measures (crude death rates, age-specific death rates and cause-specific mortality rates) are particularly relevant in general epidemiology for major diseases such as cancers and cardiovascular disease. In oral health, mortality is not commonly applied to most diseases, but it is important for cancers of the lip and oral cavity, which are a major cause of premature death in many countries (Peres et al., 2019; Watt et al., 2019).

Burden measures focus not only on case and death counts. They quantify the impact of disease on disability, quality of life, productivity and health-service use. Summary measures are widely used in modern public health, including disability-adjusted life years (DALYs), years lived with disability (YLDs) and years of life lost (YLLs). These are very pertinent to oral health because, unlike cardiovascular disease, oral diseases do not in themselves often lead to death, but they do result in significant disability, pain, social loss, and financial impact. The World Health Organization (WHO) Global Oral Health Status Report shows that 3.5 billion people worldwide are affected by oral diseases, and that they constitute a large, preventable component of the global burden of non-communicable diseases (GBD 2017 Oral Disorders Collaborators et al., 2020; Kassebaum et al., 2017).

Burden measures are useful from a population health point of view as they shift the focus not just to disease severity but also its importance in terms of public health. A disease might not be fatal but can still produce a high burden if it causes pain, chewing or speaking difficulties, recurrent treatment requirements, missed school or workdays, and impacts on quality of life. This is the case with many oral conditions. So, epidemiological analysis in oral and general health should take into account not only the presence, but the levels of pain, disability and social disadvantage, that disease creates over the life course (GBD 2017 Oral Disorders Collaborators et al., 2020; Kassebaum et al., 2017).

5.3 Scales and Indices for Oral Health and Epidemiology

Oral epidemiological studies need indices to standardize the measurement of clinical conditions. The WHO has been advocating for standardized oral health surveys for comparability, monitoring and planning (Peres et al., 2019). A particularly common indicator is the DMFT/dmft index (number of Decayed, Missing, and Filled Teeth in permanent or primary dentition). This continues to be one of the most common indicators used to assess cumulative caries experience in surveys and epidemiological research (GBD 2017 Oral Disorders Collaborators et al., 2020; Kassebaum et al., 2017) .

Other oral health indicators include the Plaque Index, Gingival Index, indices assessing oral hygiene, and indicators of periodontal status, such as the presence of pocketing, loss of attachment or screening tools for periodontal disease. These measures reflect various aspects of oral health, such as caries experience, hygiene, gingival inflammation and periodontal breakdown. Oral health is not captured completely by any one indicator, and can be assessed by different combinations of indicators, depending on research questions. For instance, a community survey might include DMFT to assess past caries experience, plaque and gingival indices to assess oral hygiene and inflammation, and periodontal indices to measure adult disease severity and need for treatment (Peres et al., 2019).

When choosing oral health indicators, it's important to consider validity, reliability, age-appropriateness, feasibility and policy relevance. Some indices offer more information but some are more feasible for large surveys. Particularly important is standardization of diagnosis and examiner training because measurement variation can confound comparisons between studies and countries (GBD 2017 Oral Disorders Collaborators et al., 2020; Peres et al., 2019).

5.4 Measures of Association and Effect

Measures of association compare the frequency of disease between groups or quantify the relationship between risk factors and disease (Peres et al., 2019). The measures of association include the risk ratio (relative risk), rate ratio, odds ratio and risk difference. The risk ratio compares the risk in two groups. The rate ratio compares incidence rates (person-time). The odds ratio compares the odds of exposure in case and control groups, or the odds of disease in exposed and unexposed groups and is commonly used in case-control studies (Peres et al., 2019; Watt et al., 2019).

Rate ratio, odds ratio and relative risk are crucial measures in oral and general health epidemiology, used to describe and quantify associations between risk factors and health outcomes. For instance, exposure effect measures may include the relative risk of periodontal disease in smokers, the odds ratio for oral cancer in tobacco or alcohol users, or the rate ratio for incident caries in children with varying levels of sugar intake. All measures have contextual uses. Risk ratios might be easier to interpret with cohort studies and trials while odds ratios are particularly useful for case-control studies and logistic regression. The interpretation should take into account the study design, the frequency of the outcome, and whether the measure is relative or absolute (Peres et al., 2019).

Relative measures of effect can be presented in absolute terms. Risk difference (or attributable risk) refers to the excess of disease in the exposed group. This is particularly relevant to public health decision making as it represents excess burden rather than relative increase. A low relative effect may reflect many preventable cases if the exposure is frequent. A high relative risk may be less important in the population if the exposure is rare. Thus, relative and absolute measures should be reported wherever possible to inform clinical and public health practice (Peres et al., 2019; Watt et al., 2019).

5.5 Understanding Epidemiological Measures in Oral and General Health

The interpretation of epidemiological measures is more than a mathematical exercise. Researchers need to take into account the study design, the population under investigation, the timing of the measures, the case definition, and the potential for bias, confounding and chance. The prevalence measure from a cross-sectional study is not the same as the incidence measure from a cohort study, and the odds ratio from a case-control study should not be the same as the risk ratio, particularly if the disease is common (Peres et al., 2019; Watt et al., 2019).

In oral health, it's also important to consider issues related to the cumulative and multifactorial nature of disease. For instance, DMFT indicators are measures of cumulative caries, rather than just current untreated caries. Likewise, periodontal indices can reflect current inflammation and previous destruction. So, oral epidemiological data are typically cumulative and current. So researchers need to be cautious not to over interpret the results of single measures as causal and to interpret the results in line with the biological and clinical relevance of the index (GBD 2017 Oral Disorders Collaborators et al., 2020; Peres et al., 2019).

6. BIAS, VALIDITY, CONFOUNDING & INTERACTION

6.1 Validity, Reliability and Epidemiological Error

The trustworthiness of epidemiological studies is determined by the validity, reliability and interpretability of findings. Validity is the extent to which a study measures, or infers, what it sets out to and the extent to which findings represent the source population (Thacker & Centers for Disease Control and Prevention, 2006; Thiébaut & Thiessard, 2017). This can be internal, referring to the correctness of the study findings, and external, referring to the transferability of the study findings to other populations (GBD 2017 Oral Disorders Collaborators et al., 2020; Peres et al., 2019). Validity is essential in oral and general health epidemiology, since the results can be used to develop health policies and guidelines and implement large population-based programs.

Reliability, also known as reproducibility or precision, refers to the consistency of measurement. Reliability can be achieved without validity, but validity usually requires reliability (Peres et al., 2019; Watt et al., 2019). This is especially relevant in oral epidemiology, where the outcomes are based on clinical indices like DMFT, Plaque Index (PI) and Gingival Index (GI). There are standardized measurement procedures and examiner calibration to ensure comparable results between studies (GBD 2017 Oral Disorders Collaborators et al., 2020; Peres et al., 2019; Silness & Loe, 1964).

Random error and systematic error can lead to epidemiological error. Random error arises from chance and is more prevalent in small samples, while systematic error leads to systematic distortion and is a greater threat to validity (GBD 2017 Oral Disorders Collaborators et al., 2020; Peres et al., 2019; Silness & Loe, 1964). It is important to understand and avoid these errors when generating epidemiological findings.

6.2 Types and Sources of Bias

Bias is a systematic error in research that causes a departure from the truth and the wrong estimate of association between exposure and outcome. Bias may occur at any point in the research process, such as study design, data collection, analysis and interpretation ((Delgado-Rodríguez & Llorca, 2004; Peres et al., 2019). Bias is especially important in oral and general health research because of the use of self-reported exposures and outcomes, and the possibility of social patterning of exposures.

Selection bias occurs when the association between exposure and outcome varies between study participants and those who are not in the study. This can occur through nonresponse, attrition, or sampling from certain venues (e.g. clinics) (Delgado-Rodríguez & Llorca, 2004). For instance, oral health studies conducted in clinics may overlook people with limited access to care, and underestimate disease burden.

Information bias occurs when there are inaccuracies in the measurement or classification of exposures or outcomes. This encompasses recall bias, interviewer bias and observer bias. In the context of oral epidemiology, information bias can arise from over-reporting toothbrushing or inconsistencies in early lesion diagnosis ((Delgado-Rodríguez & Llorca, 2004; Peres et al., 2019). Using validated tools, standardized approaches and blinding can minimize information bias (Delgado-Rodríguez & Llorca, 2004).

6.3 Confounding: Definition, Origins and Prevention

Confounding happens when the relationship between exposure and outcome is biased by a third factor that is associated with exposure and outcome but is not on the causal path (Delgado-Rodríguez & Llorca, 2004; Peres et al., 2019; VanderWeele, 2019) . It can mask or create associations, or produce spurious associations.

In oral and general health research, confounding is common due to shared behavioral and social determinants. For instance, associations between oral hygiene and cardiovascular disease may be confounded by smoking, diet, or socioeconomic status. Similarly, the relationship between sugar intake and dental caries may be influenced by fluoride exposure and access to care (Delgado-Rodríguez & Llorca, 2004; Peres et al., 2019; VanderWeele, 2019).

Confounding can be controlled at both the design and analysis stages. Design strategies include randomization, restriction, and matching, while analytical methods include stratification and multivariable regression (Delgado-Rodríguez & Llorca, 2004; Peres et al., 2019; VanderWeele, 2019). Advanced methods such as propensity scores are also increasingly used. However, residual confounding may persist due to unmeasured or poorly measured variables, requiring cautious interpretation of results. Bradford Hill's criteria support the evaluation of causal relationships, while Directed Acyclic Graphs (DAGs) help identify confounding pathways and appropriate analytical adjustments in epidemiological research.

6.4 Interaction and Effect Modification

Interaction (or effect modification) is when the association between an exposure and an outcome varies by levels of another factor (Rothman et al., 2008; Vander-Weele, 2015). Interaction is a genuine phenomenon, whereas confounding should be removed, and can shed light on disease processes and population sub-groups.

Interactions can be present between age, sex, socioeconomic status, smoking, and fluoride exposure in oral and general health. For instance, the impact of sugar consumption on dental caries may differ in those without fluoride exposure, and the link between periodontal disease and systemic diseases may be influenced by diabetes or smoking. These differences point to the need to identify at-risk groups and target interventions (Delgado-Rodríguez & Llorca, 2004; Peres et al., 2019; VanderWeele, 2019) .

Interaction can be evaluated on additive and multiplicative scales, with additive interaction being more important from a public health perspective as it reveals additive effects that are greater than the sum of individual risks. This is crucial in integrated oral-systemic health, where multiple risk factors can interact to increase disease in vulnerable groups.

6.5 Implications for Oral and General Health

Bias, validity, confounding, and interaction are fundamental to the interpretation of epidemiological data in oral and general health. Observational data, self-reporting, and social determinants of health are common in oral health research, and these are prone to systematic error and confounding. Meanwhile, interaction is critical to understanding inequalities and informing interventions (Peres et al., 2019; Watt et al., 2019).

Rigorous methodology includes appropriate study design, standardized measurements, examiner training, appropriate analysis and reporting of limitations. It is critical to note that statistical significance does not always mean validity, and lack of significance does not always mean no effect. Thorough evaluation of the potential impact of bias and confounding is therefore important.

In integrated epidemiology, these epidemiological principles also inform equity analysis. Oral and systemic diseases are influenced by complex biological, behavioral and social factors, and so understanding the way bias and confounding work, and how effects vary across populations is important for effective and equitable public health interventions. Ultimately, rigorous epidemiology is essential for both scientific and policy/practice.

7. MODELS OF DISEASE CAUSATION AND DETERMINANTS

7.1 Evolution of Concepts of Disease Causation

Epidemiology has always had a focus on disease causation. The initial explanations for disease were often philosophical and supernatural, but with the emergence of science and scientific medicine, there was a greater focus on biological and environmental factors. During the 19th century, the germ theory of disease revolutionized public health by showing how specific germs could cause specific infectious diseases. This approach was very successful because it provided a direct causal link and led to the great improvements in sanitation, vaccination and infection control (Peres et al., 2019; Watt et al., 2019) . Yet while germ theory was very successful in explaining many infectious diseases, it was not sufficient to explain chronic diseases, which are not generally caused by a single necessary agent.

As the field of epidemiology developed, it became increasingly clear that many outcomes are the result of several causes, rather than one in isolation. Rather, they result from complex processes that are influenced by cumulative exposures (Peres et al., 2019; Watt et al., 2019). So, modern epidemiology has shifted from single causes to multiple and systems-based models of disease.

7.2 Pathways and the Web of Causation

The web of causation is a common model used for chronic diseases. This model does not propose disease as being caused by a single factor, but rather that disease results from a web of causal factors. This includes biological, behavioral, environmental, social and economic factors, which combine in a complex manner. The web of causation is important because it is consistent with the true nature of disease processes and not reductionist (Peres et al., 2019; Watt et al., 2019) .

Multifactorial models are necessary in oral and general health. So, caries are not just due to sugar, or the bacteria, or poor oral hygiene. It is caused by the chewing of carbohydrates, interactions with oral microorganisms, fluoride intake, individual susceptibility, oral hygiene, social determinants and time. Likewise, periodontal disease is a result of microbial insult, host inflammation, smoking, diabetes, oral hygiene and other structural factors. Similarly, chronic diseases like heart disease and diabetes stem from exposures to diet, physical activity, smoking, stress, genetics, social determinants, and health care (Peres et al., 2019; Watt et al., 2019).

Multifactorial models therefore offer a more realistic underpinning to integrated epidemiology than single-cause models.

Rothman's pie model of causality further developed multifactorial models by proposing that disease is caused by a combination of component causes that make up a sufficient cause. In this model, all of the component causes need not be present for disease to occur; the same disease may result from different combinations of exposures (Peres et al., 2019; Watt et al., 2019). This concept is important in oral and general health as it helps to explain how the same disease can be caused by different component causes in different populations. It also supports the public health maxim that eliminating one key component cause can prevent disease even in the presence of other causes.

7.3 Determinants of Oral and General Health

Determinants of health is a term used to describe the many factors that contribute to health, disease and well-being. These go beyond biological factors and include individual behaviour, social, economic, environmental, cultural, commercial and health system factors. The determinants of oral and general health are highly interlinked and shared. Consumption of sugar, smoking, excessive drinking, poor personal hygiene, lack of access to preventive services and health literacy, for example, are factors that contribute to oral diseases but also obesity, diabetes, heart disease and cancers (Peres et al., 2019; Watt et al., 2019) .

Biological determinants include age, sex, genetics, immune response, and underlying physiological vulnerability. These factors may influence susceptibility to disease, response to exposure, and progression of illness. Behavioral determinants include diet, oral hygiene practices, tobacco use, alcohol use, physical activity, and adherence to preventive care. Social and economic determinants include education, income, occupation, housing, and social exclusion. Environmental determinants include access to clean water, fluoridation, food environments, pollution, and living conditions. Health-system determinants include service availability, affordability, workforce capacity, and quality of care. Together, these factors shape patterns of both oral and systemic disease across the life course (Peres et al., 2019; Watt et al., 2019).

In recent years, increasing attention has also been given to the commercial determinants of health, which refer to the ways in which private-sector practices influence health through marketing, product availability, pricing, and policy influence. In oral health, aggressive promotion of sugary foods and beverages, tobacco products, and alcohol contributes substantially to disease burden. These same industries also affect broader NCDs patterns, reinforcing the idea that oral and general health are linked by common upstream determinants (Peres et al., 2019; Watt et al., 2019).

Understanding disease causation, therefore requires attention not only to individual behavior but also to the wider systems that shape exposure and choice.

7.4 Life-Course and Socioecological Perspectives

The **life-course perspective** emphasizes that health and disease are shaped by exposures acting across different stages of life, from preconception and early childhood to adulthood and old age. Early-life conditions can have long-lasting consequences, and repeated or cumulative disadvantage may increase risk over time. In oral health, childhood nutrition, oral hygiene habits, fluoride exposure, parental care, and early access to dental services can strongly influence later dental and periodontal outcomes. Likewise, in general health, early-life adversity, malnutrition, and poor living conditions may affect later risk of chronic disease, disability, and premature mortality (Peres et al., 2019; Watt, 2012).

This perspective is especially relevant to integrated epidemiology because many oral and systemic diseases are cumulative. A life-course framework helps epidemiologists understand that disease is not simply the result of recent exposure, but of accumulated experiences, biological embedding, and changing vulnerability across time (Peres et al., 2019; Watt, 2012).

The socioecological model complements the life-course approach by emphasizing that health is shaped across multiple levels, including the individual, interpersonal, community, institutional, and policy environments. By situating disease causation within layered contexts, socioecological thinking strengthens the ability of epidemiology to explain inequalities and to design multilevel interventions that go beyond individual education alone (Peres et al., 2019; Watt, 2012).

7.5 Causal Pathways Linking Oral and Systemic Health

An integrated understanding of disease causation must also account for the pathways linking oral and systemic health. Some links reflect shared determinants, meaning that the same risk factors drive both oral and general diseases. For instance, sugar intake is linked to both dental caries and metabolic disease, while tobacco use contributes to periodontal disease, oral cancer, cardiovascular disease, and respiratory illness. In such cases, the association between oral and systemic conditions may not be direct but may instead arise because both are caused by overlapping exposures (Peres et al., 2019; Watt, 2012).

Other pathways may involve biological interaction. Periodontal inflammation, for example, has been investigated as a possible contributor to systemic inflammatory burden, insulin resistance, and adverse pregnancy outcomes. At the same time, oral conditions may affect general health indirectly through pain, reduced chewing ability, poor nutrition, social distress, impaired school performance, or delayed care-seeking. These consequences demonstrate that oral health is not a separate domain but part of broader population health and quality of life (Peres et al., 2019; Watt, 2012).

For epidemiology, the key implication is that causal interpretation must remain cautious but comprehensive. Researchers must distinguish between direct causal effects, shared risk structures, confounding, mediation, and effect modification. Yet even when precise mechanisms are still being refined, the public health importance of oral-systemic links is clear. Disease causation models and determinants frameworks, therefore, provide an essential foundation for integrating oral health into mainstream epidemiology, prevention, and health-systems planning (Figure 3).

Figure 3. Web of causation for oral and general health

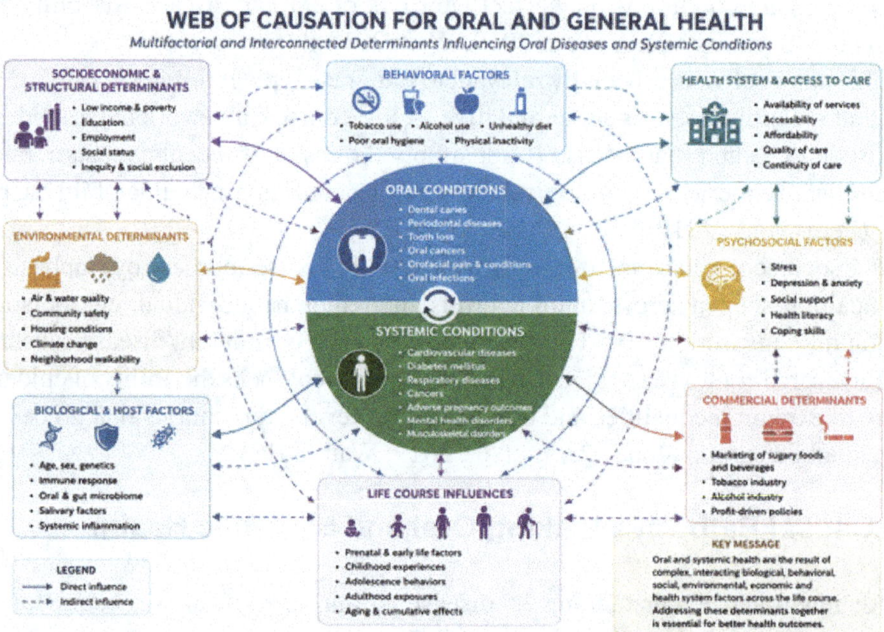

8. EPIDEMIOLOGICAL SURVEILLANCE SYSTEMS FOR ORAL DISEASES

8.1 Definition, Purpose, and Principles of Surveillance

Epidemiological surveillance is the ongoing and systematic gathering, analysis, interpretation and communication of health information for action. It's not just about describing health events, but also planning, prevention, control, evaluation, and policy (Thacker & Centers for Disease Control and Prevention, 2006; Thiébaut & Thiessard, 2017). For oral health, surveillance is especially crucial as oral diseases are common, socially determined, and largely avoidable, but tend to be neglected by health policy and practice. This enables the measurement of burden, recognition of risk factors, tracking over time, and allocation of resources (Kassebaum et al., 2017; Petersen et al., 2005).

Principles of good surveillance include clear definitions of cases, representativeness, quality, simplicity, timeliness, flexibility, acceptability, and usefulness for action (Thiébaut & Thiessard, 2017). In oral epidemiology, these are particularly relevant given that data sources are often multiple and may be periodic surveys or service-based data rather than ongoing surveillance. The World Health Organization stresses the need for oral health surveillance to be integrated with monitoring of other non-communicable diseases, and to provide information useful for planning and evaluation (Kassebaum et al., 2017; Petersen et al., 2005).

Surveillance is a continuous process that informs an ongoing public health response, unlike surveys. Surveys are cross-sectional, but surveillance enables trends and disparities to be tracked. This is especially important for chronic oral diseases, which take a long time to develop and reflect long-term exposures and the effectiveness of health systems (Peres et al., 2019; Thiébaut & Thiessard, 2017).

8.2 Types of Surveillance Systems

Surveillance systems can be categorized according to their design. Passive surveillance is based on regular reporting from health-care facilities or administrative data. They are cost-effective and simple to administer, but can have biases due to underreporting. In dentistry, passive data sources may be clinic-based, insurance-based, or hospital reports. They can be used to track service use and severe disease, but may underestimate disease burden as they do not include people who don't seek care (Thacker & Centers for Disease Control and Prevention, 2006; Thiébaut & Thiessard, 2017).

Active surveillance includes active collection of data, such as provider interviews, record reviews, or field investigations. It's more costly, but offers more reliable data. Active surveillance in oral health could be applied to track high-risk populations, identify potential oral cancer lesions, or assess the oral health status of at-risk populations (Thacker & Centers for Disease Control and Prevention, 2006; Thiébaut & Thiessard, 2017).

Sentinel surveillance involves monitoring trends and obtaining representative information using certain populations or sites. Sentinel sites for monitoring caries, periodontal disease, or dental care needs might include schools, dental hospitals, and community clinics. It's a valuable method in resource-poor settings where a national surveillance program is challenging to establish (Thiébaut & Thiessard, 2017).

Syndromic surveillance relies on symptoms or other proxies, rather than definitive diagnosis; this is more frequently applied in infectious disease surveillance. In oral health, it has limited use, but may be used to identify trends in oral lesions, trauma, or acute conditions as part of a public health event (Thacker & Centers for Disease Control and Prevention, 2006; Thiébaut & Thiessard, 2017).

8.3 Local, National, and International Oral Health Surveillance

There are several levels of oral health surveillance. At the local level, it informs school health and community-based interventions and planning for service delivery. Local surveillance can detect local inequalities, gaps in services, and local factors. School screening, community surveys, or clinic reporting can inform local policy and practice when collected regularly (Thacker & Centers for Disease Control and Prevention, 2006; Thiébaut & Thiessard, 2017). Large national datasets enable AI to identify behavioral and socioeconomic determinants, supporting targeted public health interventions and surveillance (M et al., 2025).

On a national scale, surveillance supports policy and workforce planning and tracks health targets. At the national level, data sources are commonly a combination of surveys, administrative data, and health databases. For instance, organized systems such as national oral health surveillance systems monitor the patterns of disease, use of services, and preventive measures such as fluoridation. National surveillance is crucial to highlight inequalities among populations (Thacker & Centers for Disease Control and Prevention, 2006; Thiébaut & Thiessard, 2017).

On a global scale, surveillance gives us an overview of the global burden of oral diseases and enables country comparisons. Global reports, such as those produced by the World Health Organization, compile information from various sources to draw attention to trends, issues, and areas for policy action. These systems are essential for global benchmarking, advocacy, and accountability, and highlight the importance of integrating oral health into surveillance of non-communicable diseases (Peres et al., 2019; Watt, 2012).

8.4 Linking Oral Health to General Health Surveillance

A key focus today is on embedding oral health in health surveillance systems. Traditionally, oral health data have been gathered in isolation, resulting in fragmentation and invisibility to policy-making. The World Health Organization calls for oral health to be integrated into chronic disease surveillance and universal health coverage (Peres et al., 2019). This practice is supported by the shared risk factors for other non-communicable diseases between oral diseases and sugar, tobacco, alcohol, and social determinants (Peres et al., 2019; Watt, 2012).

Integration offers several advantages. It boosts efficiency by avoiding duplication, increasing policy attention on oral health, and supporting the examination of common determinants and comorbidities. For instance, integrated data can be used to explore the relationship between oral health, diabetes, nutrition, and health care. Integrated systems also enable more people-centered and preventive health planning (Peres et al., 2019).

But integration needs to be carefully planned to include suitable indicators, training of the health workforce, data interoperability, and governance. Oral health indicators need to be well-defined and collectable as part of integrated systems. Effectively integrated surveillance enhances the monitoring of oral health and health system performance.

8.5 Applying Surveillance Data for Planning, Policy, and Evaluation

The most important use of surveillance data is for public health action. Surveillance data inform program planning through the prioritization of key conditions, risk groups, and needs. They support prevention efforts by providing information on risk factors such as sugar intake, smoking, and lack of access to health care. They also inform evaluation, by monitoring the impact of interventions and policies on health outcomes (Hajat, 2011; Peres et al., 2019).

For oral health, surveillance data are crucial to transform treatment-oriented health systems. Trends in oral caries, periodontal diseases, oral cancer and service use can be tracked over time, and disparities across socioeconomic strata can be monitored. This allows evaluation of health systems to determine whether they are getting more equitable and efficient (Thiébaut & Thiessard, 2017). It is also in line with universal health coverage (Arshed, Kazi, Kiran, et al., 2025).

Surveillance also has a vital role in advocacy and accountability. Documenting the burden of oral diseases, it facilitates the recognition of the importance of the diseases and supports the need for action. International strategies include enhancing surveillance to track progress in meeting oral health objectives and integration into universal health coverage (Thiébaut & Thiessard, 2017). Surveillance is needed to track progress in reducing disease burden, reducing inequalities, and the impact of investments. Artificial intelligence and data science complement, rather than replace, traditional epidemiological methods by enhancing disease surveillance, risk prediction, and evidence-informed decision-making. Figure 4 illustrates an epidemiological surveillance and learning health system for integrated oral and general health.

Figure 4. Modern epidemiological surveillance and learning health system or integrated oral and general health

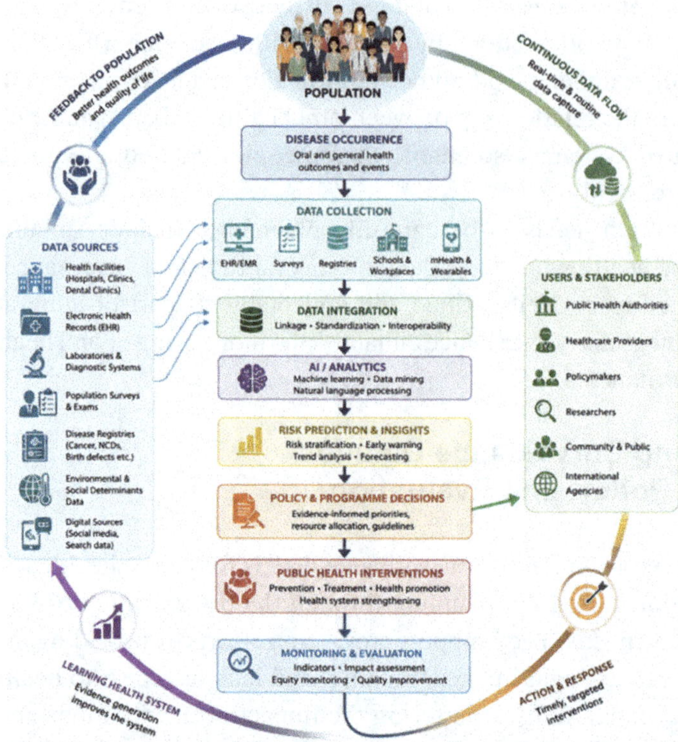

9. DATA, DATA SCIENCE, AND AI IN EPIDEMIOLOGY

9.1 Conventional Sources of Data in Oral and General Health Epidemiology

Traditionally, epidemiological research has been based on several key sources of data - population surveys, disease registers, census data, vital statistics, health facility data, and cohort studies. These continue to be critical sources of structured data on disease prevalence, risk factors, health-care use, and population profiles. In particular, standardized survey methods have been critical to assess population oral health in terms of dental caries, periodontal disease, oral hygiene, tooth loss, and dental treatment needs (Peres et al., 2019; Watt et al., 2019). The World Health Organization has been instrumental in facilitating the standardization of oral epidemiological data via survey approaches and indicators (Beam & Kohane, 2018; Topol, 2019).

Traditional data sources are particularly important because they are typically designed for population studies or surveillance. National health surveys and cohort studies are representative, can be used to compare sub-groups, and can be used to determine social gradients of disease. In oral health and general health, these data sources are crucial for examining inequalities by age, sex, income, education, and geographical location, and to understand the association of disease with determinants of health (Beam & Kohane, 2018; Topol, 2019) But they can be costly, discontinuous, and take time to produce results, which can restrict their use for decision-making.

9.2 Electronic Health Records, Registries, and Health Data

The rise of electronic health has led to new sources of epidemiological data beyond surveys. Electronic health records, claims data, laboratory information systems, and registries provide large amounts of routine data that can be used to monitor disease, predict risk, conduct comparative effectiveness studies, and health services research (Beam & Kohane, 2018; Topol, 2019) . These data are appealing as they are obtained from routine clinical care, may have broad population coverage, and can be accessed sooner than field-collected survey data.

Electronic health records and routine data provide huge opportunities, but also challenges, for oral and general health epidemiological research. These have the potential to be timely, large, longitudinal, and able to link medical data with procedures, prescriptions, laboratory data, and demographic data. But these data are not collected for research, which means they can be missing information, inconsistently coded, have variable practices for making a diagnosis, and selection bias (depending on who is receiving care) (Beam & Kohane, 2018; Salathé et al., 2012; Topol, 2019). As such, researchers need to carefully consider data quality, validity, and representativeness of routine digital data when making epidemiological inferences.

Registries are particularly important for tracking major and rare conditions, such as oral cancer, craniofacial malformations, or surgical complications. Registries may provide more consistent information about a disease than more general electronic records, but they may not be representative of the general population. Overall, integrated epidemiology is often best served by combining multiple data sources (such as surveys, registries, electronic health records, and administrative data) to leverage both population representation and detailed clinical information (Beam & Kohane, 2018; Topol, 2019).

9.3 Applications of Data Science in Epidemiology

Data science is simply a term that encompasses computer-based, statistical, and algorithmic approaches to draw insight from (often large) data. Data science has extended the capacity in epidemiology to work with big and diverse data sources, combine structured and unstructured data, discover patterns, build models, and provide more timely information about populations. This is extremely valuable in oral and general health, where data might originate from surveys, electronic health records, image archives, geospatial data, mobile devices, and administrative data sources (Beam & Kohane, 2018; Salathé et al., 2012; Topol, 2019).

Data science has made a number of contributions to epidemiology, beyond the management of large data. It also facilitates integration and interoperability, variable harmonization, and more sophisticated disease modeling. Epidemiology has historically been based on small, select data sets, while data science increasingly enables the use of large, multi-site data sets and data networks. These advances are critically important for comparative studies and contemporary surveillance, where data interoperability and harmonization are key to combining data across settings (Beam & Kohane, 2018; Salathé et al., 2012; Topol, 2019).

But data science does not substitute for epidemiology. Big data don't necessarily solve problems of bias, confounding, and measurement error. Indeed, systematic biases are even more difficult to detect when using large routine data. Therefore, data science should be thought of as building on, rather than replacing, epidemiology. Sound epidemiological thinking is still critical for formulating questions, selecting indicators, evaluating potential bias, and interpreting results (Beam & Kohane, 2018; Salathé et al., 2012; Topol, 2019).

9.4 Prediction, Surveillance, and Risk Stratification Using Artificial Intelligence

Artificial intelligence (AI) is a computing system that can undertake tasks such as pattern recognition, classification, prediction, and decision making. Epidemiology is increasingly using AI for risk prediction and automated image processing, pattern recognition in big data, and as a tool to support surveillance systems. International public health guidance has highlighted the potential for AI to enhance analytical power, speed, and surveillance for public health, but ensuring safe, ethical, and fair implementation is essential (Beam & Kohane, 2018; Salathé et al., 2012; Topol, 2019).

There is a rapid development of AI in oral health. Machine learning and computer vision are being experimented with for the diagnosis of dental caries, plaque, gingival inflammation, oral lesions, and oral cancer from image and multimodal data. AI is also increasingly being considered as a resource for population surveillance, inequalities mapping, integration of health and oral health data, and identification of subpopulations for targeted disease prevention (Beam & Kohane, 2018; Salathé et al., 2012; Topol, 2019). These trends indicate that AI may play a role in individual diagnosis, as well as precision public health in oral epidemiology.

Risk stratification is a promising application. Using data on demographics, behaviors, clinical and environmental factors, AI models could potentially help determine which people or populations are most at risk of oral and/or general health diseases. This may help to enable earlier treatment, more effective prevention, and prioritize scarce resources (Arshed, Kazi, Kiran, et al., 2025). But the value of these models is dependent on the quality and representativeness of the data used. An algorithm that is accurate from a technical perspective may be inaccurate from an epidemiological perspective if the data used for training it were biased, unrepresentative, or incomplete (Beam & Kohane, 2018; Salathé et al., 2012; Topol, 2019).

9.5 Opportunities, Challenges, and Ethical Considerations

The use of new data sources, data science and AI will provide significant benefits for oral and general health epidemiology. These include more timely surveillance, more complex risk modelling, earlier identification of disease trends, greater integration of oral health with broader health systems analytics and improved policies and planning (Beam & Kohane, 2018; Salathé et al., 2012; Topol, 2019). In countries with disjointed oral health information systems, these methods may help improve surveillance and tackle the longstanding invisibility of oral diseases in the public health agenda.

However, there are several caveats. Electronic routine data may be missing, inconsistent or skewed towards those who seek care. Electronic data may not include important social and behavioral factors, and AI may perpetuate or even worsen health inequities if it is built and validated using data from a population that doesn't represent the target population of interest. There's also a risk of prioritising predictive performance over interpretability, causality and accountability (Beam & Kohane, 2018; Salathé et al., 2012; Topol, 2019).

So, ethical and governance considerations are crucial. Recommendations for AI in health have emphasized preserving autonomy, ensuring transparency and explainability, promoting accountability, promoting inclusivity and equity, and being responsive to the needs of the health system (Beam & Kohane, 2018; Salathé et al., 2012; Topol, 2019). These are all pertinent to oral epidemiology, in which digital data systems may be less mature, vulnerable groups may be missing from data systems, and commercial technologies may be deployed more rapidly than ethical and regulatory processes can keep up.

In general, the future of integrated oral and general health epidemiology will be based on sound epidemiological principles and appropriate application of contemporary data tools. The basics of epidemiology require survey and other data sources to ensure representativeness and comparability, but digital data, data science, and AI technologies provide new opportunities for scale, speed, and integration. This means innovation should not be feared, but rather harnessed to ensure epidemiological principles, ethics, and equity are maintained. Figure 5 shows the big data ecosystem supporting oral and general health epidemiology

Figure 5. Big data ecosystem supporting oral and general health epidemiology

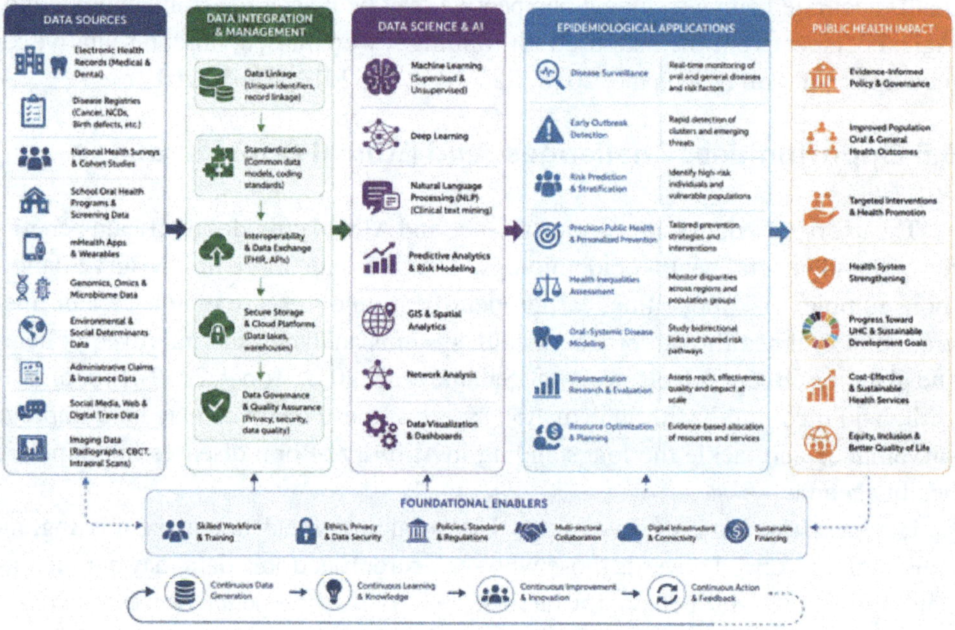

10. APPLICATIONS, CHALLENGES, AND FUTURE

10.1 Uses of Epidemiological Principles in Oral-Systemic Health

Epidemiology plays a key role in oral and general health research in describing disease patterns, determining causes, assessing interventions, tracking trends in inequalities and informing public health policies. These roles are particularly critical in the field of oral-systemic health research because of shared risk factors, social determinants, and health-care access issues for oral diseases and other non-communicable diseases. Epidemiology facilitates examination of the association between oral conditions and systemic diseases (including diabetes, cardiovascular disease, malnutrition and oral cancer), while also aiding interpretation of whether these associations may be causal (Peres et al., 2019; Thiébaut & Thiessard, 2017).

Pragmatically, epidemiology informs needs assessment, prevention planning and evaluation. Cross-sectional studies describe prevalence and treatment needs, cohort studies describe disease incidence and progression, and intervention studies (randomized or quasi-experimental studies) test behavioral, clinical and community-level interventions (Thacker & Centers for Disease Control and Prevention, 2006; Thiébaut & Thiessard, 2017). These uses are particularly important for oral health because many oral diseases are prevalent, accumulate over time, and are socially stratified. Epidemiological findings thus help to priorities groups and guide equitable resource allocation (Peres et al., 2019; Watt, 2012).

Epidemiology is also increasingly used to inform implementation and health-systems research. The current global oral health policy context is focused on prevention, surveillance, strengthening the workforce, governance and integration into health systems (Peres et al., 2019). This means epidemiological studies are expected to not only report the burden of disease, but also determine the feasibility, acceptability, scalability and equity of interventions in practice.

10.2 Challenges

But there still remain significant challenges in the area of oral and general health epidemiology. Firstly, data are not always of high quality, complete or comparable. Oral health surveillance systems are often lacking or under-developed in many countries and oral health indicators are often not included in broader surveillance. This makes it difficult to compare over time and between different settings, and may also hide inequalities in surveillance systems (Peres et al., 2019).

A further challenge is causal inference with complex, multifactorial diseases. Biological, behavioral, social and commercial factors influence the development of oral and systemic diseases, and confounding, mediation, and interaction continues to be a challenge. Many associations between oral and systemic health are significant, but they're hard to interpret because they are likely to be confounded by other factors such as cigarette smoking, diet, low socioeconomic status, and access to health care (Thacker & Centers for Disease Control and Prevention, 2006; Thiébaut & Thiessard, 2017). So better longitudinal designs, measurement, and analytic methods are required.

There are many practical challenges. Oral health services are often poorly integrated with primary health care, and inadequately funded and oriented to treatment. Lack of human resources, geographical access, referral mechanisms and affordability limit the collection of high-quality data and delivery of preventive interventions (Peres et al., 2019; Thiébaut & Thiessard, 2017). This is especially the case in low- and middle-income countries.

10.3 Equity, Policy Relevance and Health-Systems Impact

Epidemiology has a major role in assessing and tackling health inequalities. Oral diseases are heavily socially stratified, with disadvantaged populations being more exposed to risk factors, have less access to preventive care and have unmet treatment needs. Epidemiology can help to measure these inequalities, compare groups, and determine whether interventions increase or decrease inequalities (Thacker & Centers for Disease Control and Prevention, 2006; Thiébaut & Thiessard, 2017). This is of particular importance in oral public health, where health is closely linked to social determinants such as income, education, geographical location, and social exclusion.

Policy translation depends on producing evidence that is meaningful to decision-makers. Measures of burden, preventability, cost, and inequality are often more influential in policy settings than etiological detail alone. Recent WHO policy has explicitly linked oral health to universal health coverage, non-communicable disease prevention, health promotion, and stronger surveillance systems (Thacker & Centers for Disease Control and Prevention, 2006; Thiébaut & Thiessard, 2017). Oral epidemiology must therefore generate evidence that can support service planning, primary care integration, workforce development, and monitoring of health targets.

Health-systems relevance also requires implementation-focused evidence. It is not enough to know that an intervention works under ideal conditions; it is also necessary to know whether it can be delivered routinely, affordably, and equitably. This is why pragmatic trials, mixed-methods studies, and implementation-oriented research are becoming increasingly important in oral epidemiology (Thacker & Centers for Disease Control and Prevention, 2006; Thiébaut & Thiessard, 2017).

10.4 Future Directions in Integrated Oral and General Health Epidemiology

The future of oral and general health epidemiology will likely depend on stronger integration across disciplines, data systems, and levels of prevention. One important direction is the development of integrated surveillance systems that include oral health alongside broader non-communicable disease indicators. This would improve data visibility, comparability, and policy relevance while reflecting the shared determinants of oral and systemic diseases (Kassebaum et al., 2017; Petersen et al., 2005).

A second major direction is the growing use of data science and artificial intelligence to strengthen surveillance, prediction, and risk stratification. These tools may improve public health intelligence and help identify high-risk populations more efficiently. However, their use must remain transparent, ethical, and aligned with equity, human oversight, and public trust (Peres et al., 2019; Watt et al., 2019).

A third direction is the increasing importance of implementation science, systems thinking, and precision public health. Future epidemiology must address not only whether disease exists or whether an intervention can work, but also how interventions can be adapted, sustained, and scaled across diverse settings. This is particularly important in oral health, where preventive needs remain high and equitable delivery remains a challenge (Kassebaum et al., 2017; Petersen et al., 2005).

Overall, future progress will depend on balancing methodological rigor with practical relevance. The field must improve surveillance, causal inference, and data integration while remaining attentive to ethics, equity, and health-system realities. The most valuable advances will come from approaches that connect oral health with wider public health priorities and generate evidence that is scientifically robust, implementable, and policy relevant.

CONCLUSION

Epidemiology provides the conceptual and methodological foundation for understanding oral and general health as interconnected population health concerns. This chapter has shown that oral diseases are not isolated clinical conditions; they are among the most common global health problems, share major determinants with other non-communicable diseases, and reflect broader patterns of social inequality and health-system performance. Core epidemiological principles—including study design, disease measurement, bias, confounding, causation models, and surveillance—are therefore essential for generating valid evidence and guiding prevention, policy, and practice.

The chapter has also highlighted the importance of integrated approaches that link oral health with systemic health, public health surveillance, and broader health systems. Traditional epidemiological methods remain central, but emerging tools such as electronic health records, data science, and artificial intelligence are creating new opportunities for surveillance, risk prediction, and policy-relevant analysis. Their value, however, depends on strong epidemiological reasoning, ethical governance, and attention to equity.

Overall, the future of oral and general health epidemiology lies in producing evidence that is not only scientifically rigorous but also actionable. Stronger surveillance systems, improved causal understanding, and better integration of oral health into universal health coverage and non-communicable disease agendas will be critical to reducing disease burden and health inequalities. In this way, epidemiology can play a central role in advancing more preventive, integrated, and equitable health systems.

REFERENCES

Ahlbom, A. (2021). Modern Epidemiology, 4th edition. TL Lash, TJ VanderWeele, S Haneuse, KJ Rothman. Wolters Kluwer, 2021. *European Journal of Epidemiology, 36*(8), 767–768. DOI: 10.1007/s10654-021-00778-w

Arshed, M., Kazi, A. K., Ashraf, W., Kiran, M., Arshed, M., Kazi, A. K., Ashraf, W., & Kiran, M. (2025). *Universal Health Coverage: Progress Toward Achieving Universal Health Coverage and Lessons Learned* [Chapter]. Innovation and Transformation of Public Health. IGI Global Scientific Publishing. (universal-health-coverage). Https://Services.Igi-Global.Com/Resolvedoi/Resolve.Aspx?Doi=10.4018/979-8-3373-1992-6.Ch002. DOI: 10.4018/979-8-3373-1992-6.ch002

Arshed, M., Kazi, A. K., Kiran, M., Ali, S. M. F., Arshed, M., Kazi, A. K., Kiran, M., & Ali, S. M. F. (2025). *Challenges in Health Equity: Balancing Innovation With Fairness and Addressing Algorithmic Biases* [Chapter]. Innovation and Transformation of Public Health. IGI Global Scientific Publishing. (challenges-in-health-equity). Https://Services.Igi-Global.Com/Resolvedoi/Resolve.Aspx?Doi=10.4018/979-8-3373-1992-6.Ch004. DOI: 10.4018/979-8-3373-1992-6.ch004

Arshed, M., Kiran, M., Umer, M. F., Samkari, J. A., Hassan, S. M., Qamer, S., Gillani, A. H., Hameed, S., Ashraf, W., Mujtaba, H., & Khan, M. N. (2025). Prevalence and associated factors of adherence to antihypertensive medication: A nationwide cross-sectional study. *BMC Public Health, 25*(1), 2364. Advance online publication. DOI: 10.1186/s12889-025-21456-6 PMID: 40610935

Arshed, M., Mahmud, A. B., Umer, M. F., Mashhadi, F., & Kawish, A. B. (2025). Study protocol for a randomized control trial investigating the effectiveness of a multifaceted mHealth approach on adherence to antihypertensive treatment among patients in Pakistan. *Pakistan Journal of Medical Sciences, 41*(1), 1. Advance online publication. DOI: 10.12669/pjms.41.1.9272 PMID: 39867791

Beam, A. L., & Kohane, I. S. (2018). Big Data and Machine Learning in Health Care. *Journal of the American Medical Association, 319*(13), 1317–1318. DOI: 10.1001/jama.2017.18391 PMID: 29532063

Curran, G. M., Bauer, M., Mittman, B., Pyne, J. M., & Stetler, C. (2012). Effectiveness-implementation hybrid designs: Combining elements of clinical effectiveness and implementation research to enhance public health impact. *Medical Care, 50*(3), 217–226. DOI: 10.1097/MLR.0b013e3182408812 PMID: 22310560

Delgado-Rodríguez, M., & Llorca, J. (2004). Bias. *Journal of Epidemiology and Community Health, 58*(8), 635–641. DOI: 10.1136/jech.2003.008466 PMID: 15252064

Diez Roux, A. V. (2012). Conceptual approaches to the study of health disparities. *Annual Review of Public Health, 33*(1), 41–58. DOI: 10.1146/annurev-publhealth-031811-124534 PMID: 22224879

GBD 2017 Oral Disorders Collaborators, Bernabe, E., Marcenes, W., Hernandez, C. R., Bailey, J., Abreu, L. G., Alipour, V., Amini, S., Arabloo, J., Arefi, Z., Arora, A., Ayanore, M. A., Bärnighausen, T. W., Bijani, A., Cho, D. Y., Chu, D. T., Crowe, C. S., Demoz, G. T., Demsie, D. G., … Kassebaum, N. J. (2020). Global, Regional, and National Levels and Trends in Burden of Oral Conditions from 1990 to 2017: A Systematic Analysis for the Global Burden of Disease 2017 Study. *Journal of Dental Research, 99*(4), 362–373. DOI: 10.1177/0022034520908533

Gillani, A. H., Arshad, H., Arshed, M., Jairoun, A., Shukar, S., Akbar, J., Hussain, A. K., Malik, H. M. A., Ibrahim, M. I. M., & Fang, Y. (2024). Cross-sectional assessment of perception and attitude of pharmacy students towards pharmaceutical promotion: A study from developing country, Pakistan. *Frontiers in Medicine, 11*, 1424352. Advance online publication. DOI: 10.3389/fmed.2024.1424352 PMID: 39554505

Green, C. A., Duan, N., Gibbons, R. D., Hoagwood, K. E., Palinkas, L. A., & Wisdom, J. P. (2015). Approaches to Mixed Methods Dissemination and Implementation Research: Methods, Strengths, Caveats, and Opportunities. *Administration and Policy in Mental Health, 42*(5), 508–523. DOI: 10.1007/s10488-014-0552-6 PMID: 24722814

Hajat, C. (2011). An introduction to epidemiology. *Methods in Molecular Biology (Clifton, N.J.), 713*, 27–39. DOI: 10.1007/978-1-60327-416-6_3 PMID: 21153609

Kassebaum, N. J., Smith, A. G. C., Bernabé, E., Fleming, T. D., Reynolds, A. E., Vos, T., Murray, C. J. L., Marcenes, W., Abyu, G. Y., Alsharif, U., Asayesh, H., Benzian, H., Dandona, L., Dandona, R., Kasaeian, A., Khader, Y. S., Khang, Y. H., Kokubo, Y., Kotsakis, G. A., & Yonemoto, N. (2017). Global, Regional, and National Prevalence, Incidence, and Disability-Adjusted Life Years for Oral Conditions for 195 Countries, 1990-2015: A Systematic Analysis for the Global Burden of Diseases, Injuries, and Risk Factors. *Journal of Dental Research, 96*(4), 380–387. DOI: 10.1177/0022034517693566 PMID: 28792274

Khoury, M. J., Iademarco, M. F., & Riley, W. T. (2016). Precision Public Health for the Era of Precision Medicine. *American Journal of Preventive Medicine, 50*(3), 398–401. DOI: 10.1016/j.amepre.2015.08.031 PMID: 26547538

Moynihan, P. J., & Kelly, S. M. (2014). Effect on caries of restricting sugars intake: Systematic review to inform WHO guidelines. *Journal of Dental Research, 93*(1), 8–18. DOI: 10.1177/0022034513508954 PMID: 24323509

Peres, M. A., Macpherson, L. M. D., Weyant, R. J., Daly, B., Venturelli, R., Mathur, M. R., Listl, S., Celeste, R. K., Guarnizo-Herreño, C. C., Kearns, C., Benzian, H., Allison, P., & Watt, R. G. (2019). Oral diseases: A global public health challenge. *Lancet, 394*(10194), 249–260. DOI: 10.1016/S0140-6736(19)31146-8 PMID: 31327369

Petersen, P. E., Bourgeois, D., Ogawa, H., Estupinan-Day, S., & Ndiaye, C. (2005). The global burden of oral diseases and risks to oral health. *Bulletin of the World Health Organization, 83*(9), 661–669. PMID: 16211157

Proctor, E., Silmere, H., Raghavan, R., Hovmand, P., Aarons, G., Bunger, A., Griffey, R., & Hensley, M. (2011). Outcomes for implementation research: Conceptual distinctions, measurement challenges, and research agenda. *Administration and Policy in Mental Health, 38*(2), 65–76. DOI: 10.1007/s10488-010-0319-7 PMID: 20957426

Salathé, M., Bengtsson, L., Bodnar, T. J., Brewer, D. D., Brownstein, J. S., Buckee, C., Campbell, E. M., Cattuto, C., Khandelwal, S., Mabry, P. L., & Vespignani, A. (2012). Digital epidemiology. *PLoS Computational Biology, 8*(7), e1002616. DOI: 10.1371/journal.pcbi.1002616 PMID: 22844241

Silness, J., & Loe, H. (1964). PERIODONTAL DISEASE IN PREGNANCY. II. CORRELATION BETWEEN ORAL HYGIENE AND PERIODONTAL CONDTION. *Acta Odontologica Scandinavica, 22*(1), 121–135. DOI: 10.3109/00016356408993968 PMID: 14158464

Thacker, S. B. & Centers for Disease Control and Prevention. (2006). Epidemiology and public health at CDC. *MMWR Supplements, 55*(2), 3–4. PMID: 17183233

Thiébaut, R., & Thiessard, F. (2017). Public Health and Epidemiology Informatics. *Yearbook of Medical Informatics, 26*(1), 248–251. DOI: 10.15265/IY-2017-036 PMID: 29063574

Tonetti, M. S., Jepsen, S., Jin, L., & Otomo-Corgel, J. (2017). Impact of the global burden of periodontal diseases on health, nutrition and wellbeing of mankind: A call for global action. *Journal of Clinical Periodontology, 44*(5), 456–462. DOI: 10.1111/jcpe.12732 PMID: 28419559

Topol, E. J. (2019). High-performance medicine: The convergence of human and artificial intelligence. *Nature Medicine, 25*(1), 44–56. DOI: 10.1038/s41591-018-0300-7 PMID: 30617339 van Seventer, J. M., & Hochberg, N. S. (2017). Principles of Infectious Diseases: Transmission, Diagnosis, Prevention, and Control. *International Encyclopedia of Public Health*, 22–39. DOI: 10.1016/B978-0-12-803678-5.00516-6

VanderWeele, T. J. (2019). Principles of confounder selection. *European Journal of Epidemiology*, *34*(3), 211–219. DOI: 10.1007/s10654-019-00494-6 PMID: 30840181

Watt, R. G. (2012). Social determinants of oral health inequalities: Implications for action. *Community Dentistry and Oral Epidemiology*, *40*(s2, Suppl 2), 44–48. DOI: 10.1111/j.1600-0528.2012.00719.x PMID: 22998304

Watt, R. G., Daly, B., Allison, P., Macpherson, L. M. D., Venturelli, R., Listl, S., Weyant, R. J., Mathur, M. R., Guarnizo-Herreño, C. C., Celeste, R. K., Peres, M. A., Kearns, C., & Benzian, H. (2019). Ending the neglect of global oral health: Time for radical action. *Lancet*, *394*(10194), 261–272. DOI: 10.1016/S0140-6736(19)31133-X PMID: 31327370

Zwarenstein, M., Treweek, S., Gagnier, J. J., Altman, D. G., Tunis, S., Haynes, B., Oxman, A. D., & Moher, D.CONSORT group. (2008). Improving the reporting of pragmatic trials: An extension of the CONSORT statement. *BMJ (Clinical Research Ed.)*, *337*(nov11 2), a2390. DOI: 10.1136/bmj.a2390 PMID: 19001484

Chapter 3
Global Burden of Oral and Systemic Diseases:
Trends, Inequalities, and Epidemiological Transitions

Muhammad Farooq Umer
http://orcid.org/0000-0001-7779-1929
Department of Preventive Dental Sciences, College of Dentistry, King Faisal University, Hofuf, Saudi Arabia

ABSTRACT

The global burden of oral and systemic diseases shows a major public health challenge, presenting intricate connections between social, biological, and environmental factors. Over recent years, epidemiological transitions have led to a change from communicable to non-communicable diseases, with oral conditions, for instance, dental caries, periodontal disease, and oral cancers remaining highly prevalent globally. They are deeply connected with systemic diseases, which include diabetes mellitus, cardiovascular illnesses, and respiratory infections, reflecting a reciprocal relationship that worsens the global burden of disease. Currently, trends reveal that there continue to be inconsistencies in the distribution of disease, which are generally affecting underdeveloped nations and marginalized communities. Inadequate healthcare facilities, socio-economic differences, insufficient knowledge regarding health issues, and imbalance in resource distribution cause these disparities.

DOI: 10.4018/979-8-3373-8402-3.ch003

1. INTRODUCTION

1.1 Interrelationship between Oral and Systemic Diseases

In the immense field of human health systems, there is an intricate chemistry that exists between various human biological systems. Dental and systemic health are tangled in a complex network of interactions. The general health is significantly influenced by the health status of teeth, gums, and overall oral hygiene. In the modern period, the relationship between oral and systemic health is gaining recognition as a crucial part of research (Kapila, 2021). Dental disorders such as dental caries and periodontal disease affect general health and have connections with chronic diseases, for instance, diabetes and hypertension. To understand these associations, it is essential to develop integrated healthcare approaches for addressing the important causes of these systemic diseases through dental care (Sabharwal et al., 2021).

Dental caries, caused by bacterial activity within the oral cavity, progressed to systemic inflammatory reactions. Microorganisms, in case of poor oral hygiene, enter the bloodstream and propagate to distant sites, resulting in a progression of infection to various organs (Varoni & Rimondini, 2022). Likewise, periodontal disease, marked by the presence of chronic inflammation of the gingiva, has been related to uncontrolled glucose metabolism in people with diabetes. Additionally, constant inflammation may also cause other systemic illnesses such as rheumatoid arthritis, respiratory disorders, and cardiovascular disease.

1.2 Oral-Systemic Link in the Perspective of Non-Communicable Diseases

The growing incidence of non-communicable diseases (NCDs) has been established as a main global health issue and socioeconomic challenge (Beaglehole et al., 2011). Approximately two-thirds of all deaths worldwide are caused by diabetes mellitus (DM), cancer, chronic respiratory conditions, and cardiovascular diseases (CVD) (Ezzati and Riboli, 2012). A lot of risk factors, including alcohol and tobacco use; high-sugar diet; unhealthy food high in salt and saturated and trans fats; obesity; psychological pressure; genetic predisposition; and unfavorable socioeconomic circumstances, have been revealed over time to be common to oral diseases along with NCDs (Beaglehole et al., 2011).

Emergent research based on clinical evidence supported the association between periodontitis and systemic diseases and revealed that there is a bidirectional relationship between diabetes mellitus and periodontal disease. Chronic hyperglycemia significantly affects the neutrophil function, collagen production, and wound recovery, enabling diabetic patients to be more vulnerable to severe periodontitis. On the contrary, increased insulin resistance is caused by the systemic inflammation from periodontal disease, complicating glycemic control. Numerous longitudinal studies have documented that periodontal treatment can decrease HbA1c levels by up to 0.4%, emphasizing the metabolic effect of oral inflammation. Cardiovascular disease (CVD) with periodontitis also shows strong associations between them. Periodontitis causes the production of inflammatory cytokines like IL-6 and CRP, responsible for endothelial dysfunction, a precursor to atherogenesis. Along with systemic inflammation, oral bacteria have been found in atherosclerotic plaques, indicating a direct microbial invasion. Regardless of other risk factors, cohort studies show that people with periodontitis are 25-50% more prone to having CVD (Jin et al., 2016). Endothelial function can be improved by treating periodontal disorders and low levels of systemic inflammatory markers, such as CRP and fibrinogen, supporting the cardiovascular health of dental care interventions (Duley et al., 2012).

In addition, evidence indicates that, even after adjusting for confounding variables, oral diseases, particularly periodontal disease, are significantly associated with common NCDs such as CVD, DM, and chronic respiratory diseases (Mainas et al., 2022). Moreover, similar relationships have been observed in different diseases such as adverse pregnancy outcomes, chronic kidney disease, dementia, rheumatoid arthritis, metabolic syndrome, and a few types of cancers (Mainas et al., 2022). Clinical evidence further recommends that effective periodontal treatment can reduce systemic inflammation, improve cardiovascular biomarkers and endothelial functioning, and reduce blood glucose levels in patients with type 2 diabetes (Mainas et al., 2022). However, a definitive fundamental relationship has yet to be established, and further large-scale, multicentre clinical trials are needed. Given the close interrelationship between oral and overall health, common oral diseases, particularly periodontal disease, should be effectively prevented, controlled, and managed through a collaborative, multidisciplinary healthcare approach (Mainas et al., 2022).

The rationale for this chapter is based on the increasing recognition of an association between systemic diseases like diabetes, heart diseases, and respiratory infections and oral diseases like tooth decay and periodontal diseases. This interconnection is further complicated by the varying trends of disease, where non-communicable diseases are becoming progressively common as compared to communicable diseases. Even with the innovations in the medical field, dental issues such as dental caries, periodontal diseases, and oral malignancies are still frequently observed and closely related to systemic disorders, which raises the burden of disease and negatively impacts quality of life. Certain variables, such as disparities in socioeconomic situations, limited access to health care facilities, insufficient health knowledge, and the unequal distribution of health facilities, contribute to the continuation of these disparities. To address these concerns, this chapter explores current worldwide trends, inequalities, and epidemiological shifts in oral and systemic diseases. It also highlights the role of social determinants of health, and the healthcare system limitations vcontinue to affect illness outcome and patterns. Moreover, this chapter highlights the implementation of integrated, preventive, and equally implemented healthcare policies, fostering interdisciplinary alliances and interventions to lessen disease load and enhance overall health outcomes.

2. GLOBAL BURDEN OF DISEASE FRAMEWORK

2.1 Key Epidemiological Indicators in Disease Burden Assessment

The global burden of disease (GBD) elucidates the clinical and social consequences of a disease, in addition to the financial burden and human costs because of inadequate treatment and management. Quantitative assessment and monitoring of these burdens enable policymakers, public health experts, and clinicians to estimate the efficiency of interventions using standardized and reliable indicators. Key metrics, including years of life lost (YLLs), years lived with disability (YLDs), and disability-adjusted life years (DALYs), which together capture the level of premature mortality and the effect of disability on quality of life (GBD 2021 Diseases and Injuries Collaborators, 2024).

These GBD indicators play an important role in managing the distribution of financial resources, along with logistical and human capacities, predominantly in low-resource regions with limited healthcare facilities. Irrespective of their importance, surgical protocols have traditionally received less funding as compared to other regions of medicine and the public health sector (Wyper, 2024).

2.2. Global Epidemiology of Major Oral Diseases

Oral conditions, for instance, untreated caries in both permanent and deciduous teeth, periodontal disorders, and edentulism contribute a significant but frequently disregarded component of the global non-communicable disease burden. Although earlier GBD studies have combined oral health within broader non-communicable disease strategies and emphasized its significance in public health and health disparities (GBD 2017 Oral Disorders Collaborators, 2020), considerable gaps remain in understanding the epidemiology of these conditions across different life phases, particularly among younger individuals aged 0–39 years.

Traditional perceptions of oral disease distribution have influenced both healthcare planning and research priorities. The condition of dental caries has traditionally been regarded as more common in younger people, while periodontal diseases and edentulism were thought to be more common in the elderly population (Guan et al., 2024). Nevertheless, emerging evidence shows that the dynamics of these conditions are changing with a slow development of caries among permanent teeth and early periodontal disease and loss of teeth in young people (Zhang et al., 2024). The differences in prevalence might vary from one region to another and depend on socio-economic disparities, enabling an analysis of oral health in young patients. Previous Global Burden of Disease studies provided valuable data concerning the disease burden caused by oral conditions, usually focusing on the group of 10-24 year-old population or wider age ranges (GBD 2017 Oral Disorders Collaborators et al., 2020; Dai et al., 2025).

Based on the report by WHO on Global Oral Health Status (2022), roughly 3.5 billion individuals, almost half the population on earth, are affected by oral diseases, where dental caries and periodontal disorders play a significant role in this enormous global burden (Jain et al., 2024). In addition to posing risks to physical health, poor dental hygiene affects social and economic well-being due to inadequate school attendance, poor academic achievement, low workplace productivity, and job opportunities (de Abreu et al., 2021).

2.3 Epidemiology of Major Systemic Diseases

Cardiovascular disorders such as heart disease and strokes continue to be the leading causes of mortality, with an estimated 17.9 million fatalities per year. Remarkably, there is a significant relationship between a higher risk of cardiovascular episodes and periodontal disease. According to studies, people with healthy gums are less prone to experiencing heart attacks, strokes, or other serious cardiovascular events than the people having periodontal diseases (Martin et al., 2025).

Likewise, diabetes also exhibits an alarming health concern, with a projected 38 million people said to be affected by diabetes and over 98 million individuals having been reported to be prediabetics with more chances to develop type 2 diabetes (Centers for Disease Control and Prevention [CDC], 2023). Globally, over 828 million adults are affected by diabetes, a figure expected to reach 1.3 billion by 2050 (GBD 2021 Diabetes Collaborators, 2023). Type 2 diabetes accounts for the vast majority of diabetes cases, and is strongly associated with a number of chronic sequelae, including cardiovascular diseases, neuropathy, retinopathy, and nephropathy, all of which reduce quality of life and raise morbidity and fatality (Verhulst et al., 2019).

Regardless of an increasing amount of data suggesting a connection between diabetes and dental health, the results are still ambiguous and dispersed, in part because of variability in study designs, study communities, and outcomes evaluated. Periodontitis frequently co-occurs with other diabetes problems, through inflammatory and metabolic pathways by sharing common risk factors Bitencourt et al., 2023). People with diabetes may reduce haemoglobin (HbA1c) levels at 12 months post-treatment by treating periodontal diseases (Simpson et al., 2022). Nonetheless, there is still little evidence linking diabetes and dental caries, edentulism, and oral malignancy. Moreover, primary health care and diabetes management systems sometimes overlook oral health issues, particularly in low socioeconomic settings with limited health facilities (Peres et al., 2019).

3. BIOLOGICAL AND EPIDEMIOLOGICAL LINKS BETWEEN ORAL AND SYSTEMIC DISEASES

3.1 Mechanisms of Oral–Systemic Interaction

A number of interconnected mechanisms elucidate the epidemiological relations between oral and systemic diseases:

1. **Chronic systemic inflammation:** Chronic systemic inflammation carries a key role in involving oral and systemic diseases. Persistent oral infections like periodontitis cause the release of inflammatory mediators, for example, TNF-α, IL-1β, IL-6, and C-reactive protein, which may go into the blood circulation, resulting in an increase in the overall inflammatory burden in the body, possibly deteriorating existing diseases or being responsible for the development of new pathologies (Brower, 2025).
2. **Bacteremia and microbial dissemination:** Disease-causing pathogens present in the oral cavity can be dispersed through the circulation throughout the body. Eventually, they can spread to distant sites, initiate immune responses, and in few cases directly cause tissue damage and disease progression (Brower, 2025).
3. **Immunological cross-reactivity:** Molecular simulation between antigens of oral microorganisms and host tissues may provoke autoimmune reactions, thereby being responsible for the development or progression of systemic diseases (Brower, 2025).
4. **Shared risk factors:** It is evidently proved that both oral and systemic diseases are caused by the similar risk factors, which can be modifiable or non-modifiable, such as smoking, excess consumption of sugar, alcohol intake, poor dietary habits (with excessive ingestion of saturated fat and sodium), fatness, psychological pressure, depression, genetic predisposition, and socio-economic disparities. The control of these risk factors is essential in the incorporation of oral health into the general public health system (Wolf et al., 2021).

3.2 Evidence Concerning Specific Oral and Systemic Conditions

3.2.1 Periodontal Disease and Systemic Health

Periodontal disorders are a long-standing inflammatory illnesses that harm the tissues supporting the teeth and are one of the most widely studied oral diseases with regard to systemic health. Globally, it is predominantly affecting adults.

• *Cardiovascular Diseases (CVD)*

A firm relationship occurs between periodontal disease and cardiovascular outcomes, including atherosclerosis, myocardial infarction, and stroke. The chances of stroke may become more than twice in individuals with periodontitis, and have a 3 to 5.7-fold greater chance of cardiac failure (Yan et al., 2022). The pathophysiology behind cardiovascular events is primarily linked to chronic systemic inflammation, in which inflammatory cytokines are produced within the periodontium, causing endothelial dysfunction and the development of atherosclerotic plaques. Moreover, transient bacteremia from periodontal pockets may enable oral microorganisms to gain access into the bloodstream, leading to thrombosis and vascular damage. Epidemiological research strongly recommends that patients with moderate to severe periodontitis have a significantly increased probability of developing CVD, irrespective of other CVD risk factors.

• *Diabetes mellitus*

A strong reciprocal relationship exists between periodontal disease and diabetes. Periodontitis is often considered the sixth complication of diabetes and tends to be more severe in diabetic individuals. On the contrary, periodontal disease increases the chances of insulin resistance and type 2 diabetes by supporting systemic inflammation that impedes insulin signaling and glucose metabolism. Studies also reveal that periodontal therapy can be responsible for improved glycemic control. Diabetes, in turn, impairs immune response and increases susceptibility to oral infections, further worsening periodontal health, thereby reinforcing a two-way relationship (Preshaw et al., 2012).

• *Adverse Pregnancy Outcomes*

Periodontal disease is connected to adverse events, including preterm labor, low birth weight babies, and pre-eclampsia. Although the exact biological pathways remain under investigation, systemic inflammatory responses and hematogenous transfer of oral bacteria and their products to the placenta are considered key mechanisms.

Periodontal infection has been associated with a higher risk of preterm delivery, emphasizing the importance of maternal oral health in pregnancy outcomes (Vidmar Šimic et al., 2023).

• *Respiratory Diseases*

Oral pathogens can be inhaled into the lower respiratory tract, causing critical conditions such as aspiration pneumonia, chronic obstructive pulmonary disease (COPD), and bronchitis to develop. This risk is particularly elevated in hospitalized, elderly, or immune-compromised individuals. Periodontitis has also been associated with an increased risk of COPD, with affected individuals showing approximately a 2.1-fold higher likelihood of developing the condition (Scales et al., 2015).

• *Rheumatoid Arthritis (RA)*

Evidence increasingly supports a connection between periodontal disease and rheumatoid arthritis. The microorganism Porphyromonas gingivalis is known to produce peptidylarginine deiminase (PAD), which is responsible for the development of autoimmune responses found in patients with rheumatoid arthritis (Brower, 2025).

• *Neurodegenerative Diseases*

Some emerging epidemiological studies have provided evidence for the connection between periodontitis and neurodegenerative diseases, such as Alzheimer's disease, with mechanisms like systemic inflammation causing neuroinflammation and the translocation of oral bacteria to the brain via the blood-brain barrier (Brower, 2025).

3.2.2 Poor Oral Hygiene and Systemic Health

Poor dental hygiene, as evidenced by poor plaque control and lack of dental visits, is one of the significant risk factors for the development of periodontal diseases and dental caries, respectively. (Brower, 2025).

• *Bacteremia and Infection*

Poor oral hygiene results in an increased accumulation of bacteria within the oral cavity. Everyday activities such as chewing and toothbrushing can cause transient bacteremia, allowing oral microorganisms to enter the bloodstream. Even though these bacteria are naturally killed by the immune system of our body, recurrent or extreme incidents of bacteremia may raise the possibility of infective endocarditis, particularly in patients with underlying cardiac illnesses (Brower, 2025).

• *Gastrointestinal Tract*

A robust relationship found between the microbial groups of the oral cavity and the gastrointestinal system. Poor oral hygiene may cause bacterial imbalances that may affect gut bacteria, probably leading to many diseases, for example, inflammatory bowel disease and colorectal carcinoma. While the fundamental mechanisms are still unclear, the concept of an oral–gut axis is becoming more and more supported by research (Brower, 2025).

• *Obesity*

Oral disease-causing pathogens can disturb both the oral and gut microorganisms by the ingestion of bacteria and the release of inflammatory mediators, probably leading to gut dysbiosis associated with oral infections. Utilization of energy is affected by gut dysbiosis, which results in fat deposition, therefore increasing the potential of obesity (Patra et al., 2023). Likewise, inflammation because of oral microorganisms can disturb the activity of adipocytes, leading to disturbances in lipids metabolism and increasing the discharge of extra leptin and other adipokines and supporting fat accumulation (Clemente-Suárez et al., 2023). Therefore, these findings support the robust connection between oral and systemic health and emphasized the potential role of obesity and chronic systemic conditions (Patra et al., 2023).

3.2.3 Tooth Caries and Systemic Health

Dental caries denotes a common infectious disease caused by acid-producing bacteria that destroys mineral substances in teeth. However, it remains confined within the mouth; severe forms can progress to systemic illnesses.

• *Hypertension*

Inflammation is a key underlying cause of both dental issues and hypertension. Initial vascular changes related to hypertension may arise as a result of systemic inflammation and endothelial dysfunction. Nevertheless, more complex cardiovascular conditions like stroke and coronary heart disease are usually caused by various risk factors, suggesting that inflammation of the oral cavity is not enough to cause such diseases (Gualtero et al., 2023).

• *Systemic Infection*

If untreated, dental caries may cause pulpitis, abscess formation, and cellulitis. These infections can progress away from the oral cavity, resulting in systemic complications, for instance, pyrexia, swelling on the face, and, in severe cases, critical conditions such as Ludwig's angina or cavernous sinus thrombosis, particularly in individuals with compromised immune systems (Brower, 2025).

4. EPIDEMIOLOGICAL TRANSITION AND CHANGING DISEASE PATTERNS

4.1 Concept of Epidemiological Transition

A major change in the leading causes of death, along with increased life expectancy and a growing proportion of older adults, has been a defining feature of the epidemiological transition observed in Western countries. Recently, renewed attention has been given to this transition model due to the availability of more detailed cause-specific mortality data from lower- and middle-income countries (LMICs) (Santosa et al., 2014). It has also been suggested that combining this approach with the socio-ecological approach in the field of epidemiology would offer a more holistic framework to analyze and understand the shifting trends in the realm of health and diseases (Zuckerman et al., 2014).

4.2 Shift from Communicable to Non-Communicable Diseases

Globally, patterns of morbidity and mortality have shifted over the past century from infectious communicable diseases toward non-communicable diseases (NCDs) and injuries. This long-term transformation in disease patterns is referred to as the "epidemiological transition". The concept originally emerged within demography, where population changes were first systematically studied. Ultimately, it became a part of epidemiology and public health, resulting in the development of the broader term "global health transition" (Rockett, 1999). The global health transition is indicated by increased life expectancy and a change from communicable to degenerative illnesses that have significantly impacted the demand for and provision of health care services. Attaining the goal of "Health for All" needs a clear understanding of epidemiological transition and its related variations in disease patterns and health trends (Krenz & Strulik, 2023).

4.3 Demographic Transition and Population Ageing

One of the major global demographic trends is population ageing, which is mainly influenced by increased longevity because of better health care practices, better socioeconomic conditions, and easy availability of innovative technology (Suzman et al., 2015). Increased longevity is being noticed in developed countries along with low- and middle-income countries, mainly because of better public health infrastructure, extensive immunization programs, and a decline in mortality rate due to infectious diseases (Kowal et al., 2010). Nonetheless, longer lifespans may not necessarily translate to an extended healthspan, which is the amount of time spent in good health without chronic diseases or functional impairment.

4.4 Impact of Urbanization and Lifestyle Changes

A complicated interaction of individual, social, and environmental elements can affect urban health consequences. Urban health inequalities included socio-economic disparities, which influence access to healthcare services, education, job opportunities, and healthy living environments. The socioeconomic stratification commonly noticed in urban populations greatly affects health status. Socially and economically deprived communities are more likely to have earlier development of chronic conditions and a higher prevalence of multiple concomitant diseases (Álvarez-Gálvez et al., 2023).

Urban settings impact dietary habits by the variations in food access, cultural standards, and financial restrictions. Residents of more prosperous urban areas generally have access to a wide variety of healthy food selections, whereas those living in lower-income communities often face challenges in obtaining a nutritious diet. This is mainly because of the limited and inaccessibility of reasonable and healthy foods, for instance, fresh fruits, vegetables, and whole grains. The shortage of supermarkets in these areas has a crucial role in making food choices and is related to worse health outcomes among marginalized populations (Vilar-Compte et al., 2021).

Another key factor affecting dietary patterns of urban areas is the ongoing "westernization" of diets, which has been identified as a key driver of the increasing prevalence of non-communicable diseases. Longitudinal studies have demonstrated that urbanization and rising income levels are associated with a gradual shift away from traditional dietary patterns toward increased consumption of ultra-processed foods, refined sugars, unhealthy fats, and red or processed meats (Howard et al., 2021).

5. GLOBAL INEQUALITIES IN ORAL AND SYSTEMIC HEALTH

5.1 Overview of Health Inequalities

Oral health disparities still remain a serious health problem and are mostly experienced by underprivileged communities. Health disparities are commonly recognized as a major challenge confronting healthcare systems globally (Shadmi et al., 2020). The Centers for Disease Control and Prevention (CDC) describes health disparities as "preventable differences in the burden of disease, injury, violence, or in opportunities to achieve optimal health that are experienced by socially disadvantaged racial, ethnic, and other population groups and communities" (Centers for Disease Control and Prevention, 2024). Disparities in health play a critical role not only on an individual level but also in communities because they have a direct effect on the health and well-being of individuals (Cogburn, 2019). These preventable differences in health-related problems such as diseases, opportunities, and injuries persistently affect the marginalized groups of the population. The World Health Organization (WHO) has emphasized the importance of achieving universal oral health coverage, as reflected in the 2024 Bangkok Declaration, which calls for reasonable access to necessary oral healthcare services by 2030 (World Health Organization, 2025).

Effective global health planning is imperative for the precise understanding of the changing burden of oral diseases, mainly in the context of growing populations in low-income countries and population ageing in high-income communities (Peres et al., 2019). Additionally, since oral diseases, for example, periodontitis, carious teeth, and oral malignancy, have shared risk factors and their health status influences the overall bodily system, it makes increasing sense to view these diseases comprehensively. Hence, this integrated approach reveals the rising recognition of oral health as a difficult, multisystem public health issue (Baima et al., 2023).

5.2 Key Dimensions of Health Disparities

5.2.1 Income and Financial Constraints

An essential factor that affects oral health access is income status. Lower socioeconomic individuals have restricted access to good healthcare facilities, nutritional imbalances, and unhealthy environments that lead to health disparities. Low Income affects diet varieties; people tend to eat more sugary, unhealthy foodstuffs that put them at risk for dental cavities. Besides, the high prices of restorative dental treatments further encourage oral health disparities, inciting many individuals to delay or avoid necessary care. One of the studies has revealed that uninsured individuals are about twice as likely to experience untreated dental caries than those with private insurance (Vujicic et al., 2016).

5.2.2 Education and Health Literacy

Health outcomes are significantly influenced by certain factors such as educational attainment and occupational status. Higher educated people are more likely to seek dental care quickly, are more knowledgeable regarding oral hygiene practices, and are better at identifying early signs of oral disease. Conversely, poor oral hygiene practices, delayed diagnosis, and non-compliance with treatment are linked to low literacy about health. Improved oral hygiene practices and a decreased incidence of periodontal disease have been associated with higher educational status. Furthermore, effective public health initiatives enhance oral health literacy in underprivileged populations (Yu et al., 2024).

5.2.3 Occupation and Work Environment

Occupational conditions, including job-related stress, irregular working schedules, and access to employer-provided dental benefits, have a considerable impact on oral health status. Individuals engaged in physical work often tend to be less covered by dental insurance or have the low flexibility to attend dental appointments. Moreover, stress at work can cause negative practices like bruxism and poor nutrition, damaging teeth (Sato et al., 2021).

5.2.4 Geographic Location

Rural and urban underprivileged communities face distinctive health care barriers, which include weak health care facilities, lack of access to services, and insufficient health care personnel (Dopelt et al., 2021). Rural-dwelling populations have a high probability of experiencing long travel distances to receive their oral care treatment, along with a higher prevalence rate of untreated cases of oral diseases (Skillman et al., 2010). In this regard, teledentistry has been identified as an approach that is likely to facilitate bridging geographic gaps and expand access to oral healthcare services (Fitzpatrick, 2023).

5.2.5 Gender and Sexual Orientation

Gender inequalities remain prevalent in regions pertaining to health, while people who belong to underdeveloped populations may be subjected to additional difficulties, such as discrimination and a lack of access to culture-specific healthcare, which hinders their ability to seek suitable medical assistance (Lampe et al., 2024).

5.3 Relationship between Socioeconomic Factors and Health Outcomes

5.3.1 Cultural Beliefs and Practices

Cultural attitudes and beliefs related to oral health widely vary across populations and are often closely linked with socioeconomic conditions. Indigenous populations in many countries tend to experience poorer oral health effects, mainly owing to the combined impact of cultural practices and obstacles to accessing proper healthcare services (Jamieson et al., 2020). Nevertheless, culturally sensitive, community-based interventions have revealed promising outcomes, improving patient engagement along with overall oral health status (Nghayo et al., 2024).

5.3.2 Oral Health and Systemic Diseases

Socioeconomic inequalities in oral health raise the prevalence of systemic diseases such as diabetes and cardiovascular disease. Oral health problems are related to chronic systemic diseases, leading to a vicious cycle that impacts more significantly individuals from lower socioeconomic backgrounds. The connection between periodontal disease and cardiovascular disease is well-documented in deprived populations lacking access to dental care prevention and treatment options (Herrera et al., 2024).

5.4 Inequalities in Ageing Populations

Health equity continues to be an important issue for older people, and inequities are observed among different races, ethnicities, geographies, and socio-economic statuses, leading to disparities in ageing experiences.

Ethnic and racial minorities are also at higher risk of chronic diseases and early death among the elderly due to multiple social and economic factors (Wallace et al., 2016). Elderly individuals in rural areas do not have much access to health care facilities and other resources as compared to those who reside in urban areas, contributing to the health disparities between the two regions. Other factors like lack of adequate food and restricted mobility also affect the health of economically vulnerable older individuals (Henning-Smith et al., 2019).

5.5 Healthcare Access Challenges

The challenges faced by elderly patients accessing healthcare services include inadequate transport services, a shortage of experts in geriatric medicine, and fragmented service provision processes.

The problem of restricted mobility and lack of adequate transport services makes it impossible for many elderly patients to access medical care, especially those living in rural or underdeveloped communities, thereby causing a delay in diagnosis and worsening of their health condition (Syed et al., 2013). Workforce shortages in geriatrics and primary care further reduce the availability and quality of age-appropriate healthcare services. Besides, the fact that many elderly patients suffer from various illnesses necessitates collaboration between many practitioners, which is hindered by fragmented care models (Bierman et al., 2021). (Fig. 1).

Figure 1. Trends and inequalities in oral and systemic disorders.

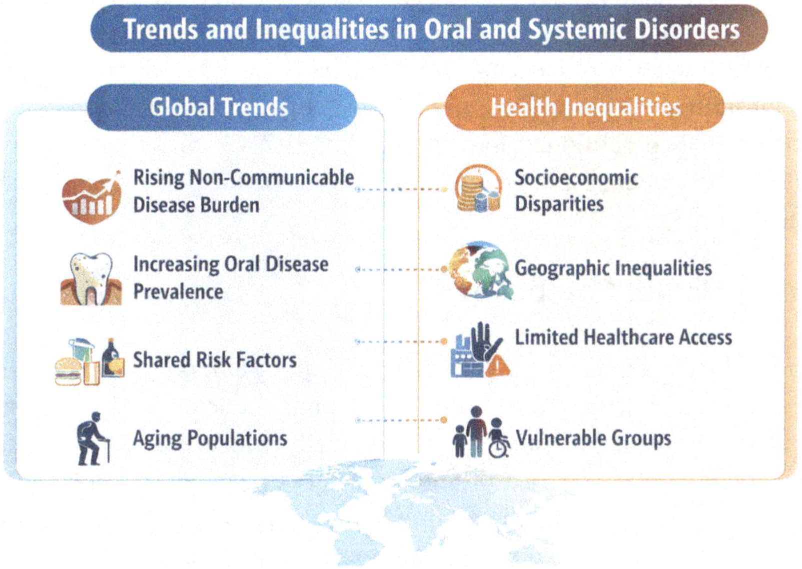

6. PUBLIC HEALTH STRATEGIES FOR INTEGRATED DISEASE PREVENTION

Integrating effective clinical and community-based interventions within a multi-level socio-ecological framework can improve the availability of health care services across different levels of influence, thus increasing the likelihood that individuals will utilize available resources. Greater engagement with services such as community health programs also improves their sustainability by enhancing cost-effectiveness and reducing the risk of underutilization (Castillo et al., 2019).

To support integration across all levels of prevention, several key considerations must be addressed. Significant financial investment and supportive policy frameworks are required to transform existing systems or develop new, coordinated networks that efficiently link available resources (Castillo et al., 2019). Moreover, proper training is necessary to guarantee successful application, maintenance, and sustainability of these systems. Evidenced-based approaches, cost-effectiveness, and acceptance are crucial for setting priorities of such strategies in both health care and community environments; yet, reaching consensus on these issues may not always be an easy task (Caron et al., 2023).

Overcoming these barriers needs strong leadership dedicated to encouraging integrated clinical and community-based strategies, accompanied by securing necessary financial and policy support. It also requires the development of educational curricula that highlight collaboration between clinical and community health services. Conventionally, health professional education has focused primarily on specialization within individual disciplines; nonetheless, there is increasing recognition of the need to prepare practitioners to work collaboratively in planning, implementing, and assessing comprehensive health strategies for major public health challenges (Bhati et al., 2023).

6.1 Public Health Perspective

From a public health perspective, oral health among elders signifies an increasing yet often ignored concern. Regardless of the high occurrence of oral diseases in this population, oral health remains unsatisfactorily prioritized within public health strategies, mainly in the context of chronic disease management and ageing policies. The issues become more distressing; the aged people under constant medical treatment are more liable to develop oral consequences because of persistent use of polypharmacy and the existence of concomitant diseases (Lipsky et al., 2024).

There are substantial disparities in oral health among the elderly, which are affected by such variables as housing conditions, education, socioeconomic standing, and availability of healthcare services (Lowenstein et al., 2025). The availability of dental care services is highly inadequate among residents of long-term facilities, those with economic hardships, and people who are mobility impaired (Rani et al., 2025). Many healthcare systems fail to provide adequate integration of dental care within their healthcare services, thus causing avoidable deterioration of patients' conditions (Ghoneim et al., 2022).

Basic prevention measures can be implemented in community-based programs, primary health care, and competent care centers, minimizing the use of special dentistry services (Abimbola, 2023). Education campaigns aimed at elderly individuals, their caregivers, and health care providers have achieved positive effects in improving oral self-care practices and overall oral health status. Combining oral self-care into general health promotion may result in higher rates of compliance and emphasize the importance of oral self-care as part of general health (Bashirian et al., 2023). Public health approaches that include carer-delivered oral hygiene procedures can greatly decrease the prevalence of oral diseases in long-term care centers (Rani et al., 2025).

Moreover, incorporation oral care into general medicine and geriatrics is another important part of a holistic approach to prevent poor health outcomes. Synchronization across disciplines can be effective regarding identifying medication side effects in the oral cavity and conducting preventive interventions (Prasad et al., 2019). With respect to the public health perspective, practicing oral self-care might assist in the preparation of recommendations, education programs, and incentive structures (Anyikwa & Ogwo, 2025).

In many countries, financing preventive dental care for senior citizens continues to be a significant problem. In some healthcare systems, access to dental care facilities is restricted where dental services are only partially covered under public programs. Accessibility and long-term sustainability could be enhanced by the integration of oral health promotion strategies and self-care techniques into insurance frameworks, community programs, and primary care services (Prasad et al., 2019; Anyikwa & Ogwo, 2025).

In spite of variations in financing strategies across nations, improved preventive measures combined with the integration of oral care and ageing guidelines are some steps to decrease the deleterious impact of medications on the systemic health of the ageing population (Ghoneim et al., 2022).

Strengthening public health care approaches that emphasize oral self-care has the potential to reduce oral health disparities. By recognizing oral self-care as both an individual responsibility and a public health priority, healthcare systems can move toward more comprehensive, preventive, and sustainable models of care for older adults receiving long-term treatment (Chan et al., 2023).

7. FUTURE DIRECTIONS AND PREVENTIVE STRATEGIES

7.1 Personalized and Risk-Based Preventive Approaches

Future preventive approaches to oral health care in medicated older persons must become more personalized and risk-oriented. Research advances on genetic predisposition, inflammatory processes, and oral microbiome activity have assisted the recognition of people who are more vulnerable to developing oral diseases (Khan et al., 2025). Despite the impracticality of applying genetic testing on a routine basis in clinical practice, combining clinical evidence, medication, and biological markers will help introduce more patient-oriented preventive actions. Individuals who are more prone to oral issues associated with systemic drug therapy need to be involved in practicing for better oral hygiene, go through more visits for consultations, and obtain personalized prevention measures (Maranville & Di Rienzo, 2014).

7.2 Technological and Interdisciplinary Innovations

For older people, advancements in technology like teledentistry, portable dental applications, and telemonitoring can be used to ease access to oral healthcare, particularly in cases where an individual is unable to leave home. These innovations enable early detection of health problems and encourage self-management (Beltrán et al., 2025).

Interdisciplinary collaboration is also necessary for the implementation of preventive strategies successfully. Integrating oral health assessments into primary care and geriatric services, along with the involvement of physicians, nurses, and pharmacists, can improve the identification and management of oral side effects related to medication. Pharmacists, in particular, play a crucial role in recognizing xerogenic medications and providing preventive guidance due to their involvement in medication management (Nelson et al., 2023).

7.3 Research and Policy Priorities

Research in the future must focus on the assessment of preventive measures that include the use of technology, involvement of caregivers, and education in oral care. Studies involving a longitudinal analysis of the effect of preventive measures are required for older patients under medication therapy. From a policy perspective, focusing on the oral health of older persons and those with chronic diseases could help develop policies, educational programs, and reimbursement mechanisms for prevention strategies (Kocher et al., 2024).

8. CONCLUSION

The emerging global burden of oral and systemic diseases emphasizes the critical need for a more integrated and equitable approach to healthcare systems. With epidemiological trends indicating that disease burdens are characterized by non-communicable diseases, the link between oral and systemic health is becoming ever more evident. Socio-economic differences and restricted access to prevention and medical facilities, as well as disparities in health knowledge, continue to create disparities among population groups, specifically in low-and middle-income countries. Addressing these challenges requires a change from segmented care models to comprehensive, patient-centered systems that incorporate oral health into general healthcare structures. Establishing public health infrastructure, encouraging interdisciplinary collaboration, and prioritizing prevention through community-based policies are mandatory to alleviate disease burden. Health policymakers need to adopt health care policies that emphasize inclusivity, surveillance mechanisms, and health resource allocation that will ensure everyone is provided with health care services.

FUNDING STATEMENT

"The Deanship of Scientific Research, Vice Presidency supported this Book for Graduate Studies and Scientific Research, King Faisal University, Saudi Arabia. [Project Number: KFU262220].

REFERENCES

Abimbola, O. Y. (2023). Evaluating the impact of community-based oral health education programs on preventive dental behaviors among adults in the United States. *International Journal of Medical and Health Research, 1*(1), 68–99. DOI: 10.61424/ijmhr.v1i1.605

Álvarez-Gálvez, J., Ortega-Martín, E., Carretero-Bravo, J., Pérez-Muñoz, C., Suárez-Lledó, V., & Ramos-Fiol, B. (2023). Social determinants of multimorbidity patterns: A systematic review. *Frontiers in Public Health, 11*, 1081518. DOI: 10.3389/fpubh.2023.1081518 PMID: 37050950

Anyikwa, C. L., & Ogwo, C. E. (2025). Enhancing oral health outcomes through public health policy reform. *Frontiers in Oral Health, 6*, 1604465. DOI: 10.3389/froh.2025.1604465 PMID: 40551851

Baima, G., Shin, H. S., Arrica, M., Laforí, A., Cordaro, M., & Romandini, M. (2023). The co-occurrence of the two main oral diseases: Periodontitis and dental caries. *Clinical Oral Investigations, 27*(11), 6483–6492. DOI: 10.1007/s00784-023-05253-2 PMID: 37714978

Bashirian, S., Khoshravesh, S., Ayubi, E., Karimi-Shahanjarini, A., Shirahmadi, S., & Solaymani, P. F. (2023). The impact of health education interventions on oral health promotion among older people: A systematic review. *BMC Geriatrics, 23*(1), 548. DOI: 10.1186/s12877-023-04259-5 PMID: 37697260

Beaglehole, R., Bonita, R., Horton, R., Adams, C., Alleyne, G., Asaria, P., Baugh, V., Bekedam, H., Billo, N., Casswell, S., Cecchini, M., Colagiuri, R., Colagiuri, S., Collins, T., Ebrahim, S., Engelgau, M., Galea, G., Gaziano, T., Geneau, R., & Watt, J. (2011). Priority actions for the non-communicable disease crisis. *Lancet, 377*(9775), 1438–1447. DOI: 10.1016/S0140-6736(11)60393-0 PMID: 21474174

Beltrán, V., López, L., Acuña-Mardones, P., Silva, R., Acevedo, C., Bustos, J., Alarcón, C., von Marttens, R., Espinoza, I., & Mariño, R. (2025). A teledentistry care model for older populations in remote settings in Chile using satellite communication technology. *Frontiers in Oral Health*, *6*, 1699401. DOI: 10.3389/froh.2025.1699401 PMID: 41424661

Bhati, D., Deogade, M. S., & Kanyal, D. (2023). Improving Patient Outcomes through Effective Hospital Administration: A Comprehensive Review. *Cureus*, *15*(10), e47731. DOI: 10.7759/cureus.47731 PMID: 38021686

Bierman, A. S., Wang, J., O'Malley, P. G., & Moss, D. K. (2021). Transforming care for people with multiple chronic conditions: Agency for Healthcare Research and Quality's research agenda. *Health Services Research*, *56*(S1, Suppl 1), 973–979. DOI: 10.1111/1475-6773.13863 PMID: 34378192

Bitencourt, F. V., Nascimento, G. G., Costa, S. A., Andersen, A., Sandbæk, A., & Leite, F. R. M. (2023). Co-occurrence of Periodontitis and Diabetes-Related Complications. *Journal of Dental Research*, *102*(10), 1088–1097. DOI: 10.1177/00220345231179897 PMID: 37448314

Brower, T. (2025). Systemic diseases linked to oral health: A review of the epidemiology of periodontal disease, poor oral hygiene, and tooth caries. *Dental Science and Innovative Research*, *4*(1). Advance online publication. DOI: 10.61148/3065-7008/DSIR/051

Caron, R. M., Noel, K., Reed, R. N., Sibel, J., & Smith, H. J. (2023). Health Promotion, Health Protection, and Disease Prevention: Challenges and Opportunities in a Dynamic Landscape. *AJPM Focus*, *3*(1), 100167. DOI: 10.1016/j.focus.2023.100167 PMID: 38149078

Castillo, E. G., Ijadi-Maghsoodi, R., Shadravan, S., Moore, E., Mensah, M. O.III, Docherty, M., Aguilera Nunez, M. G., Barcelo, N., Goodsmith, N., Halpin, L. E., Morton, I., Mango, J., Montero, A. E., Rahmanian Koushkaki, S., Bromley, E., Chung, B., Jones, F., Gabrielian, S., Gelberg, L., & Wells, K. B. (2019). Community Interventions to Promote Mental Health and Social Equity. *Current Psychiatry Reports*, *21*(5), 35. DOI: 10.1007/s11920-019-1017-0 PMID: 30927093

Centers for Disease Control and Prevention. (2023). *National diabetes statistics report*. U.S. Department of Health and Human Services. https://www.cdc.gov/diabetes/php/data-research/index.html

Centers for Disease Control and Prevention. (2024). *Health disparities*. https://www.cdc.gov/healthy-youth/health-disparities/index.html

Chan, A. K. Y., Chu, C. H., Ogawa, H., & Lai, E. H. H. (2023). Improving oral health of older adults for healthy ageing. *Journal of Dental Sciences*, *19*(1), 1–7. DOI: 10.1016/j.jds.2023.10.018 PMID: 38303786

Clemente-Suárez, V. J., Redondo-Flórez, L., Beltrán-Velasco, A. I., Martín-Rodríguez, A., Martínez-Guardado, I., Navarro-Jiménez, E., Laborde-Cárdenas, C. C., & Tornero-Aguilera, J. F. (2023). The Role of Adipokines in Health and Disease. *Biomedicines*, *11*(5), 1290. DOI: 10.3390/biomedicines11051290 PMID: 37238961

Cogburn, C. D. (2019). Culture, Race, and Health: Implications for Racial Inequities and Population Health. *The Milbank Quarterly*, *97*(3), 736–761. DOI: 10.1111/1468-0009.12411 PMID: 31512293

Dai, X., Dai, M., Liang, Y., Li, X., & Zhao, W. (2025). Global burden and trends of oral disorders among adolescent and young adults (10–24 years old) from 1990 to 2021. *BMC Oral Health*, *25*(1), 486. DOI: 10.1186/s12903-025-05864-z PMID: 40186217

de Abreu, M. H. N. G., Cruz, A. J. S., Borges-Oliveira, A. C., Martins, R. C., & Mattos, F. F. (2021). Perspectives on Social and Environmental Determinants of Oral Health. *International Journal of Environmental Research and Public Health*, *18*(24), 13429. DOI: 10.3390/ijerph182413429 PMID: 34949037

Dopelt, K., Avni, N., Haimov-Sadikov, Y., Golan, I., & Davidovitch, N. (2021). Telemedicine and eHealth Literacy in the Era of COVID-19: A Cross-Sectional Study in a Peripheral Clinic in Israel. *International Journal of Environmental Research and Public Health*, *18*(18), 9556. DOI: 10.3390/ijerph18189556 PMID: 34574480

Duley, S. I., Fitzpatrick, P. G., Zornosa, X., & Barnes, W. G. (2012). A center for oral health promotion: Establishing an inter-professional paradigm for dental hygiene, health care management and nursing education. *Journal of Dental Hygiene*, *86*(2), 63–70. PMID: 22584443

Ezzati, M., & Riboli, E. (2012). Can noncommunicable diseases be prevented? Lessons from studies of populations and individuals. *Science*, *337*(6101), 1482–1487. DOI: 10.1126/science.1227001 PMID: 22997325

Fitzpatrick, P. J. (2023). Improving health literacy using the power of digital communications to achieve better health outcomes for patients and practitioners. *Frontiers in Digital Health*, *5*, 1264780. DOI: 10.3389/fdgth.2023.1264780 PMID: 38046643

. GBD 2017 Oral Disorders Collaborators, Bernabé, E., Marcenes, W., Hernandez, C. R., Bailey, J., Abreu, L. G., Alipour, V., Amini, S., Arabloo, J., Arefi, Z., Arora, A., Ayanore, M. A., Bärnighausen, T. W., Bijani, A., Cho, D. Y., Chu, D. T., Crowe, C. S., Demoz, G. T., Demsie, D. G., Dibaji Forooshani, Z. S., … Kassebaum, N. J. (2020). Global, regional, and national levels and trends in burden of oral conditions from 1990 to 2017: A systematic analysis for the Global Burden of Disease 2017 study. *Journal of Dental Research, 99*(4), 362–373. https://doi.org/.DOI: 10.1177/0022034520908533

. GBD 2021 Diabetes Collaborators (2023). Global, regional, and national burden of diabetes from 1990 to 2021, with projections of prevalence to 2050: a systematic analysis for the Global Burden of Disease Study 2021. *Lancet (London, England), 402*(10397), 203–234. https://doi.org/.DOI: 10.1016/S0140-6736(23)01301-6

. GBD 2021 Diseases and Injuries Collaborators. (2024). Global incidence, prevalence, years lived with disability (YLDs), disability-adjusted life-years (DALYs), and healthy life expectancy (HALE) for 371 diseases and injuries in 204 countries and territories and 811 subnational locations, 1990–2021: A systematic analysis for the Global Burden of Disease Study 2021. *The Lancet, 403*(10440), 2133–2161. https://doi.org/.DOI: 10.1016/S0140-6736(24)00757-8

Ghoneim, A., Ebnahmady, A., D'Souza, V., Parbhakar, K. K., He, H., Gerbig, M., Singhal, S., & Quiñonez, C. (2022). The impact of dental care programs on healthcare system and societal outcomes: A scoping review. *BMC Health Services Research, 22*(1), 1574. DOI: 10.1186/s12913-022-08951-x PMID: 36564768

Gualtero, D. F., Lafaurie, G. I., Buitrago, D. M., Castillo, Y., Vargas-Sanchez, P. K., & Castillo, D. M. (2023). Oral microbiome mediated inflammation, a potential inductor of vascular diseases: A comprehensive review. *Frontiers in Cardiovascular Medicine, 10*, 1250263. DOI: 10.3389/fcvm.2023.1250263 PMID: 37711554

Guan, W., Li, J., Liang, Q., Huang, Y., Li, S., Xu, X., Zhang, Y., Wang, F., & Xu, X. (2024). Disease burden and health inequality of older adults with edentulism and the projected trend until 2040: Based on the Global Burden of Disease study 2021. *Clinical Oral Investigations, 29*(1), 22. DOI: 10.1007/s00784-024-06111-5 PMID: 39699767

Henning-Smith, C., Moscovice, I., & Kozhimannil, K. (2019). Differences in social isolation and its relationship to health by rurality: Rural–urban differences in social isolation. *The Journal of Rural Health : Official Journal of the American Rural Health Association and the National Rural Health Care Association, 35*(4), 540–549. DOI: 10.1111/jrh.12344 PMID: 30609155

Herrera, D., Sanz, M., Shapira, L., Brotons, C., Chapple, I., Frese, T., Graziani, F., Hobbs, F. D. R., Huck, O., Hummers, E., Jepsen, S., Kravtchenko, O., Madianos, P., Molina, A., Ungan, M., Vilaseca, J., Windak, A., & Vinker, S. (2024). Periodontal diseases and cardiovascular diseases, diabetes, and respiratory diseases: Summary of the consensus report by the European Federation of Periodontology and WONCA Europe. *The European Journal of General Practice*, *30*(1), 2320120. DOI: 10.1080/13814788.2024.2320120 PMID: 38511739

Howard, A. G., Attard, S. M., Herring, A. H., Wang, H., Du, S., & Gordon-Larsen, P. (2021). Socioeconomic gradients in the Westernization of diet in China over 20 years. *SSM - Population Health*, *16*, 100943. DOI: 10.1016/j.ssmph.2021.100943 PMID: 34703875

Jain, N., Dutt, U., Radenkov, I., & Jain, S. (2024). WHO's global oral health status report 2022: Actions, discussion and implementation. *Oral Diseases*, *30*(2), 73–79. DOI: 10.1111/odi.14516 PMID: 36680388

Jamieson, L., Haag, D., Schuch, H., Kapellas, K., Arantes, R., & Thomson, W. M. (2020). Indigenous Oral Health Inequalities at an International Level: A Commentary. *International Journal of Environmental Research and Public Health*, *17*(11), 3958. DOI: 10.3390/ijerph17113958 PMID: 32503229

Jin, L. J., Lamster, I. B., Greenspan, J. S., Pitts, N. B., Scully, C., & Warnakulasuriya, S. (2016). Global burden of oral diseases: Emerging concepts, management and interplay with systemic health. *Oral Diseases*, *22*(7), 609–619. DOI: 10.1111/odi.12428 PMID: 26704694

Kapila, Y. L. (2021). Oral health's inextricable connection to systemic health: Special populations bring to bear multimodal relationships and factors connecting periodontal disease to systemic diseases and conditions. *Periodontology 2000*, *87*(1), 11–16. DOI: 10.1111/prd.12398 PMID: 34463994

Khan, A., Barapatre, A. R., Babar, N., Doshi, J., Ghaly, M., Patel, K. G., Nawaz, S. M., Hasana, U. M., Khatri, S. P. M., Pathange, S. M., Pesaru, A. R., Puvvada, C. S., Billoo, M., & Jamil, U. (2025). Genomic medicine and personalized treatment: A narrative review. *Annals of Medicine and Surgery (London)*, *87*(3), 1406–1414. DOI: 10.1097/MS9.0000000000002965 PMID: 40213198

Kocher, T., Meisel, P., Baumeister, S., & Holtfreter, B. (2024). Impact of public health and patient-centered prevention strategies on periodontitis and caries as causes of tooth loss in high-income countries. *Periodontology 2000*, *98*(1), 65–99. DOI: 10.1111/prd.12592 PMID: 39323071

. Kowal, P., Kahn, K., Ng, N., Naidoo, N., Abdullah, S., Bawah, A., Binka, F., Chuc, N. T., Debpuur, C., Ezeh, A., Xavier Gómez-Olivé, F., Hakimi, M., Hirve, S., Hodgson, A., Juvekar, S., Kyobutungi, C., Menken, J., Van Minh, H., Mwanyangala, M. A., Razzaque, A., … Tollman, S. M. (2010). Ageing and adult health status in eight lower-income countries: the INDEPTH WHO-SAGE collaboration. *Global health action, 3*, . https://doi.org/.DOI: 10.3402/gha.v3i0.5302

Krenz, A., & Strulik, H. (2023). Physiological aging in India: The role of the epidemiological transition. *PLoS One*, *18*(7), e0287259. DOI: 10.1371/journal.pone.0287259 PMID: 37467173

Lampe, N. M., Barbee, H., Tran, N. M., Bastow, S., & McKay, T. (2024). Health Disparities among Lesbian, Gay, Bisexual, Transgender, and Queer Older Adults: A Structural Competency Approach. *International Journal of Aging & Human Development*, *98*(1), 39–55. DOI: 10.1177/00914150231171838 PMID: 37122150

Lipsky, M. S., Singh, T., Zakeri, G., & Hung, M. (2024). Oral health and older adults: A narrative review. *Dentistry Journal*, *12*(2), 30. DOI: 10.3390/dj12020030 PMID: 38392234

Lowenstein, A., Singh, M. L., & Papas, A. S. (2025). Addressing disparities in oral health access and outcomes for aging adults in the United States. *Frontiers in Dental Medicine*, *6*, 1522892. DOI: 10.3389/fdmed.2025.1522892 PMID: 40236738

Mainas, G., Ide, M., Rizzo, M., Magan-Fernandez, A., Mesa, F., & Nibali, L. (2022). Managing the systemic impact of periodontitis. *Medicina (Kaunas, Lithuania)*, *58*(5), 621. DOI: 10.3390/medicina58050621 PMID: 35630038

Maranville, J. C., & Di Rienzo, A. (2014). Combining genetic and nongenetic biomarkers to realize the promise of pharmacogenomics for inflammatory diseases. *Pharmacogenomics*, *15*(15), 1931–1940. DOI: 10.2217/pgs.14.129 PMID: 25495413

Martin, S. S., Aday, A. W., Allen, N. B., Almarzooq, Z. I., Anderson, C. A. M., Arora, P., Avery, C. L., Baker-Smith, C. M., Bansal, N., Beaton, A. Z., Commodore-Mensah, Y., Currie, M. E., Elkind, M. S. V., Fan, W., Generoso, G., Barone Gibbs, B., Heard, D. G., Hiremath, S., Johansen, M. C., & Palaniappan, L. P. (2025). 2025 heart disease and stroke statistics: A report of US and global data from the American Heart Association. *Circulation*, *151*(8), e41–e660. DOI: 10.1161/CIR.0000000000001303 PMID: 39866113

Nelson, S., Kim, E. G. R., & Kaelber, D. C. (2023). Integrating oral health into primary care: Perspectives for older adults. *Journal of Dental Research*, *102*(8), 849–853. DOI: 10.1177/00220345231165011 PMID: 37085982

Nghayo, H. A., Palanyandi, C. E., Ramphoma, K. J., & Maart, R. (2024). Oral health community engagement programs for rural communities: A scoping review. *PLoS One*, *19*(2), e0297546. DOI: 10.1371/journal.pone.0297546 PMID: 38319914

Patra, D., Banerjee, D., Ramprasad, P., Roy, S., Pal, D., & Dasgupta, S. (2023). Recent insights of obesity-induced gut and adipose tissue dysbiosis in type 2 diabetes. *Frontiers in Molecular Biosciences*, *10*, 1224982. DOI: 10.3389/fmolb.2023.1224982 PMID: 37842639

Peres, M. A., Macpherson, L. M. D., Weyant, R. J., Daly, B., Venturelli, R., Mathur, M. R., Listl, S., Celeste, R. K., Guarnizo-Herreño, C. C., Kearns, C., Benzian, H., Allison, P., & Watt, R. G. (2019). Oral diseases: A global public health challenge. *Lancet*, *394*(10194), 249–260. DOI: 10.1016/S0140-6736(19)31146-8 PMID: 31327369

Prasad, M., Manjunath, C., Murthy, A. K., Sampath, A., Jaiswal, S., & Mohapatra, A. (2019). Integration of oral health into primary health care: A systematic review. *Journal of Family Medicine and Primary Care*, *8*(6), 1838–1845. DOI: 10.4103/jfmpc.jfmpc_286_19 PMID: 31334142

Preshaw, P. M., Alba, A. L., Herrera, D., Jepsen, S., Konstantinidis, A., Makrilakis, K., & Taylor, R. (2012). Periodontitis and diabetes: A two-way relationship. *Diabetologia*, *55*(1), 21–31. DOI: 10.1007/s00125-011-2342-y PMID: 22057194

Rani, H., Azizan, A. A., Walad, N. I. A., Hassan, S. A. A., Dom, T. N. M., Yeoh, D. S. H., Tay, J. W. C., Rosli, M. S. A., Aun, N. S. M., Aziz, A. F. A., Thwin, K. M., & Tew, I. M. (2025). Challenges and recommendations for oral healthcare of older adults in a long-term care facility. *Health Care*, *13*(20), 2642. DOI: 10.3390/healthcare13202642 PMID: 41154320

Rockett, I. R. (1999). Population and health: An introduction to epidemiology (2nd ed.). *Population Bulletin, 54*(4), 1–44.

Sabharwal, A., Stellrecht, E., & Scannapieco, F. A. (2021). Associations between dental caries and systemic diseases: A scoping review. *BMC Oral Health*, *21*(1), 472. DOI: 10.1186/s12903-021-01803-w PMID: 34563194

Santosa, A., Wall, S., Fottrell, E., Högberg, U., & Byass, P. (2014). The development and experience of epidemiological transition theory over four decades: A systematic review. *Global Health Action*, *7*(1), 23574. DOI: 10.3402/gha.v7.23574 PMID: 24848657

Sato, Y., Saijo, Y., & Yoshioka, E. (2021). Work stress and oral conditions: A systematic review of observational studies. *BMJ Open*, *11*(5), e046532. DOI: 10.1136/bmjopen-2020-046532 PMID: 34049917

Scales, B. S., Erb-Downward, J. R., Huffnagle, I. M., LiPuma, J. J., & Huffnagle, G. B. (2015). Comparative genomics of Pseudomonas fluorescens subclade III strains from human lungs. *BMC Genomics*, *16*(1), 1032. DOI: 10.1186/s12864-015-2261-2 PMID: 26644001

Shadmi, E., Chen, Y., Dourado, I., Faran-Perach, I., Furler, J., Hangoma, P., Hanvoravongchai, P., Obando, C., Petrosyan, V., Rao, K. D., Ruano, A. L., Shi, L., de Souza, L. E., Spitzer-Shohat, S., Sturgiss, E., Suphanchaimat, R., Uribe, M. V., & Willems, S. (2020). Health equity and COVID-19: Global perspectives. *International Journal for Equity in Health*, *19*(1), 104. DOI: 10.1186/s12939-020-01218-z PMID: 32586388

Simpson, T. C., Clarkson, J. E., Worthington, H. V., MacDonald, L., Weldon, J. C., Needleman, I., Iheozor-Ejiofor, Z., Wild, S. H., Qureshi, A., Walker, A., Patel, V. A., Boyers, D., & Twigg, J. (2022). Treatment of periodontitis for glycaemic control in people with diabetes mellitus. *Cochrane Database of Systematic Reviews*, *4*(4), CD004714. Advance online publication. DOI: 10.1002/14651858.CD004714 PMID: 35420698

Skillman, S. M., Doescher, M. P., Mouradian, W. E., & Brunson, D. K. (2010). The challenge to delivering oral health services in rural America. *Journal of Public Health Dentistry*, *70*(s1, Suppl 1), S49–S57. DOI: 10.1111/j.1752-7325.2010.00178.x PMID: 20806475

Suzman, R., Beard, J. R., Boerma, T., & Chatterji, S. (2015). Health in an ageing world—What do we know? *Lancet*, *385*(9967), 484–486. DOI: 10.1016/S0140-6736(14)61597-X PMID: 25468156

Syed, S. T., Gerber, B. S., & Sharp, L. K. (2013). Traveling towards disease: Transportation barriers to health care access. *Journal of Community Health*, *38*(5), 976–993. DOI: 10.1007/s10900-013-9681-1 PMID: 23543372

Varoni, E. M., & Rimondini, L. (2022). Oral microbiome, oral health and systemic health: A multidirectional link. *Biomedicines*, *10*(1), 186. DOI: 10.3390/biomedicines10010186 PMID: 35052865

Verhulst, M. J. L., Loos, B. G., Gerdes, V. E. A., & Teeuw, W. J. (2019). Evaluating all potential oral complications of diabetes mellitus. *Frontiers in Endocrinology*, *10*, 56. DOI: 10.3389/fendo.2019.00056 PMID: 30962800

Vidmar Šimic, M., Maver, A., Zimani, A. N., Hočevar, K., Peterlin, B., Kovanda, A., & Premru-Sršen, T. (2023). Oral microbiome and preterm birth. *Frontiers in Medicine*, *10*, 1177990. DOI: 10.3389/fmed.2023.1177990 PMID: 37608830

Vilar-Compte, M., Burrola-Méndez, S., Lozano-Marrufo, A., Ferré-Eguiluz, I., Flores, D., Gaitán-Rossi, P., Teruel, G., & Pérez-Escamilla, R. (2021). Urban poverty and nutrition challenges associated with accessibility to a healthy diet: A global systematic literature review. *International Journal for Equity in Health*, *20*(1), 40. DOI: 10.1186/s12939-020-01330-0 PMID: 33472636

Vujicic, M., Buchmueller, T., & Klein, R. (2016). Dental Care Presents The Highest Level Of Financial Barriers, Compared To Other Types Of Health Care Services. *Health Affairs (Project Hope)*, *35*(12), 2176–2182. DOI: 10.1377/hlthaff.2016.0800 PMID: 27920304

Wallace, S., Nazroo, J., & Bécares, L. (2016). Cumulative effect of racial discrimination on the mental health of ethnic minorities in the United Kingdom. *American Journal of Public Health*, *106*(7), 1294–1300. DOI: 10.2105/AJPH.2016.303121 PMID: 27077347

Wolf, T. G., Cagetti, M. G., Fisher, J.-M., Seeberger, G. K., & Campus, G. (2021). Non-communicable diseases and oral health: An overview. *Frontiers in Oral Health*, *2*, 725460. DOI: 10.3389/froh.2021.725460 PMID: 35048049

World Health Organization. (2025). *Bangkok declaration—No health without oral health: Towards universal health coverage for oral health by 2030*. https://www.who.int/publications/m/item/bangkok-declaration-no-health-without-oral-health

Wyper, G. M. A. (2024). The global burden of disease study and population health metrics. *Population Health Metrics*, *22*(1), 35. DOI: 10.1186/s12963-024-00357-7 PMID: 39673070

Yan, Y., Mao, M., Li, Y. Q., Chen, Y. J., Yu, H. D., Xie, W. Z., Huang, Q., Leng, W. D., & Xiong, J. (2022). Periodontitis Is Associated With Heart Failure: A Population-Based Study (NHANES III). *Frontiers in Physiology*, *13*, 854606. DOI: 10.3389/fphys.2022.854606 PMID: 35514329

Yu, S., Huang, S., Song, S., Lin, J., & Liu, F. (2024). Impact of oral health literacy on oral health behaviors and outcomes among the older adults: A scoping review. *BMC Geriatrics*, *24*(1), 858. DOI: 10.1186/s12877-024-05469-1 PMID: 39438807

Zhang, X., Wang, X., Wu, J., Wang, M., Hu, B., Qu, H., Zhang, J., & Li, Q. (2024). The global burden of periodontal diseases in 204 countries and territories from 1990 to 2019. *Oral Diseases*, *30*(2), 754–768. DOI: 10.1111/odi.14436 PMID: 36367304

Zuckerman, M. K., Harper, K. N., Barrett, R., & Armelagos, G. J. (2014). The evolution of disease: Anthropological perspectives on epidemiologic transitions. *Global Health Action*, *7*(1), 23303. DOI: 10.3402/gha.v7.23303 PMID: 24848652

Chapter 4
Shared Risk Factor Approach in Oral-Systemic Diseases:
Common Risk Factors, Periodontal-Cardiovascular-Diabetes Triad, and Global SRFA-Based Policy

Muhammad Mohsin Javaid
http://orcid.org/0000-0003-2130-5156

School of Dentistry, Shaheed Zulfiqar Ali Bhutto Medical University, Islamabad, Pakistan & School of Public Health, Health Services Academy Islamabad, Pakistan

Hasan Mujtaba
http://orcid.org/0000-0002-1099-215X

School of Dentistry, Shaheed Zulfiqar Ali Bhutto Medical University, Islamabad, Pakistan

Najam Ul Hassan
http://orcid.org/0009-0002-6345-968X

School of Dentistry, Shaheed Zulfiqar Ali Bhutto Medical University, Islamabad, Pakistan

Muhammad Shoaib

Multan Medical and Dental College, Ibne Sina Hospital, Multan, Pakistan

Shahzad Ahmad

The University of Buckingham, Buckingham, UK

DOI: 10.4018/979-8-3373-8402-3.ch004

ABSTRACT

The shared risk factor approach (SRFA) provides a comprehensive framework that can effectively manage the growing global burden of oral and systemic diseases using a common modifiable risk factors approach. Oral health and major non-communicable diseases are closely linked risk factors such as tobacco use, unhealthy dietary patterns, physical inactivity, obesity, and inadequate oral hygiene. This chapter explores the relationship between dental health and the major NCDs, especially the periodontal-cardiovascular-diabetes complex. The chapter also discusses the problem of global differences in terms of disease occurrence and availability of healthcare services, highlighting the need for equity-based interventions. It suggests a global policy framework based on SRFA, which involves the integration of oral health in health systems, the enhancement of primary health care, and inter-sectoral cooperation. Therefore, optimal resource allocation and adherence to global health priorities are possible.

1. INTRODUCTION

1.1 Concept of Oral-Systemic Health Integration

Oral health is one of the basic aspects of human health and wellbeing, and the link between oral health and systemic diseases is widely recognized. The Global Burden of Disease Study (2019) stated that more than 3.5 billion people suffer from oral disorders, with untreated dental caries being the most widespread disease on a global scale. Oral diseases such as periodontitis, oral cancers, and edentulism reduce the quality of life and worsen existing socioeconomic disparities (GBD 2019 Diseases and Injuries Collaborators, 2020). Additionally, the United Nations' World Health Organization highlights the importance of universal health coverage and the association between oral health and several chronic diseases, such as cardiovascular diseases, diabetes, and cancers (Lamster, 2021).

The connection between oral health and overall systemic health has received increasing recognition above the last two decades. Numerous researchers have been explored the link between periodontal disease and various systemic disorders, including cardiovascular problems, ischemic strokes, diabetes mellitus, respiratory illnesses, low birth weight, premature birth, dementia, and even cancer. The major factors responsible for such a connection include infection by microorganisms, cross-reactivity of the immune system, and the secretion of inflammatory factors. Moreover, systemic conditions like diabetes and cyclic neutropenia greatly increase the susceptibility to periodontal infection (Schwarz et al., 2023).

Dysfunction of the immune system is one of the significant predisposing factors not only in gingivitis and periodontitis but also in other oral diseases, such as candidiasis. This two-way relationship indicates that a healthy oral condition is necessary to achieve good overall health and a high standard of living. Periodontitis is one of the major health problems affecting a vast number of individuals, as it causes adverse impacts on their oral health. Its impact on the body can lead to nutritional problems, as well as lowering a person's quality of life. Its systemic consequences may also contribute to starvation and a decline in overall quality of life, alongside significant psychosocial and economic burdens.

1.2 Evolution of the Shared Risk Factor Approach (SRFA)

The rise in NCDs (non-communicable diseases) around the world poses significant health and socio-economic burdens in various societies. Systemic diseases like cardiovascular disorders, diabetes mellitus, cancer, and chronic respiratory conditions contribute to nearly two-thirds of all deaths globally. There have been multiple pieces of evidence indicating an overlap in the risk factors that cause both NCDs and oral diseases that are highly common. The common risk factors associated with both include excessive consumption of sugary foods, alcohol consumption, smoking, diets loaded with fats and sodium, obesity, psychological pressure, depression, genetic predispositions, and social influences. To address these risk factors becomes imperative in incorporating oral health care preventive measures in extensive medical practices. The significance of executing effective programs that overcome the above risk factors cannot be exaggerated in preventing disease incidence and obtaining successful treatment and health outcomes (Wolf et al., 2021).

1.3 Rationale for SRFA in Modern Public Health

The Shared Risk Factor Approach (SRFA) has emerged as a significant tool in modern public health care owing to the developing insight that most of the oral and systemic disorders occur due to a common set of adjustable risk factors. A main foundation for SRFA lies in the increasing incidence of NCDs globally, such as cardiovascular diseases, diabetes mellitus, cancers, and chronic respiratory disorders, together with oral diseases such as dental caries and periodontal disease. These conditions share major behavioral risk factors, for instance use of tobacco, harmful diet (mainly high sugar intake), physical inactivity, and excessive alcohol consumption. By directing the shared determinants of these diseases, public health programs can achieve a broader scope of influence on multiple health outcomes and decrease the disease burden effectively. Contrasting the disease-specific methods that have been conventionally implemented, SRFA emphasizes an integrated prevention-based approach that aims the underlying causes, thereby giving a more effective and reliable means of promoting health.

1.4 Scope of the Chapter

This chapter explores the relationship between systemic illnesses and oral diseases through examining their shared risk factors, microbiology, and socio-economic concerns. By integrating evidence from contemporary research and public health efforts, it targets the need for cooperative interdisciplinary approaches, effective preventive approaches, and policy developments to alleviate global inequalities in oral health.

2. COMMON RISK FACTORS IN ORAL AND SYSTEMIC DISEASES

2.1 Behavioral Risk Factors

Tobacco use has long been related to periodontitis and edentulism. In smokers and consumers of smokeless tobacco, the oral cavity is exposed to raise nicotine levels, with concentrations in gingival crevicular fluid observed to be up to 300 times greater in comparison with the bloodstream. Owing to its vaso-constrictive properties, nicotine may alleviate blood loss on probing (a hallmark of periodontal disease), enabling disease detection to be more challenging in smokers. In spite of this, nicotine exerts harmful effects on periodontal tissues by impairing the multiplication and attachment of human gingival fibroblasts to root surfaces, consequently compromising gingival attachment. Moreover, it aggravates the formation and activity of osteoclasts, causing increased resorption of alveolar bone. Nicotine also regulates the expression of advanced glycation end products and their receptors in periodontal tissues that can reduce healing and the success of periodontal surgical procedures in smokers (Javed et al., 2019).

Stress, a psychophysiological response to internal or external stimuli, is vital for survival as it makes the body fight acute challenges like infection or surgical procedures. This reaction involves mechanisms such as redistribution of immune cells, intensified alertness, and rearrangement of energy resources. However, short-term (acute) stress can enhance immune system function, while persistent or chronic stress may disrupt immune homeostasis and cause adverse health outcomes. Stress can originate from physical factors, such as infection, in addition to psychological effects, including major life incidents and everyday pressures. Continuous stress can initiate depression, nervousness, cognitive impairment, and changes in self-respect, with its overall impact affected by managing strategies, social support, and life routine aspects (Alotiby, 2024).

Numerous research studies indicate a positive relationship between stress and periodontal disorders. Chronic stress can be assessed through self-reported measures or biomarkers such as cortisol and has been linked to increased attachment loss, deeper periodontal pockets, and enhanced alveolar bone resorption. Financial stress and depression also serve to increase the likelihood of development of this disease, according to results from large population studies. In addition, it is evidently supported that depression is associated with higher levels of serum IgG antibodies, along with poor periodontal status. This highlights the importance of psychological health and stress management in preventing and controlling periodontal disease (Knight et al. 2016).

Excessive alcohol consumption is recognized as a shared risk factor that adversely impacts both oral and overall health. Persons who consume high amounts of alcohol tend to exhibit a greater number of decayed tooth surfaces as well as an increased prevalence of periapical lesions. (Joseph et al., 2016).

2.2 Biological and Metabolic Risk Factors

The increasing global occurrence of obesity has led to an increase in metabolic syndrome and type 2 diabetes, with diabetes accounting for about 2.6% of global disability-adjusted life years (DALYs) in 2019 (GBD 2019 Diseases and Injuries Collaborators, 2020). The relationship between periodontal disease and metabolic syndrome is believed to stem from common inflammatory pathways and the buildup of advanced glycation end products. These situations are shaped by many factors, involving obesity, insulin resistance, genetic predisposition, and oral infections, all of which can weaken endothelial function and interrupt glucose metabolism (Meurman & Bascones-Martínez, 2021).

There is a reciprocal association between diabetes mellitus and periodontal diseases, as DM increases the probability of infections in the oral cavity, whereas periodontal infections may have a negative impact on the blood glucose levels. Recent findings show that the successful management of periodontal diseases positively impacts the glucose level in patients with type 2 DM, whereas better glucose metabolism may improve the periodontal health of the patient. This bidirectional association underscores the importance of integrated healthcare strategies. Robust interdisciplinary alliance and precise communication between medical and dental experts are imperative to heighten patient outcomes and improve overall quality of life (Meurman & Bascones-Martínez, 2021).

2.3 Environmental and Social Determinants

The environment exhibits a key role in defining health outcomes, including both social and built factors. Social determinants, for instance, income differences, entrance to social support, and exposure to discrimination, along with environmental conditions created by humans, considerably impact overall health. Concerning oral health, conditions such as dental caries and fluorosis are strongly associated with environmental parameters, mainly water fluoridation. Dental caries, one of the most prevalent chronic diseases globally, excessively impacts underprivileged populations, specifically children from ethnic minorities, rural areas, and lower socioeconomic classes. Robust evidence reveals that water fluoridation and fluoride-based preventions successfully reduce caries in underdeveloped communities, emphasizing the requirement for equitable public health policies (De Abreu et al., 2021).

Additionally, environmental changes intensify prevalent health inconsistencies through both indirect and direct effects. The changes in severe weather patterns, combined with the insufficient food and water supplies and vector-borne diseases, show the intimate relationship between climate change and health. It is particularly difficult for susceptible groups, as they experience limited access to healthcare facilities and emerging levels of social inequalities. Effectual approaches to considering these problems include developing policies which are aimed at decreasing carbon dioxide releases and sustaining climate stability, and reinforcement of healthcare systems. It is important to employ a multidisciplinary approach that requires the collaboration of the local community members, the government support, and the international organizations. There is sufficient evidence revealing the direct connection between environmental variables and human well-being that impacts all types of health concerns, from cardiovascular disorders to psychological ailments. Maintainable development involves the integration of economic progress, social justice, and environmental protection, playing a pivotal role in managing these challenges. The United Nations' 17 Sustainable Development Goals (SDGs) for 2030 offer a strategic framework for achieving inclusive and sustainable improvement. These goals underscore poverty and starvation reduction, universal access to education, healthcare, and uncontaminated water, along with gender impartiality and environmental protection. These harmonized movements are necessary in dealing with the disparities in oral health and other systemic disorders (De Abreu et al., 2021).

3. PATHOPHYSIOLOGICAL LINKS BETWEEN ORAL AND SYSTEMIC DISEASES

3.1 Role of Chronic Inflammation

Chronic infection in the oral cavity, particularly in periodontal tissues, is closely linked to imbalances in the oral microbiota and may elevate the overall systemic inflammatory load (Yekani et al., 2025). In the older population, periodontal disease has been linked to various systemic conditions, including fragility, diabetes mellitus, respiratory and cardiovascular disorders (Öçbe et al., 2025). Taking into account that systemic inflammation shows a vital role in disease pathogenesis in elder people, the interaction between them possesses great clinical significance (Acipinar & Yalcin, 2025).

3.2 Microbial Dysbiosis and Oral Microbiome

Infections arising in any part of the body increase the level of chemokines, cytokines, and other inflammatory factors, eventually resulting in inflammation. Oral and dental infections are quite prevalent and are often associated with continuous bacterial activity, which results in inflammation of the surrounding tissues. Oral microorganisms have the potential to spread to cause infections in the jaw bones, face and deeper anatomical spaces such as the Para pharyngeal or peri-tonsillar areas. For chronic conditions, infections may progress to involve the brain or lungs through aspiration. In addition to local and distant spread, oral diseases can also affect other organs due to bacterial toxins and a compromised immune response, leading to conditions such as viridans streptococcal endocarditis and glomerulonephritis. Furthermore, oral infections may interfere with the coagulation process, contributing to systemic inflammatory conditions (Meurman & Bascones-Martínez, 2021).

At a broader level, evidence indicates that approximately 20% of circulating small molecules are derived from microbial sources. Considering its abundant diversity in microorganisms, the oral cavity can play a key role as a system exposing the body to different microbes. The area of inflamed gums in case of gingivitis can resemble that of a person's palm in terms of dimensions. This allows microorganisms to enter the blood or lymph circulation, where their presence causes stimulation of immune and epithelial cells, for instance, B and T lymphocytes, which in turn have an impact on DNA damage and repair. To address dysbiosis associated with oral diseases, strategies aimed at restoring microbial balance such as probiotic therapy have been proposed, as they may support oral health and help limit disease progression (Meurman & Bascones-Martínez, 2021).

3.3 Immune Response and Systemic Dissemination

Diabetes and periodontitis share a strong bidirectional relationship, where diabetes increases the likelihood of developing chronic periodontitis by approximately two to three times, while periodontal disease, in turn, worsens systemic inflammation and interferes with glycemic control. Microorganisms exist in periodontal pockets and affect the host immune system, instigating persistent inflammation with extensive systemic consequences.

3.4 Oxidative Stress and Endothelial Dysfunction

Specific pathogens, such as *P. gingivalis*, stimulate inflammatory signaling pathways like NF-κB, leading to decreased insulin sensitivity, heightened insulin resistance, and disturbances in glucose metabolism. Furthermore, periodontal infections induce oxidative stress, causing the production of reactive oxygen species (ROS) that further disrupt insulin signaling and amplify systemic inflammation (Jia et al., 2023).

4. THE PERIODONTAL–CARDIOVASCULAR–DIABETES TRIAD

4.1 Periodontal Disease and Diabetes Mellitus

The periodontal pathogens can get into the bloodstream, causing bacteremia and increasing the concentration of systemic markers of inflammation, which include C-reactive protein and pentraxin-3. It is important to mention that the treatment for periodontal disease has helped to decrease these markers, thus stressing the significance of good oral hygiene in the successful management of diabetes and systemic inflammation in general (Jia et al., 2023).

According to meta-analyses, diabetic patients have a two- to three-fold higher risk of having periodontitis when compared with non-diabetic people (Xie et al., 2023). On the other hand, one of the studies shows that NSPT can positively influence glycemic status, causing an improvement in the hemoglobin HbA1c level by 0.3%-0.6% within 3-6 months (Simpson et al., 2022).

Additionally, a randomized control trial study conducted on more than 1000 patients suffering from type 2 diabetes revealed that there was an improvement in the HbA1c level, irrespective of the modifications in their antidiabetic drugs; hence, stressing the importance of proper oral hygiene (Wojtkowska et al., 2021).

4.2 Periodontal Disease and Cardiovascular Diseases

Periodontal disease is known to be associated with an increased risk of heart attack and stroke, especially in young people, smokers, and poor socio-economic families. The connection between periodontal infections and CVD can be elucidated through both indirect and direct mechanisms. Directly, the oral bacteria and their endotoxins can move into the bloodstream, stimulating hypercoagulability and atherosclerosis formation. Indirectly, periodontal infections provoke systemic inflammation, as presented by raised levels of markers such as C-reactive protein in affected individuals (Pietiäinen et al., 2018).

Periodontal pathogens, especially P. gingivalis, and their metabolic products, can spread into the systemic circulation through unhealthy periodontal tissues. This results in systemic inflammation and eventually predisposes to atherosclerotic plaque formation. Research evidence originating from human trials and animal experiments shows that P. gingivalis infection is related to gut dysbiosis, resulting in endo-toxemia and increasing the inflammatory cytokines levels, for instance, C-reactive protein (CRP), IL-1β, IL-6, and TNF-α. These inflammatory processes have a crucial role to play in endothelial dysfunction and the development of atherosclerosis.

Furthermore, oral bacteria such as Streptococcus gordonii and Streptococcus sanguis, usually found in dental plaque, have contributed to infective endocarditis because of their capability to adhere to thrombus-like deposits on the endothelium lining the blood vessels. Moreover, there is proof that periodontal treatment decreases levels of serum CRP and reduces systemic inflammation, consequently supporting the link between periodontal condition and inflammation burden. Likewise, periodontal disease has also been associated with new biomarkers like Galectin-3 and suPAR, which indicate inflammation of the heart and cardiac fibrosis. These outcomes illustrate the significance of periodontal disease in predicting cardiovascular diseases and reducing its incidence (Pietiäinen et al., 2018; Meurman & Bascones-Martínez, 2021).

4.3 Diabetes Mellitus and Cardiovascular Diseases

The CVD-DM relationship is well demonstrated, which includes the most important risk factors such as hyperglycemia, insulin resistance, endothelial dysfunction, dyslipidemia, and chronic inflammation. Cardiovascular disease is one of the leading causes of high mortality rates among patients with diabetes, since more than 65% of deaths are caused by cardiovascular complications in patients with DM (de Carvalho et al., 2021).

Persistent hyperglycemia has a detrimental effect on cardiovascular damage by impairing endothelial function. Hyperglycemia is caused by the increased production of reactive oxygen species (ROS), unavailability of nitric oxide, and increased AGEs production (Gatto et al., 2025). They cause enhanced permeability of vascular walls, increased bonding of white blood cells, and smooth muscle proliferation that activate atherosclerosis development (Gatto et al., 2025).

Insulin resistance is a main indicator of type 2 diabetes, which triggers an even more rapid onset of atherosclerosis due to specific processes. It stimulates the release of free fatty acids, activates the liver to produce very-low-density lipoproteins (VLDL), and decreases the levels of high-density lipoproteins (HDL), resulting in an atherogenic lipid profile (Aalizadeh et al., 2024). At the cellular level, insulin resistance causes the inflammatory process via triggering such mechanisms as NF-κB and increasing the amounts of ICAM-1 and VCAM-1 adhesion molecules. Moreover, pro-inflammatory cytokines, including IL-6 and TNF-α, increase vascular inflammation, whereas reduced endothelial nitric oxide synthase (eNOS) activity causes unavailability of nitric oxide (NO).

Simultaneously, pro-thrombotic factors like plasminogen activator inhibitor-1 (PAI-1) become activated in insulin resistance, leading to increased risks of thrombosis. Hence, insulin resistance disturbs the functioning of the endothelium and causes the processes of inflammation and thrombosis in the cardiovascular and diabetic patients. This notion is further supported by the fact that people suffering from insulin resistance have increased thickness of carotid intima-media layers and coronary artery calcification, which are both strong predictors of cardiovascular consequences (Fig. 1) (Fuster et al., 2024).

Figure 1. Periodontal-Cardiovascular-Diabetes Triad.

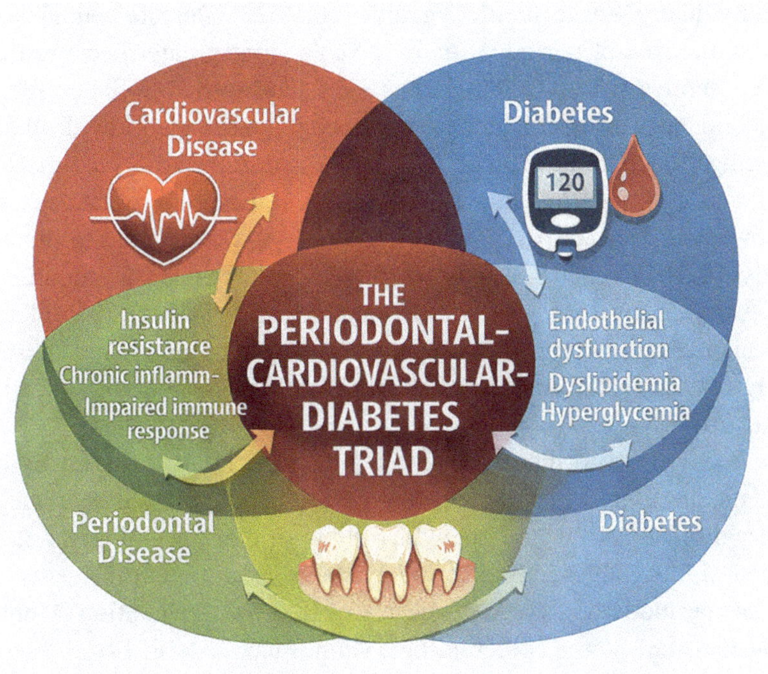

5. EPIDEMIOLOGICAL EVIDENCE SUPPORTING ORAL AND SYSTEMIC DISEASES

5.1 Global Burden of Oral and Systemic Diseases

Worldwide, billions of people are affected by oral diseases, with untreated dental caries being the most widespread among all such illnesses. According to a 2022 estimation, the global average prevalence of caries in permanent teeth is about 29%, representing over 2 billion cases. The highest incidence is found in low- and middle-income areas, including around 816 million cases in lower-middle-income nations and 690 million cases in upper-middle-income nations, accounting for around 75% of the global burden. Clear regional variations are equally evident, with the prevalence rate predicted to be around 25% for the Western Pacific Region but reaching around 34% in the European State (World Health Organization, 2022).

Periodontitis has also become a progressively more important public health issue, with the incidence of the condition showing a dramatic rise. Though an untreated carious tooth remains the most common oral health problem, affecting about 2 billion individuals, severe periodontitis stands as a close second, affecting approximately 1 billion individuals (World Health Organization, 2022). Despite being less common than caries, the role of periodontitis in DALYs is far greater because the disease is relatively more severe (GBD 2021 Diseases and Injuries Collaborators, 2024).

Xerostomia (dry mouth) is increasingly recognized as a worldwide phenomenon due to aging, rheumatoid arthritis, Sjögren's syndrome, diabetes mellitus, HIV infection, and drug therapy with radiotherapy and medication that causes reduced saliva flow (Anil et al., 2016). According to a report conducted in the Newcastle 85+ Study, which included 853 subjects, 57% had experienced dry mouth symptoms (Albani et al., 2021). Likewise, a cross-sectional survey of 1,226 elderly people living in institutions (average age 83.9 years) showed a higher chance of suffering from drug-related xerostomia based on an increasing dosage of medication (Janssens et al., 2017).

It has been observed that there is a higher association between oral diseases and systemic diseases, which include heart diseases; diabetes; cerebrovascular and respiratory diseases, among others, which show similar physiological mechanisms (Khadka et al., 2021). Specifically, the existence of a mutual influence of type 2 diabetes and periodontitis is recognized as a well-known correlation (Montero et al., 2024). Furthermore, some epidemiologic studies have established the associations between periodontitis and metabolic syndrome and obesity (Jepsen et al., 2020).

In addition, in a recent extensive systematic review of 294 meta-analyses and 856 comparisons, there were found 59 associations with robust evidence for a two-way association between oral diseases and NCDs. Among oral health situations, periodontitis presented the strongest association, followed by tooth loss (Botelho et al., 2022).

5.2 Trends and Epidemiological Transitions

The epidemiologic transition theory (Omran, 2005) describes a shift from declining mortality due to infectious diseases toward a growing predominance of chronic, non-communicable diseases (Oni & Unwin, 2015). This transition is also accompanied by demographic changes, particularly population aging, which (along with evolving disease patterns across age groups) requires health systems to adjust their service delivery and social care frameworks.

Consequently, national health systems are needed to simultaneously manage infectious diseases that predominantly affect children and infants while also addressing the increasing burden of chronic conditions (Frenk & Moon, 2013).

The Global Burden of Diseases, Risk Factors, and Injuries project promoted the DALY approach by adding the years of life lost (YLL) as early mortality and years of disability (YLD) to form a single measure for health analysis by employing two different angles (GBD 2023 Disease and Injury and Risk Factor Collaborators, 2025). From a public health standpoint, YLL reflects the effectiveness of a health system in preventing early death and extending life expectancy, whereas YLD offers insight into the overall health status and quality of life of a population over time (Martinez et al., 2019).

In simpler terms, YLL indicates how effectively a healthcare system diagnoses and treats conditions to reduce premature mortality, while YLD reflects its ability to promote health, prevent disease, minimize complications, and deliver adequate rehabilitation services. In terms of concepts, differences in the prevalence and mortality rates of acute illnesses will have an impact on the years of life lost. However, it is also based on the degree of prevention since primary prevention decreases the years lived with disability, while secondary and tertiary prevention will increase the years lived with disability (Martinez et al., 2019).

5.3 Inequalities in Disease Distribution

Health inequalities continue to exist in the global community today. Studies have revealed that poor health is still experienced among marginalized communities even in developed nations (Taha et al., 2022; Love-Koh et al., 2020). In LMICs, access and service use-related inequalities are more common, with maternal and child health services facing the most inequities. This is more evident in parts of Asia and Africa where internal inequalities remain high (Yaya & Ghose, 2019).

Additionally, there is a global health problem that includes diseases that spread through communicable diseases, non-communicable diseases (NCDs), and injury-related issues (Emadi et al., 2021). This systematic problem has been made even worse through structures such as globalization and neoliberalism, where power, resources, and opportunities have been divided along existing inequalities (Haldane et al., 2023).

6. GLOBAL FRAMEWORK AND POLICY IMPLICATIONS FOR SRFA-BASED PREVENTION

6.1 Need for Integrated Health Policies

Oral health sustainability in relation to the SRFA approach is about creating health policies aimed at fostering integration in health care by engaging stakeholders from various fields in tackling common risk factors such as smoking, improper dietary habits, alcohol intake, and poor personal hygiene practices (National Institute of Dental and Craniofacial Research [NIDCR], 2021; Glick et al., 2023).

Coordination between governmental bodies, dentistry services, educational organizations, and community-based entities will lead to optimized allocation of resources and innovation. Through such cooperation, an integrated approach can be developed that aims to solve problems related to oral as well as general health, ensuring a more comprehensive response to existing and emerging public health challenges (Junaid et al., 2022; Alderwick et al., 2021; Kreuter et al., 2021).

6.2 Health System Strengthening and Universal Health Coverage

Effective and sustainable SRFA-based policies require adequate monitoring, evaluation, and continuous measures to enhance health systems and advance Universal Health Coverage (UHC) goals (Simpson, 2011). Application of measurable indicators facilitates policymakers to assess the efficacy of the proposed intervention approaches and address any limitations in the distribution of health services (Sreedharan et al., 2024). This adaptive approach enables health systems to remain responsive to changing disease trends, demographic changes, and innovations in technology and simultaneously support equal access to prevention and treatment services.

6.3 National and Regional Policy Initiatives

Another crucial aspect of policy development through the SRFA method is enabling environmental sustainability as part of oral health initiatives. There is a need for national and sub-national guidelines that support environmental practices in healthcare that include friendly obtaining of dental products, clinical waste reduction, and energy-efficient services in dentistry. Incorporating environmental considerations in the field of public health facilitates the provision of dental services in harmony with sustainability principles by addressing both ecological and economic dimensions (Martin & Mulligan, 2022; Martínez-Peláez et al., 2023).

6.4 The Contribution of Primary Care to the Implementation of SRFA

Sustainable oral health development via SRFA is a continuous and evolving process that requires well-developed primary health care systems. By integrating oral health care into primary health care, oral health care practitioners are able to provide preventive and interventional services focused on common risk factors within the community. These initiatives make sure there is better access to healthcare services along with enhancing the quality of service provision in the healthcare industry and making it more resilient in dealing with future challenges (NIDCR, 2021; Martin & Mulligan, 2022; Varzakas & Antoniadou, 2024).

7. EQUITY IN ACCESS TO ORAL HEALTHCARE: ADDRESSING DISPARITIES

7.1 Integrating Cultural Competence Into Oral Health Systems

Impartial access to oral health care services will need strategies that align with the particular requirements of the respective communities (Foláyan et al., 2025). This will entail implementing approaches that consider cultural nuances in tackling barriers that arise in dealing with various minority groups (Nair & Adetayo, 2019; Stubbe, 2020). Moreover, certain policies can help to address issues associated with the health care system (Nair & Adetayo, 2019; Singh et al., 2023).

7.2 Policy Interventions to Combat Economic and Structural Barriers

Moreover, structural barriers can be addressed through improvements in transportation systems along with teledentistry applications (Jindal et al., 2023). These approaches might be valuable in alleviating the disparities present among urban and rural/remote areas, ensuring oral care delivery is more stable (Chen et al., 2019).

7.3 Community-Centered Approaches and Social Mobilization

Developing partnerships with community organizations, faith-based institutions, and service providers is critical in raising awareness about oral health (Gwathmey et al., 2024). Active community engagement helps in building an understanding of preventative oral hygiene practices and promotes collaboration to create supportive environments that maintain oral health (Molete et al., 2024).

8. ORAL HEALTH DISEASE BURDEN: ADVANCING POPULATION-SPECIFIC, HIGH-IMPACT SRFA INTERVENTIONS

8.1 Adopting a Life-Course and Risk-Based Strategy

Worldwide, oral diseases, for instance, dental caries, periodontal disorders, and oral cancer, carry a significant burden on healthcare systems. Dental caries remains the most commonly observed condition among children and adolescents, indicating the significance of preventive measures like implementation of fluoride varnishes in schools, water fluoridation, and less sugar consumption. On the other hand, periodontal diseases are more common in working adults, prompting the need for interventions such as promoting oral hygiene awareness, quitting smoking, and helping in early detection of periodontal disease. In older age groups, oral cancers are also more likely to occur in heavy smokers and drinkers. Consequently, routine screening for these cancers should be included in primary health care (World Health Organization, 2025; Peres et al., 2019). Adapting policies to particular age groups and risk profiles enables interventions to align with disease patterns, leading to better efficiency in resource allocation.

8.2 Improving Epidemiological Intelligence and Surveillance Systems

The innovative approaches towards effective public health strategies are based on the use of interventions that are supported by scientific and factual successful evidence (Thomson et al., 2018). Identifying and prioritizing the problems associated with oral health requires a systematic approach involving the use of needs assessments, including disease burden and inadequate services. Continuous monitoring of the trends in terms of oral health is essential in making timely decisions. Under such perspectives, the implementation of population-based preventive measures becomes important for decreasing the burden of the disease and improving oral health status (Shahzad et al., 2019).

8.3 Integrating Prevention and Early Detection Within Primary Care

Besides the preventive strategies, prompt detection is equally important in controlling the extent and progression of oral diseases. Routine oral health check-ups along with general examination ensure the timely identification of problems, make it easier to identify any possible issues early and take preventive measures before the condition worsens to a point where it could become fatal (Betts & Moravec,

2023). Such a proactive approach not only benefits individuals but also economically better because costly treatment procedures can be avoided through early intervention (Abdul Raheem, 2023).

8.4 Equity-Orientated Resource Allocation and Service Planning

Effective resource distribution is influenced by robust epidemiologic research, which is imperative in assessing the best means to address issues through preventive interventions (Fairchild et al., 2018). This enables preventive measures, and healthcare delivery can target those at risk, thus improving the quality of results and effective use of healthcare facilities (Kruk et al., 2018; Hoagland & Kipping, 2024).

8.5 Leveraging Digital Health and Innovative Service Delivery Models

Effective interventions comprise innovative methods, like community screening programs, portable dental facilities, and teledentistry services (Niknam et al., 2023). These models expand the influence of conventional health care systems, particularly in remote areas with insufficient dental care services (Niknam et al., 2023). The use of teledentistry systems facilitates early diagnosis, risk prediction, and remote sorting, thus encouraging a shift toward preventive and minimally invasive treatment procedures and addressing challenges related to travel restrictions and overcrowding in health care facilities. Incorporation of epidemiological information and the support of public-private partnerships provide more efficient resource allocation, improve equity in access to care, and help in reducing the overall burden of oral diseases (Jindal et al., 2023).

8.6 Multi-Sectoral and Public–Private Partnerships for Sustainable Implementation

Moreover, effective collaboration may be achieved through public-private partnership scheme that combines technical expertise with funding support in order to establish sustainable oral health programs (Strasser et al., 2021).

9. PUBLIC HEALTH STRATEGIES FOR SRFA IMPLEMENTATION

The population health approach is an attempt to shift from a traditional model of acute care treatment to the new model, which places emphasis on the health and wellness of a whole population. Activities of public health organizations, especially activities focused on the prevention of chronic illnesses, operate in collaboration with clinical services to offer a broad spectrum of services, comprising preventive and curative care, thereby enhancing overall population health (Cohen et al., 2014).

Globally, healthcare systems are increasingly faced with challenges by persistent pressures that contribute to suboptimal performance and health disparities (Frenk et al., 2010). These challenges involve the rising burden of chronic diseases, along with increasing expenses and raising complications in healthcare delivery. A cross-sectoral collaboration has been widely identified as a critical element of the population health approach (Washington et al., 2016; Etches et al., 2006) in order to respond effectively and move beyond the traditional biomedical model toward a population-centered framework (Berwick et al., 2008).

In particular, many researchers have demonstrated the significance of integrating primary care (PC) and public health (PH) systems to acquire maintainable improvements in health outcomes. Their results point out that some of the most important public health concerns, such as non-communicable disease management, child and maternal health, and cancer prevention, lie in the domain of both sectors. However, despite this overlap, primary care and public health systems often operate independently, limiting their potential to deliver coordinated and effective care (Huynh & Cohen, 2013; Gosling et al., 2016).

10. POLICY RECOMMENDATIONS: STRENGTHENING SRFA-ORIENTATED ORAL HEALTH SYSTEMS

10.1 Incorporating Oral Health Into Universal Health Coverage and Primary Care Systems

Sustainability, equity, and decreasing the burden of oral diseases can form the basis for developing strong policy frameworks that will ensure the establishment of facilities to deliver oral healthcare in public health settings (Abodunrin et al., 2023). The provision of such policy frameworks is important because of the need to incorporate oral health into the general healthcare system such that it is recognized as an integral part of the whole process of healthcare provision (Prasad et al., 2019). Integration makes it possible to recognize the connection between oral health problems and systemic diseases like diabetes and heart-related conditions (Fu et al., 2025). Furthermore, oral health examinations can be incorporated into medical examinations to diagnose and timely manage conditions effectively at reduced cost and prevent further progression of disease (Prasad et al., 2019; Amaya et al., 2024).

10.2 Strengthening Cross-Sectoral Governance and Multi-Stakeholder Collaboration

Collaboration between various government agencies, institutions of higher learning, community organizations, and the private sector is key in harnessing both human and material resources (Obi et al., 2024). Cross-sector partnerships promote knowledge and technology transfer, together with resource mobilization, enabling the development of holistic models of care, particularly in underprivileged areas (Hoagland & Kipping, 2024; Alderwick et al., 2021). Moreover, such collaborations help to develop multidisciplinary educational frameworks that prepare oral healthcare providers to handle various dental health issues (Glick et al., 2023). Coordination can lead to creativity and adaptability of policies (Kruk et al., 2018; Alderwick et al., 2021).

10.3 Promoting Research, Innovation, and Digital Health Transformation

Investment in research and innovation has an extremely critical part to play in the facilitation of preventive procedures, diagnostic tools, and sustainable means of managing oral health care. Such innovations like telehealth and digital diagnostics offer great potential for improving service delivery and enhancing availability, particularly in under-resourced areas (de Carvalho & Zanatta, 2024). Additionally, these technologies also aid in early detection and allow for the creation of specific interventions that address the unique requirements of different populations (Kruk et al., 2018).

10.4 Community Empowerment and Context-Sensitive Oral Health Programming

Community- orientated activities play a pivotal role towards ensuring equity in oral health care (Yuan et al., 2021). Community participation in the development of programs for improving health contributes significantly to fostering ownership and cultural relevance, which also takes into consideration the specific socio-economic and geographical environment (Alderwick et al., 2021). Examples of these initiatives are campaigns promoting health awareness, mobile dental services, and implementing teledentistry programs to serve remote and underdeveloped communities (Bala et al., 2023).

Furthermore, the establishment of robust monitoring and evaluation frameworks becomes vital to assess the effectiveness of implemented policies and recognize areas for improvement (Danforth et al., 2023). Systematic data collection and analysis provide timely responses in order to allow for quicker responses and better resource utilization for enhancing health outcomes (Cascini et al., 2021). These systems also encourage responsibility and help disseminate knowledge of best practices across regions. Evaluation helps maintain policies that are aligned with the goals of sustainability, equity, and reducing the burden of oral diseases (Abodunrin et al., 2023; Mathur et al., 2025).

11. CONCLUSION

The SRFA approach can be considered innovative and revolutionary, as it offers a holistic approach to managing the burden of both oral and systemic diseases and, more precisely, periodontal-cardiovascular-diabetes triad. By recognizing the fact that oral diseases and some non-communicable diseases have common modifiable risk factors such as unhealthy lifestyles (poor nutrition, tobacco use, alcohol consumption, poor dental hygiene, and socioeconomic inequities), SRFA departs from traditional and fragmented approaches towards an innovative one. In particular, SRFA includes equitable access to oral healthcare services, designing population-specific interventions aimed at prevention, and integrating oral health into general healthcare to facilitate early diagnosis and management as well as minimize further complications. In addition, the implementation of innovative strategies (teledentistry, mobile dental units, and digital health technologies) can significantly improve the availability and efficiency of care, especially in underserved and remote areas. Integration with multisectoral collaboration and public–private partnerships enhances the long-term sustainability and scalability of oral health initiatives.

REFERENCES

Aalizadeh, Y., Khamisi, N., Asghari, P., Safari, A., Mottaghi, M., Taherkhani, M. H., Alemi, A., Ghaderi, M., & Rahmanian, M. (2024). The Mediterranean diet and periodontitis: A systematic review and meta-analysis. *Heliyon, 10*(15), e35633. DOI: 10.1016/j.heliyon.2024.e35633 PMID: 39170303

AbdulRaheem, Y.AbdulRaheem Y. (2023). Unveiling the Significance and Challenges of Integrating Prevention Levels in Healthcare Practice. *Journal of Primary Care & Community Health, 14*, 21501319231186500. DOI: 10.1177/21501319231186500 PMID: 37449436

Abodunrin, O. R., Olagunju, M. T., Alade, O. T., & Foláyan, M. O. (2023). Relationships between oral health and the sustainable development goals: A scoping review. *BioMed, 3*(4), 460–470. DOI: 10.3390/biomed3040037

Acipinar, S., & Yalcin, M. (2025). Correlation between aging, periodontal diagnoses and systemic diseases: A retrospective analysis of 3,000 patients. *BMC Oral Health, 25*(1), 1832. DOI: 10.1186/s12903-025-07228-z PMID: 41291667

Albani, V., Nishio, K., Ito, T., Kotronia, E., Moynihan, P., Robinson, L., Hanratty, B., Kingston, A., Abe, Y., Takayama, M., Iinuma, T., Arai, Y., & Ramsay, S. E. (2021). Associations of poor oral health with frailty and physical functioning in the oldest old: Results from two studies in England and Japan. *BMC Geriatrics, 21*(1), 187. DOI: 10.1186/s12877-021-02081-5 PMID: 33736595

Alderwick, H., Hutchings, A., Briggs, A., & Mays, N. (2021). The impacts of collaboration between local health care and non-health care organizations and factors shaping how they work: A systematic review of reviews. *BMC Public Health, 21*(1), 753. DOI: 10.1186/s12889-021-10630-1 PMID: 33874927

Alotiby, A. (2024). Immunology of Stress: A Review Article. *Journal of Clinical Medicine, 13*(21), 6394. DOI: 10.3390/jcm13216394 PMID: 39518533

Amaya, A., Medina, I., Mazzilli, S., D'Arcy, J., Cocco, N., Van Hout, M. C., Stöver, H., & Moazen, B. (2024). Oral health services in prison settings: A global scoping review of availability, accessibility, and model of delivery. *Journal of Community Psychology, 52*(8), 1108–1137. DOI: 10.1002/jcop.23081 PMID: 37566403

Anil, S., Vellappally, S., Hashem, M., Preethanath, R. S., Patil, S., & Samaranayake, L. P. (2016). Xerostomia in geriatric patients: A burgeoning global concern. *Journal of Investigative and Clinical Dentistry, 7*(1), 5–12. DOI: 10.1111/jicd.12120 PMID: 25175324

Bala, R., Sargaiyan, V., Rathi, S. A., Mankar, S. S., Jaiswal, A. K., & Mankar, S. A. (2023). Mobile dental clinic for oral health services to underserved rural Indian communities. *Bioinformation, 19*(13), 1383–1387. DOI: 10.6026/973206300191383 PMID: 38415028

Berwick, D. M., Nolan, T. W., & Whittington, J. (2008). The triple aim: Care, health, and cost. *Health Affairs (Project Hope), 27*(3), 759–769. DOI: 10.1377/hlthaff.27.3.759 PMID: 18474969

Betts, K. J., & Moravec, L. (2023). Integration of oral health screening, intervention, and referral into the pediatric well-child visit. *Journal of Pediatric Health Care : Official Publication of National Association of Pediatric Nurse Associates & Practitioners, 37*(6), 609–615. DOI: 10.1016/j.pedhc.2023.05.007 PMID: 37330729

Botelho, J., Mascarenhas, P., Viana, J., Proença, L., Orlandi, M., Leira, Y., Chambrone, L., Mendes, J. J., & Machado, V. (2022). An umbrella review of the evidence linking oral health and systemic noncommunicable diseases. *Nature Communications, 13*(1), 7614. DOI: 10.1038/s41467-022-35337-8 PMID: 36494387

Carvalho, L. F. D. C. E. S., & Zanatta, R. F. (2024). Editorial: Technological innovations for improved prevention and diagnosis of oral disease. *Frontiers in Oral Health, 5*, 1481890. DOI: 10.3389/froh.2024.1481890 PMID: 39355782

Cascini, F., Santaroni, F., Lanzetti, R., Failla, G., Gentili, A., & Ricciardi, W. (2021). Developing a data-driven approach in order to improve the safety and quality of patient care. *Frontiers in Public Health, 9*, 667819. DOI: 10.3389/fpubh.2021.667819 PMID: 34095071

Chen, X., Orom, H., Hay, J. L., Waters, E. A., Schofield, E., Li, Y., & Kiviniemi, M. T. (2019). Differences in Rural and Urban Health Information Access and Use. *The Journal of Rural Health : Official Journal of the American Rural Health Association and the National Rural Health Care Association, 35*(3), 405–417. DOI: 10.1111/jrh.12335 PMID: 30444935

Cohen, D., Huynh, T., Sebold, A., Harvey, J., Neudorf, C., & Brown, A. (2014). The population health approach: A qualitative study of conceptual and operational definitions for leaders in Canadian healthcare. *SAGE Open Medicine, 2*, 2050312114522618. DOI: 10.1177/2050312114522618 PMID: 26770704

Danforth, K., Ahmad, A. M., Blanchet, K., Khalid, M., Means, A. R., Memirie, S. T., Alwan, A., & Watkins, D. (2023). Monitoring and evaluating the implementation of essential packages of health services. *BMJ Global Health, 8*(Suppl 1), e010726. DOI: 10.1136/bmjgh-2022-010726 PMID: 36977532

De Abreu, M. H. N. G., Cruz, A. J. S., Borges-Oliveira, A. C., Martins, R. D. C., & Mattos, F. D. F. (2021). Perspectives on social and environmental determinants of oral health. *International Journal of Environmental Research and Public Health, 18*(24), 13429. https://www.mdpi.com/1660-4601/18/24/13429. DOI: 10.3390/ijerph182413429 PMID: 34949037

de Carvalho, R. D. P., Casarin, R. C. V., de Lima, P. O., & Cogo-Müller, K. (2021). Statins with potential to control periodontitis: From biological mechanisms to clinical studies. *Journal of Oral Biosciences, 63*(3), 232–244. DOI: 10.1016/j.job.2021.06.002 PMID: 34146687

Emadi, M., Delavari, S., & Bayati, M. (2021). Global socioeconomic inequality in the burden of communicable and non-communicable diseases and injuries: An analysis on global burden of disease study 2019. *BMC Public Health, 21*(1), 1771. DOI: 10.1186/s12889-021-11793-7 PMID: 34583668

Etches, V., Frank, J., Di Ruggiero, E., & Manuel, D. (2006). Measuring population health: A review of indicators. *Annual Review of Public Health, 27*(1), 29–55. DOI: 10.1146/annurev.publhealth.27.021405.102141 PMID: 16533108

Fairchild, G., Tasseff, B., Khalsa, H., Generous, N., Daughton, A. R., Velappan, N., Priedhorsky, R., & Deshpande, A. (2018). Epidemiological Data Challenges: Planning for a More Robust Future Through Data Standards. *Frontiers in Public Health, 6*, 336. DOI: 10.3389/fpubh.2018.00336 PMID: 30533407

Foláyan, M. O., Bernard, O. T., Titus, O. S., Alade, O., Aliyu, T. K., Bhayat, A., Ndembi, N., Fasiku, G., & El Tantawi, M. (2025). Cultural practices, oral health service utilisation and oral health policy and guidelines development in Africa: Insights from the yorùbá ethnic group. *Frontiers in Oral Health, 6*, 1539827. DOI: 10.3389/froh.2025.1539827 PMID: 40045959

Frenk, J., Chen, L., Bhutta, Z., Cohen, J., Crisp, N., Evans, T., Fineberg, H., Garcia, P., Ke, Y., Kelley, P., Kistnasamy, B., Meleis, A., Naylor, D., Pablos-Mendez, A., Reddy, S., Scrimshaw, S., Sepulveda, J., Serwadda, D., & Zurayk, H. (2010). Health professionals for a new century: Transforming education to strengthen health systems in an interdependent world. *Lancet, 376*(9756), 1923–1958. DOI: 10.1016/S0140-6736(10)61854-5 PMID: 21112623

Frenk, J., & Moon, S. (2013). Governance challenges in global health. *The New England Journal of Medicine, 368*(10), 936–942. DOI: 10.1056/NEJMra1109339 PMID: 23465103

Fu, D., Shu, X., Zhou, G., Ji, M., Liao, G., & Zou, L. (2025). Connection between oral health and chronic diseases. *MedComm*, *6*(1), e70052. DOI: 10.1002/mco2.70052 PMID: 39811802

Fuster, V., García-Álvarez, A., Devesa, A., Mass, V., Owen, R., Quesada, A., Fuster, J. J., García-Lunar, I., Pocock, S., Sánchez-González, J., Sartori, S., Peyra, C., Andres, V., Muntendam, P., & Ibanez, B. (2024). Influence of Subclinical Atherosclerosis Burden and Progression on Mortality. *Journal of the American College of Cardiology*, *84*(15), 1391–1403. DOI: 10.1016/j.jacc.2024.06.045 PMID: 39357937

Gatto, A., Liu, K., Milan, N., & Wong, S. (2025). The Effects of GLP-1 Agonists on Musculoskeletal Health and Orthopedic Care. *Current Reviews in Musculoskeletal Medicine*, *18*(10), 469–480. DOI: 10.1007/s12178-025-09978-3 PMID: 40372699

GBD 2019 Diseases and Injuries Collaborators (2020). Global burden of 369 diseases and injuries in 204 countries and territories, 1990-2019: a systematic analysis for the Global Burden of Disease Study 2019. *Lancet (London, England)*, *396*(10258), 1204–1222. https://doi.org/.DOI: 10.1016/S0140-6736(20)30925-9

GBD 2021 Diseases and Injuries Collaborators (2024). Global incidence, prevalence, years lived with disability (YLDs), disability-adjusted life-years (DALYs), and healthy life expectancy (HALE) for 371 diseases and injuries in 204 countries and territories and 811 subnational locations, 1990-2021: a systematic analysis for the Global Burden of Disease Study 2021. *Lancet (London, England)*, *403*(10440), 2133–2161. https://doi.org/DOI: 10.1016/S0140-6736(24)00757-8

GBD 2023 Disease and Injury and Risk Factor Collaborators (2025). Burden of 375 diseases and injuries, risk-attributable burden of 88 risk factors, and healthy life expectancy in 204 countries and territories, including 660 subnational locations, 1990-2023: a systematic analysis for the Global Burden of Disease Study 2023. *Lancet (London, England)*, *406*(10513), 1873–1922. https://doi.org/DOI: 10.1016/S0140-6736(25)01637-X

Glick, M., Urquhart, O., Bhosale, A. S., Carrasco-Labra, A., & Edelson, J. T. (2023). A unified voice to drive global improvements in oral health. *BMC Global and Public Health*, *1*(1), 19. DOI: 10.1186/s44263-023-00019-0 PMID: 39681896

Gosling, R., Davies, S. M., & Hussey, J. A. (2016). How integrating primary care and public health could improve population health outcomes: A view from Liverpool, UK. *Public Health Research & Practice*, *26*(1), e2611602. DOI: 10.17061/phrp2611602 PMID: 26863165

Gwathmey, T. M., Williams, K. L., Caban-Holt, A., Starks, T. D., Foy, C. G., Mathews, A., & Byrd, G. S. (2024). Building a Community Partnership for the Development of Health Ministries Within the African American Community: The Triad Pastors Network. *Journal of Community Health*, *49*(3), 559–567. DOI: 10.1007/s10900-023-01315-4 PMID: 38265538

Haldane, V., Ariyarajah, A., Berry, I., Loutet, M., Salamanca-Buentello, F., & Upshur, R. E. G. (2023). Global inequity creates local insufficiency: A qualitative study of COVID-19 vaccine implementation challenges in low-and-middle-income countries. *PLoS One*, *18*(2), e0281358. DOI: 10.1371/journal.pone.0281358 PMID: 36780502

Hoagland, A., & Kipping, S. (2024). Challenges in promoting health equity and reducing disparities in access across new and established technologies. *The Canadian Journal of Cardiology*, *40*(6), 1154–1167. DOI: 10.1016/j.cjca.2024.02.014 PMID: 38417572

Huynh, T. M., & Cohen, D. (2013). Innovators and early adopters of population health in healthcare: Real and present opportunities for healthcare-public health collaboration. *Healthcare Papers*, *13*(3), 53–89. DOI: 10.12927/hcpap.2014.23683 PMID: 24524572

Janssens, B., Vanobbergen, J., Petrovic, M., Jacquet, W., Schols, J. M. G. A., & De Visschere, L. (2017). The oral health condition and treatment needs assessment of nursing home residents in Flanders (Belgium). *Community Dental Health*, *34*(3), 143–151. DOI: 10.1922/CDH_4086Janssens09 PMID: 28872808

Javed, F., Rahman, I., & Romanos, G. E. (2019). Tobacco-product usage as a risk factor for dental implants. *Periodontology 2000*, *81*(1), 48–56. DOI: 10.1111/prd.12282 PMID: 31407428

Jepsen, S., Suvan, J., & Deschner, J. (2020). The association of periodontal diseases with metabolic syndrome and obesity. *Periodontology 2000*, *83*(1), 125–153. DOI: 10.1111/prd.12326 PMID: 32385882

Jia, S., Li, X., & Du, Q. (2023). Host insulin resistance caused by *Porphyromonas gingivalis*—Review of recent progresses. *Frontiers in Cellular and Infection Microbiology*, *13*, 1209381. DOI: 10.3389/fcimb.2023.1209381 PMID: 37520442

Jindal, M., Chaiyachati, K. H., Fung, V., Manson, S. M., & Mortensen, K. (2023). Eliminating health care inequities through strengthening access to care. *Health services research, 58 Suppl 3*(Suppl 3), 300–310. .DOI: 10.1111/1475-6773.14202

Joseph, B. K., Kullman, L., & Sharma, P. N. (2016). The oral-systemic disease connection: A retrospective study. *Clinical Oral Investigations*, *20*(8), 2267–2273. DOI: 10.1007/s00784-016-1725-3 PMID: 26841905

Junaid, S. B., Imam, A. A., Balogun, A. O., De Silva, L. C., Surakat, Y. A., Kumar, G., Abdulkarim, M., Shuaibu, A. N., Garba, A., Sahalu, Y., Mohammed, A., Mohammed, T. Y., Abdulkadir, B. A., Abba, A. A., Kakumi, N. A. I., & Mahamad, S. (2022). Recent Advancements in Emerging Technologies for Healthcare Management Systems: A Survey. *Healthcare (Basel)*, *10*(10), 1940. DOI: 10.3390/healthcare10101940 PMID: 36292387

Khadka, S., Khan, S., King, A., Goldberg, L. R., Crocombe, L., & Bettiol, S. (2021). Poor oral hygiene, oral microorganisms and aspiration pneumonia risk in older people in residential aged care: A systematic review. *Age and Ageing*, *50*(1), 81–87. DOI: 10.1093/ageing/afaa102 PMID: 32677660

Knight, E. T., Liu, J., Seymour, G. J., Faggion, C. M.Jr, & Cullinan, M. P. (2016). Risk factors that may modify the innate and adaptive immune responses in periodontal diseases. *Periodontology 2000*, *71*(1), 22–51. DOI: 10.1111/prd.12110 PMID: 27045429

Kreuter, M. W., Thompson, T., McQueen, A., & Garg, R. (2021). Addressing Social Needs in Health Care Settings: Evidence, Challenges, and Opportunities for Public Health. *Annual Review of Public Health*, *42*(1), 329–344. DOI: 10.1146/annurev-publhealth-090419-102204 PMID: 33326298

Kruk, M. E., Gage, A. D., Arsenault, C., Jordan, K., Leslie, H. H., Roder-DeWan, S., Adeyi, O., Barker, P., Daelmans, B., Doubova, S. V., English, M., García-Elorrio, E., Guanais, F., Gureje, O., Hirschhorn, L. R., Jiang, L., Kelley, E., Lemango, E. T., Liljestrand, J., & Pate, M. (2018). High-quality health systems in the sustainable development goals era: Time for a revolution. *The Lancet. Global Health*, *6*(11), e1196–e1252. DOI: 10.1016/S2214-109X(18)30386-3 PMID: 30196093

Lamster, I. B. (2021). The 2021 WHO Resolution on Oral Health. *International Dental Journal*, *71*(4), 279–280. DOI: 10.1016/j.identj.2021.06.003 PMID: 34256923

Love-Koh, J., Griffin, S., Kataika, E., Revill, P., Sibandze, S., & Walker, S. (2020). Methods to promote equity in health resource allocation in low- and middle-income countries: An overview. *Globalization and Health*, *16*(1), 6. DOI: 10.1186/s12992-019-0537-z PMID: 31931823

Martin, N., & Mulligan, S. (2022). Environmental sustainability through good-quality oral healthcare. *International Dental Journal*, *72*(1), 26–30. DOI: 10.1016/j.identj.2021.06.005 PMID: 34412896

Martinez, R., Soliz, P., Caixeta, R., & Ordunez, P. (2019). Reflection on modern methods: Years of life lost due to premature mortality-a versatile and comprehensive measure for monitoring non-communicable disease mortality. *International Journal of Epidemiology*, *48*(4), 1367–1376. DOI: 10.1093/ije/dyy254 PMID: 30629192

Martínez-Peláez, R., Ochoa-Brust, A., Rivera, S., Félix, V. G., Ostos, R., Brito, H., Félix, R. A., & Mena, L. J. (2023). Role of Digital Transformation for Achieving Sustainability: Mediated Role of Stakeholders, Key Capabilities, and Technology. *Sustainability (Basel)*, *15*(14), 11221. DOI: 10.3390/su151411221

Mathur, M. R., Bhosale, A. S., Abel, S. N., Fisher, J., Listl, S., Carrasco-Labra, A., Urquhart, O., & Glick, M. (2025). Envisioning sustainable oral health through effective advocacy. *BMC Global and Public Health*, *3*(1), 15. DOI: 10.1186/s44263-025-00133-1 PMID: 39972337

Meurman, J. H., & Bascones-Martínez, A. (2021). Oral infections and systemic health—More than just links to cardiovascular diseases. *Oral Health & Preventive Dentistry*, *19*(1), 441–448. DOI: 10.3290/j.ohpd.b1993965 PMID: 34505498

Molete, M. M., Malele-Kolisa, Y., Thekiso, M., Lang, A. Y., Kong, A., & George, A. (2024). The role of community health workers in promoting oral health at school settings: A scoping review. *Journal of Public Health Dentistry*, *84*(2), 175–186. DOI: 10.1111/jphd.12612 PMID: 38558304

Montero, E., Bujaldón, R., Montanya, E., Calle-Pascual, A. L., Rojo-Martínez, G., Castaño, L., Franch-Nadal, J., Delgado, E., Chaves, F., Alonso, B., Sanz, M., & Herrera, D. (2024). Cross-sectional association between severe periodontitis and diabetes mellitus: A nation-wide cohort study. *Journal of Clinical Periodontology*, *51*(4), 368–379. DOI: 10.1111/jcpe.13937 PMID: 38140803

Nair, L., & Adetayo, O. A. (2019). Cultural competence and ethnic diversity in healthcare. *Plastic and Reconstructive Surgery. Global Open*, *7*(5), e2219. DOI: 10.1097/GOX.0000000000002219 PMID: 31333951

National Institute of Dental and Craniofacial Research (US). (2021). *Oral health in America: Advances and challenges*. Bethesda, MD: Author. https://www.ncbi.nlm.nih.gov/books/NBK576535/

Niknam, F., Sharifian, R., Bashiri, A., Mardani, M., Akbari, R., Tuffaha, H., Do, L., & Bastani, P. (2023). Tele-dentistry, its trends, scope, and future framework in oral medicine; a scoping review during January 1999 to December 2021. *Archives of public health = Archives belges de sante publique, 81*(1), 104. https://doi.org/.DOI: 10.1186/s13690-023-01128-w

Obi, C. O., Jiakor, I. E., Etiaba, E., & Onwujekwe, O. (2024). Collaborations and networks within communities for improved utilization of primary healthcare centers: On the road to universal health coverage. *International Journal of Public Health, 69*, 1606810. DOI: 10.3389/ijph.2024.1606810 PMID: 38887723

Öçbe, M., Çelebi, E., & Öçbe, Ç. B. (2025). An overlooked connection: Oral health status in patients with chronic diseases. *BMC Oral Health, 25*(1), 314. DOI: 10.1186/s12903-025-05673-4 PMID: 40016657

Omran, A. R. (2005). The epidemiologic transition: A theory of the epidemiology of population change. 1971. *The Milbank Quarterly, 83*(4), 731–757. DOI: 10.1111/j.1468-0009.2005.00398.x PMID: 16279965

Oni, T., & Unwin, N. (2015). Why the communicable/non-communicable disease dichotomy is problematic for public health control strategies: Implications of multimorbidity for health systems in an era of health transition. *International Health, 7*(6), 390–399. DOI: 10.1093/inthealth/ihv040 PMID: 26103981

Peres, M. A., Macpherson, L. M. D., Weyant, R. J., Daly, B., Venturelli, R., Mathur, M. R., Listl, S., Celeste, R. K., Guarnizo-Herreño, C. C., Kearns, C., Benzian, H., Allison, P., & Watt, R. G. (2019). Oral diseases: A global public health challenge. *Lancet, 394*(10194), 249–260. DOI: 10.1016/S0140-6736(19)31146-8 PMID: 31327369

Pietiäinen, M., Liljestrand, J. M., Kopra, E., & Pussinen, P. J. (2018). Mediators between oral dysbiosis and cardiovascular diseases. *European Journal of Oral Sciences, 126*(S1), 26–36. DOI: 10.1111/eos.12423 PMID: 30178551

Prasad, M., Manjunath, C., Murthy, A. K., Sampath, A., Jaiswal, S., & Mohapatra, A. (2019). Integration of oral health into primary health care: A systematic review. *Journal of Family Medicine and Primary Care, 8*(6), 1838–1845. DOI: 10.4103/jfmpc.jfmpc_286_19 PMID: 31334142

Schwarz, C., Hajdu, A. I., Dumitrescu, R., Sava-Rosianu, R., Bolchis, V., Anusca, D., Hanghicel, A., Fratila, A. D., Oancea, R., Jumanca, D., Galuscan, A., & Leretter, M. (2023). Link between Oral Health, Periodontal Disease, Smoking, and Systemic Diseases in Romanian Patients. *Healthcare (Basel), 11*(16), 2354. DOI: 10.3390/healthcare11162354 PMID: 37628551

Shahzad, M., Upshur, R., Donnelly, P., Bharmal, A., Wei, X., Feng, P., & Brown, A. D. (2019). A population-based approach to integrated healthcare delivery: A scoping review of clinical care and public health collaboration. *BMC Public Health, 19*(1), 708. DOI: 10.1186/s12889-019-7002-z PMID: 31174501

Simpson, D. D. (2011). A framework for implementing sustainable oral health promotion interventions. *Journal of Public Health Dentistry*, *71*(s1, Suppl. 1), S84–S94. DOI: 10.1111/j.1752-7325.2011.00234.x PMID: 21499507

Simpson, T. C., Clarkson, J. E., Worthington, H. V., MacDonald, L., Weldon, J. C., Needleman, I., Iheozor-Ejiofor, Z., Wild, S. H., Qureshi, A., Walker, A., Patel, V. A., Boyers, D., & Twigg, J. (2022). Treatment of periodontitis for glycaemic control in people with diabetes mellitus. *Cochrane Database of Systematic Reviews*, *4*(4), CD004714. Advance online publication. DOI: 10.1002/14651858.CD004714.pub4 PMID: 35420698

Singh, H., Fulton, J.IV, Mirzazada, S., Saragosa, M., Uleryk, E. M., & Nelson, M. L. A. (2023). Community-based culturally tailored education programs for Black communities with cardiovascular disease, diabetes, hypertension, and stroke: Systematic review findings. *Journal of Racial and Ethnic Health Disparities*, *10*(6), 2986–3006. DOI: 10.1007/s40615-022-01474-5 PMID: 36508135

Sreedharan, J., Subbarayalu, A. V., Kamalasanan, A., Albalawi, I., Krishna, G. G., Alahmari, A. D., Alsalamah, J. A., Alkhathami, M. G., Alenezi, M., Alqahtani, A. S., Alahmari, M., Phillips, M. R., & MacDonald, J. (2024). Key Performance Indicators: A Framework for Allied Healthcare Educational Institutions. *ClinicoEconomics and Outcomes Research*, *16*, 173–185. DOI: 10.2147/CEOR.S446614 PMID: 38562567

Strasser, S., Stauber, C., Shrivastava, R., Riley, P., & O'Quin, K. (2021). Collective insights of public-private partnership impacts and sustainability: A qualitative analysis. *PLoS One*, *16*(7), e0254495. DOI: 10.1371/journal.pone.0254495 PMID: 34283847

Stubbe, D. E. (2020). Practicing cultural competence and cultural humility in the care of diverse patients. *Focus - American Psychiatric Publishing*, *18*(1), 49–51. DOI: 10.1176/appi.focus.20190041 PMID: 32047398

Taha, M. K., Martinon-Torres, F., Köllges, R., Bonanni, P., Safadi, M. A. P., Booy, R., Smith, V., Garcia, S., Bekkat-Berkani, R., & Abitbol, V. (2022). Equity in vaccination policies to overcome social deprivation as a risk factor for invasive meningococcal disease. *Expert Review of Vaccines*, *21*(5), 659–674. DOI: 10.1080/14760584.2022.2052048 PMID: 35271781

Thomson, K., Hillier-Brown, F., Todd, A., McNamara, C., Huijts, T., & Bambra, C. (2018). The effects of public health policies on health inequalities in high-income countries: An umbrella review. *BMC Public Health*, *18*(1), 869. DOI: 10.1186/s12889-018-5677-1 PMID: 30005611

Varzakas, T., & Antoniadou, M. (2024). A holistic approach for ethics and sustainability in the food chain: The gateway to oral and systemic health. *Foods, 13*(8), 1224. DOI: 10.3390/foods13081224 PMID: 38672896

Washington, A. E., Coye, M. J., & Boulware, L. E. (2016). Academic Health Systems' Third Curve: Population Health Improvement. *Journal of the American Medical Association, 315*(5), 459–460. DOI: 10.1001/jama.2015.18550 PMID: 26836726

Wojtkowska, A., Zapolski, T., Wysokińska-Miszczuk, J., & Wysokiński, A. P. (2021). The inflammation link between periodontal disease and coronary atherosclerosis in patients with acute coronary syndromes: Case-control study. *BMC Oral Health, 21*(1), 5. DOI: 10.1186/s12903-020-01356-4 PMID: 33407375

Wolf, T. G., Cagetti, M. G., Fisher, J. M., Seeberger, G. K., & Campus, G. (2021). Non-communicable diseases and oral health: An overview. *Frontiers in Oral Health, 2*, 725460. DOI: 10.3389/froh.2021.725460 PMID: 35048049

World Health Organization. (2022). *Global oral health status report: Towards universal health coverage for oral health by 2030*. https://www.who.int/publications/i/item/9789240061484

World Health Organization. Oral health. Geneva: World Health Organization (2025). Available at:https://www.who.int/news-room/fact-sheets/detail/oral-health(Accessed March 20, 2025).

Xie, H., Qin, Z., Ling, Z., Ge, X., Zhang, H., Guo, S., Liu, L., Zheng, K., Jiang, H., & Xu, R. (2023). Oral pathogen aggravates atherosclerosis by inducing smooth muscle cell apoptosis and repressing macrophage efferocytosis. *International Journal of Oral Science, 15*(1), 26. DOI: 10.1038/s41368-023-00232-5 PMID: 37380627

Yaya, S., & Ghose, B. (2019). Global Inequality in Maternal Health Care Service Utilization: Implications for Sustainable Development Goals. *Health Equity, 3*(1), 145–154. DOI: 10.1089/heq.2018.0082 PMID: 31289773

Yekani, M., Dastgir, M., Fattahi, S., Shahi, S., Maleki Dizaj, S., & Memar, M. Y. (2025). Microbiological and molecular aspects of periodontitis pathogenesis: An infection-induced inflammatory condition. *Frontiers in Cellular and Infection Microbiology, 15*, 1533658. DOI: 10.3389/fcimb.2025.1533658 PMID: 40406516

Yuan, M., Lin, H., Wu, H., Yu, M., Tu, J., & Lü, Y. (2021). Community engagement in public health: A bibliometric mapping of global research. *Archives of Public Health = Archives Belges de Santé Publique, 79*(1), 6. DOI: 10.1186/s13690-021-00525-3 PMID: 33436063

Chapter 5
The Digital Transformation of Epidemiology:
Big Data in Health, Real-Time Surveillance, Cloud Computing, IoT, Ethics, and the Future

Aidalina Mahmud
Universiti Putra Malaysia, Malaysia

Muhammad Arshed
http://orcid.org/0009-0005-0683-9610
Baqai Medical University, Karachi, Pakistan

Abdul Kabeer Kazi
http://orcid.org/0000-0001-9860-2891
Baqai Medical University, Karachi, Pakistan

Mehwish K. Kiran
Baqai Medical University, Karachi, Pakistan

Waseela Ashraf
http://orcid.org/0000-0002-2236-8581
University of Europe for Applied Sciences, UAE

ABSTRACT

Epidemiology is undergoing a revolution. Traditionally, the discipline was based on long-lagged surveys, case reporting, and data systems that were often siloed

DOI: 10.4018/979-8-3373-8402-3.ch005

and hard to integrate. This chapter describes how this transformation is playing out in four key areas. It examines the various sources of data and the issue of data integration, the phenomenon of real-time digital surveillance, and the impact of technologies such as cloud computing and the Internet of Things on how data is stored and analyzed. The considerations are presented in the context of integrated oral and general health, which is described here using the EpiDentomics model. The key concept is that, when harnessed appropriately, digital technologies can help overcome some of the traditional barriers between dentistry and medicine to create a more integrated, responsive population health approach. Moving forward, technologies such as federated learning, privacy-preserving data analysis, and the development of integrated oral and systemic health dashboards hold potential with a strong commitment to equity and ethics.

1. INTRODUCTION

Epidemiology has traditionally been a retrospective science. Epidemiologists were forced to wait for long-term cohort studies to yield results (often several years later), while surveillance reports were generally retrospective and health surveys were only done at infrequent intervals. The data were typically structured, but often incomplete, and delays were inevitable. But this is no longer the case in recent years. The growth of electronic health records, wearable devices, mobile devices and cloud computing has ushered in a new era where vast amounts of varied health data are being collected and analyzed in close to real-time. This is more than a technological change. It speaks to a shift in the scope of what epidemiology can quantify, the speed at which it can act, and the population it can reach. Clinical encounters are now being captured by electronic health records. Personal monitors capture physiological indicators such as heart rate, sleep and exercise. Meanwhile, social media platforms can give early warnings of symptom onset, days or weeks before these are reported by conventional reporting systems (Brownstein et al., 2009; Eysenbach, 2009). These advances support what is becoming known as digital epidemiology, in which health inferences are made from digital data, rather than just from conventional (and often discontinuous) data gathering approaches (Salathe et al., 2012).

These developments have important implications for oral and general health. Traditionally, data from the oral and medical professions have been housed in distinct systems, reflecting different professional structures and cultures. This has thwarted efforts to study the many well-established bidirectional associations between oral health and systemic diseases, such as the associations between periodontitis and diabetes, oral infections and cardiovascular risk, and the negative impact of poor dentition on nutritional health (Sanz et al., 2020; Chapple et al., 2022). The emergence of connected digital platforms offers the possibility of making these connections. EpiDentomics offers a new conceptual model to overcome the traditional division between oral and medical health research. This model has a more comprehensive perspective on dental disease and considers oral health as a part of the body's health. It enables the population level analysis of established two-way relationships (e.g. periodontal inflammation and glycemic control in diabetes; microbial burden in the mouth and cardiovascular risk of poor oral health; nutritional outcomes of poor dentition). Integrated usage of digital data sources and the discipline-crossing approach to removing silos and linking together shared risk factors, common pathogenic pathways and the population-level impact of coordinated prevention strategies is an important aspect of the EpiDentomics that sets it apart from traditional oral epidemiology (Kassebaum et al., 2017; Foláyan & Starr, 2024).

This chapter takes a systematic approach to this vision. Section 2 explores the variety of big health data sources and how to combine them. Section 3 considers the use of digital epidemiology to support real-time surveillance. Section 4 examines the impact of cloud computing and the Internet of Things in public health. Section 5 covers issues of ethics, privacy and governance, which are critical in the use of these technologies. Section 6 looks at the impact on integrated oral and general health epidemiology. Section 7 provides future directions and Section 8 brings together the lessons learned.

2. BIG HEALTH DATA: SOURCES AND INTEGRATION

The concept of “big data” is often reduced to large amounts of data in health research - think large numbers of patient records, images, or transactions. But useful data for epidemiologists is more than a matter of volume. This is sometimes referred to as the “5 Vs”: volume, velocity, variety, veracity, and value (Raghupathi and Raghupathi, 2014). These factors present interesting opportunities for population health research, as well as challenges for doing that research. (Figure 1).

Figure 1. 5 Vs of big data applied to oral- health systemic epidemiology. Each dimension creates both opportunities and challenges for integrated EpiDentomics research.

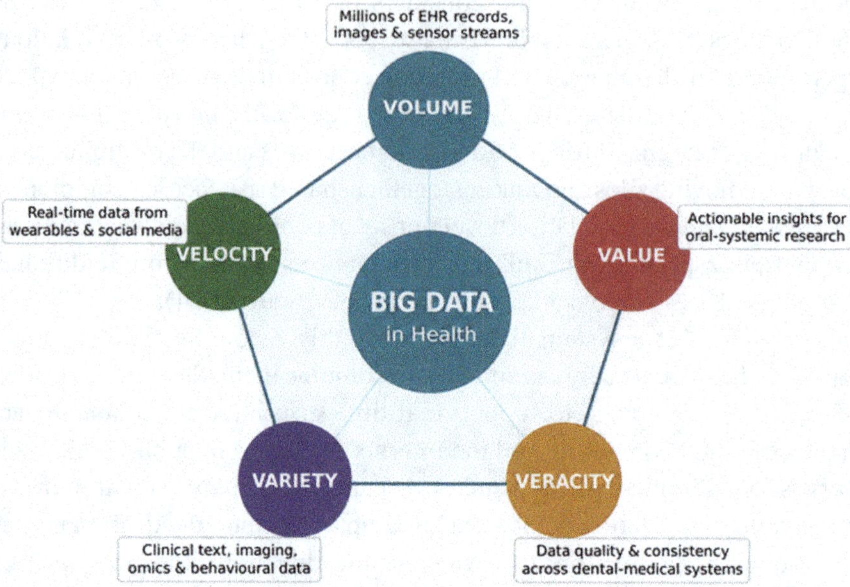

Table 1 illustrates major sources of big data used in oral–systemic epidemiology, summarizing their epidemiological strengths, limitations, and relevance to EpiDentomics. These diverse data sources enable integrated, longitudinal investigations of oral–systemic health relationships while presenting important challenges related to data quality, interoperability, and representativeness.

Table 1. Big data sources in oral health systemic epidemiology

Data Source	Examples	Epidemiologic Strengths	Key Limitations	Oral Health Relevance
EHR / EDR	Diagnoses, prescriptions, lab results, clinical notes	Longitudinal histories for millions; no primary data collection burden; enables incidence & prevalence estimates	Built for billing, not research; incomplete dental coding; quality varies by institution	When dental and medical records are linked, reveals oral-systemic comorbidities at population scale
Disease Registries	Cancer registries, periodontal disease databases, cleft lip/palate records	Large curated populations; long follow-up periods; standardized data collection protocols	Incomplete coverage in low-income settings; siloed from medical data; slow update cycles	Oral cancer burden, periodontal prevalence and congenital oral condition tracking
Imaging & Omics	CBCT, intraoral scanners, salivary microbiome, genomics, proteomics	Deep biological phenotyping; reveals mechanisms behind oral-systemic associations	High cost; large storage requirements; specialist expertise needed for analysis	Links dental imaging and salivary biomarkers to cardiovascular and metabolic disease pathways
Wearables and mHealth	Smartwatches, CGMs, connected toothbrushes, dental reminder apps	Continuous behavioural and physiological monitoring in real-world conditions; improves on self-report	Severe selection bias toward younger, wealthier, more educated populations	Objective brushing behaviour data; glycaemic patterns linked to periodontal outcomes
Social Media and Digital Trace	Search queries, social media posts, mobile phone mobility data	Near-real-time situational awareness; precedes formal reporting by days or weeks	Poor representativeness; not suitable for causal inference; platform-specific biases	Tracks dental pain complaints, oral health help-seeking behaviour and vaccination sentiment

Big data sources in oral-systemic epidemiology: characteristics, limitations, and EpiDentomics relevance. EHR = electronic health record; EDR = electronic dental record; CBCT = cone-beam computed tomography; CGM = continuous glucose monitor

2.1 Electronic Health Records and Administrative Data

Electronic health records and electronic dental records are probably the most direct sources of digital clinical data. They capture clinical histories that provide details of diagnoses, procedures, medications, laboratory findings, vital signs, and notes. For epidemiologists this presents an opportunity that has been elusive in the past: a link to long term clinical records for very large numbers of people, without the need for time and effort intensive data collection.

The potential here is considerable. These data can be analyzed for incidence and prevalence of disease from diagnostic coding, patient pathways, and associations between interventions and outcomes. They can also, when medical and dental records are linked, offer evidence of relationships between oral and systemic health that have proven difficult to identify in smaller studies (Cowie et al., 2017; Romero Laorden et al., 2022).

These data, however, have limitations. Electronic health records were not intended for research. They were designed for clinical practice and administrative uses like billing. This means that coding may differ between providers, institutions and countries. Data are also often missing and rarely random. Rather, they can be indicative of variations in access to care, patient attitudes and system capacity. Furthermore, coding frameworks such as International Classification of Diseases (ICD) and Systematized Nomenclature of Medicine Clinical Terms (SNOMED CT) are not as well developed and used for dental conditions as they are for many medical conditions (Redd et al., 2021).

To facilitate data exchange, there have been attempts to improve data integration through interoperability standards, such as HL7 Fast Healthcare Interoperability Resources (FHIR). This is an API and modular based standard that allows data integration between health systems, including the potential integration of medical and dental systems (Mandl et al., 2020). But there has been differential uptake. Specifically, the adoption of interoperable systems has lagged behind in dentistry relative to medicine, and this has a negative impact on the exchange of medical and oral health data (Zimmerman et al., 2022).

The differences found between dentistry and medicine are not only technical but also cultural and this presents another challenge for integrating data. Research with academic medical institutions in the US and Germany finds that while the vast majority of physicians and dentists agree that it's important for oral and systemic health data to be shared, they disagree about which information is valuable. For example, dentists are more interested in rich clinical data and physicians are more interested in brief standardized information about oral health status, but not procedure level data (Kalenderian et al., 2019).

These are important because they can influence how integrated systems are used. Just achieving interoperability is insufficient if the data shared doesn't match the needs and processes of each profession. For integrated records to be used effectively, the design of the interface and integration of workflows need to be aligned with the professional thought processes and decision making of clinicians from both professions.

The FAIR principles that data should be findable, accessible, interoperable, and reusable is a useful guide to determine whether dental records can be used for research and other purposes. The evidence to date indicates that electronic dental records are often not findable, accessible, interoperable or reusable and cannot be used to inform large scale epidemiological studies (Joda and Spallek, 2023).

A potential solution is to use natural language processing to structure free text notes. As much useful information in dental electronic records is captured in free text format, it is increasingly recognized as a crucial step towards making these data accessible and meaningful for large-scale research. (Table 2)

Table 2. Interoperability standards and frameworks

Standard	Purpose	Medicine Adoption	Dentistry Adoption	Key Gap for EpiDentomics
HL7 FHIR	API-based exchange of health records between institutions	High — mandated in US and EU health systems	Low — dental EHR vendors significantly lag behind	Dental procedure and diagnosis codes not yet fully mapped within FHIR profiles
OMOP CDM	Common data model enabling federated research queries across institutions without moving raw data	Widely adopted in PCORnet, OHDSI and large research networks	Minimal — OMOP dental extensions currently under development	No standardised representation of tooth-surface codes or periodontal staging data
SNOMED CT	Clinical terminology system for diagnoses, procedures and clinical findings	Broadly used; national adoption mandated in several countries	Limited and inconsistent — dental terms less granular than medical equivalents	Dental conditions frequently under-coded relative to medical diagnoses in shared systems
ICD-11	International disease classification for diagnoses and public health reporting	Global standard for mortality and morbidity reporting	Partial — dental ICD codes routinely under-utilised in hospital datasets	Dental diagnoses frequently omitted or miscoded in electronic health records
FAIR Principles	Framework for Findable, Accessible, Interoperable and Reusable research data	Promoted across research funders and academic publishing requirements	Rarely evaluated explicitly for dental records or dental research outputs	Dental EHR systems frequently fail accessibility and reusability criteria for secondary research use

Key interoperability standards and frameworks for oral-systemic health data integration. FHIR = Fast Healthcare Interoperability Resources; OMOP CDM = Observational Medical Outcomes Partnership Common Data Model; FAIR = Findable, Accessible, Interoperable, Reusable.

2.2 Registries and Population Databases

Registries of specific diseases such as cancer, congenital anomalies, stroke and rare diseases, and large population health databases, such as national surveys, vital statistics, and birth and death registrations, are still fundamental for epidemiological research. Their management and use have changed. Digital information systems allow for more timely registry updates, linkages between different registries, and easier access to registries for research.

In oral health, registries for periodontal disease, cleft lip and palate and oral cancer have significant potential. Once these databases are digitalized and linked to medical data, they can offer greater insight into the burden of oral disease and its association with systemic health. This enables researchers to look beyond individual reports from individual hospitals and gain insight into population-level trends (Listl et al., 2015).

2.3 Imaging, Omics, and High Dimensional Clinical Data

The rise of digital imaging has led to the production of many new types of data in oral health. Digital radiography, cone beam computed tomography, intraoral scanners and optical coherence tomography provide detailed imaging of the mouth. Similarly, advances in the fields of genomics, transcriptomics, microbiome, proteomics and metabolomics have provided novel approaches to examining biological systems at the molecular level.

When synthesized, these data allow so-called deep phenotyping, where individuals and populations are defined with much more granularity than is currently used in the clinical setting (Tran et al., 2021). That's where the concept of EpiDentomics gets exciting. For instance, by combining salivary microbiome data with systemic markers of inflammation, or a dental imaging diagnosis with a cardiovascular disease marker, we may be able to find underlying mechanisms that link oral and systemic disease. Likewise, analyzing gene expression in the oral tissues in combination with metabolic disease processes may reveal otherwise hidden mechanisms (Hajishengallis, 2022).

Integration of this kind, however, is not easy. It requires the creation of large scale, interoperable data platforms that can safely integrate medical and dental data and overcome technical and ethical issues.

The combination of multi omic data with clinical data is an emerging and exciting area of EpiDentomics. Specifically, the oral microbiome, or the collection of oral microorganisms, is known to be involved in systemic health. Disruptions in this microbial community have been associated with a variety of diseases, such as atherosclerosis, insulin resistance and inflammatory bowel disease, mainly through the impact on inflammatory processes (Gualtero et al., 2023).

Saliva has become an important and feasible source of biological data. It includes many markers, such as inflammatory cytokines, metabolites, and bacterial DNA, that can be measured and it can be collected non-invasively and conveniently. This makes it particularly attractive for large population based studies. When collected as part of a larger set of health information, within an integrated digital health environment, salivary measurements offer an opportunity to detect early indicators of disease risk without the need for blood sampling or clinical visits.

Meanwhile, genetic science is starting to add new dimensions. Genome wide association studies have discovered genetic variations that appear to have an influence on both the oral microbiome and metabolic health outcomes, suggesting that the association between oral and systemic health may have a genetic component (Stankevic et al., 2024). Integrating all these factors, such as genetic information, microbiome profiles, dental health and systemic health outcomes, is a long term aspiration for EpiDentomics. This will rely on data systems that are able to link records across organizations, and are interoperable, secure, and governed, as outlined in this chapter.

2.4 Mobile Health, Wearables and Patient Generated Data

The increasing adoption of wearable's devices, such as smart watches, fitness trackers, continuous glucose monitors and pulse oximeters, has created a new source of continuous, out-of-clinic health data. These wearable devices provide information on physical activity, heart rate monitoring, sleep and metabolic monitoring in the home environment. Meanwhile, mobile phone apps allow data on dietary intake, mood, medications, and even dental-related factors such as tooth brushing, reminders, and teledentistry (Meskó et al., 2017).

This is a significant advance for epidemiology in terms of measuring behavioral risk factors. Rather than surveys conducted at a point in time, patterns can now be observed in real-time and in the real world. But the data aren't without their problems. Perhaps the most obvious issue is selection bias. Wearable technology users are generally younger, better educated and better off than the rest of the population, and so the types of people most burdened by disease may not be well represented in these data (Ledger and McCaffrey, 2014).

Unless this is carefully accounted for there is a risk that research based on these data will perpetuate rather than narrow health inequalities (Arshed, Kazi, Kiran, et al., 2025). Therefore, epidemiologists must carefully balance excitement and scepticism when considering the use of patient-generated data, and carefully account for potential biases when designing studies and drawing conclusions.

2.5 Digital Trace Data: Social Media, Search Queries, and Mobility

In addition to clinical and structured data sources, increasing research has begun to use digital traces of online interactions. These include social media postings, internet searches and even users' mobile phone trajectories. These data are being used as proxy measures of health.

Perhaps the best known of these is Google Flu Trends. While it subsequently became a warning of the dangers of relying too heavily on algorithms, it demonstrated that, under certain circumstances, searches can provide an indication of infectious diseases more rapidly than conventional sources (Lazer et al., 2014). Likewise, social media platforms such as Twitter have also been used to monitor sentiment about vaccination, consumption patterns, mental health issues, and even user reports of dental pain (Paul and Dredze, 2011).

Data such as these are well-suited to extracting insights from the population in a timely fashion. But they are not without their limitations. Lack of representativeness, data validity, and platform-specific biases make them less appropriate for causal inferences. So, their real purpose is to supplement, not replace, the more traditional epidemiological data.

2.6 Integration, Interoperability, and Quality

The true power of big data in epidemiology does not lie with any one source of information, but with the ability to combine different data. When data from different systems are integrated, we can gain a better picture of person's health. For instance, a person diagnosed with diabetes in the hospital, seen for gum disease in a dental clinic and who has low activity and poor sleep according to wearable data is better understood when these factors are put together.

But combining such information is not always easy. It raises technical, legal and ethical issues. To overcome some of the challenges, common data models, such as the Observational Medical Outcomes Partnership model and the PCORnet Common Data Model, have been proposed. These models define a common structure for data, making it possible to perform analyses across multiple sites without sharing data between sites (Garza et al., 2016).

Privacy of patients is also important. Techniques such as probabilistic record linkage and tokenization allow us to link data from different sources, such as medical and dental data, without exposing personally identifiable information (Christen, 2012). But quality is important too. Software that identifies missing data, inconsistent codes, implausible data and temporal inconsistencies are essential to avoid biased or misleading analyses (Kahn et al., 2016).

For the specific case of integrating oral and general health data, a major technical challenge is the lack of established methods to represent dental data within existing data models. Work is underway to extend models like OMOP to include dental diagnoses, procedures and measurements, and this is a key step to improving integrated and comprehensive epidemiological studies (Garza et al., 2016; Zimmerman et al., 2022).

One thing that's difficult to conceptualize when considering data integration is the amount of social and institutional work that is required. The integration of dental and medical data is not a technical project. It includes legal contracts, data sharing policies and governance arrangements that can be as complicated as the technology itself.

This is evident from the experiences of Nordic countries. Their capacity to undertake large scale research into oral and systemic health is not just because of their technical capabilities, but also because of their long term investment in national registries, universal health identification and data governance. What is notable is the level of sustained political and institutional support for these systems (Sandlund et al., 2021).

Where this type of infrastructure is not already in place, the digital transformation underway presents another opportunity. Rather than having to retrofit existing siloed systems, there is an opportunity to develop integrated dental and medical data systems. The trick will be to make sure that the governance systems grow alongside the technology. It's not enough to have robust technical systems. They have to be complemented by equally robust institutional frameworks. (Figure 2)

Figure 2. Moving from fragmented dental-medical data siloes to an integrated research platform

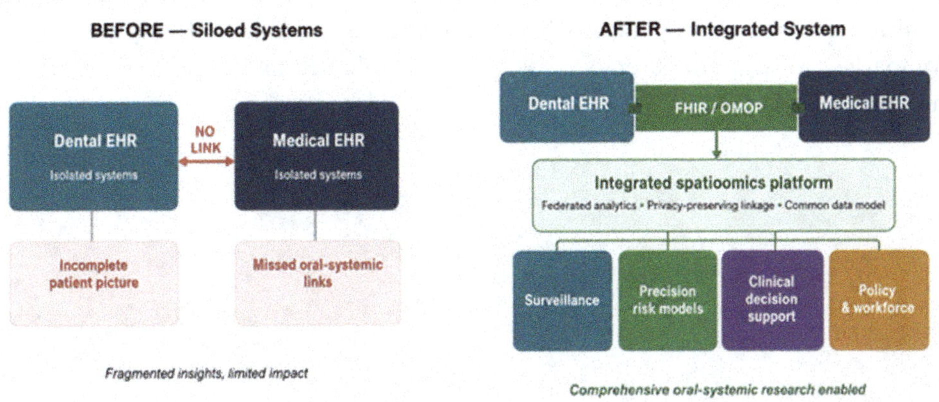

FHIR = Fast Healthcare Interoperability Resources; OMOP = Observational Medical Outcomes Partnership Common Data Model.

3. DIGITAL EPIDEMIOLOGY AND REAL-TIME SURVEILLANCE

Real-time surveillance is an example of digital epidemiology. When time is of the essence, such as in the case of a new infectious disease, the delivery of a tainted food or drug, or the detection of unusual clinical signs, the time taken to detect and respond can be critical. Digital systems have started to reduce this time considerably, from weeks to days, and even hours.

3.1 Traditional to Digital Surveillance

Epidemiological surveillance has always emphasized the importance of completeness and accuracy. This guarantees quality, but sacrifices timeliness. For instance, the process for reporting a case of a notifiable disease involves a number of steps, from initial presentation to a health professional, to diagnosis, reporting, and aggregation at a local and national level before being incorporated into the data. This can take up to four weeks (Buehler et al., 2003). This can be a serious problem during outbreaks, as it means transmission continues unchecked.

Electronic surveillance systems seek to resolve this problem by removing the need to collect data and using algorithms to interpret a stream of data. Syndromic surveillance systems are a good example. These are now in widespread use in many high-income countries, and monitor measures such as emergency department presentations, over-the-counter drug sales and school absenteeism in close to real-time. They look for patterns that won't necessarily be diagnoses, but could be indicators of new diseases (Henning, 2004). Examples in the US include BioSense, globally HealthMap, and in Europe, EuroNORM (Brownstein et al., 2008). Figure 3 shows comparison of traditional epidemiological surveillance and digital real-time surveillance systems.

Figure 3. Comparison of traditional epidemiological surveillance and digital real-time surveillance systems

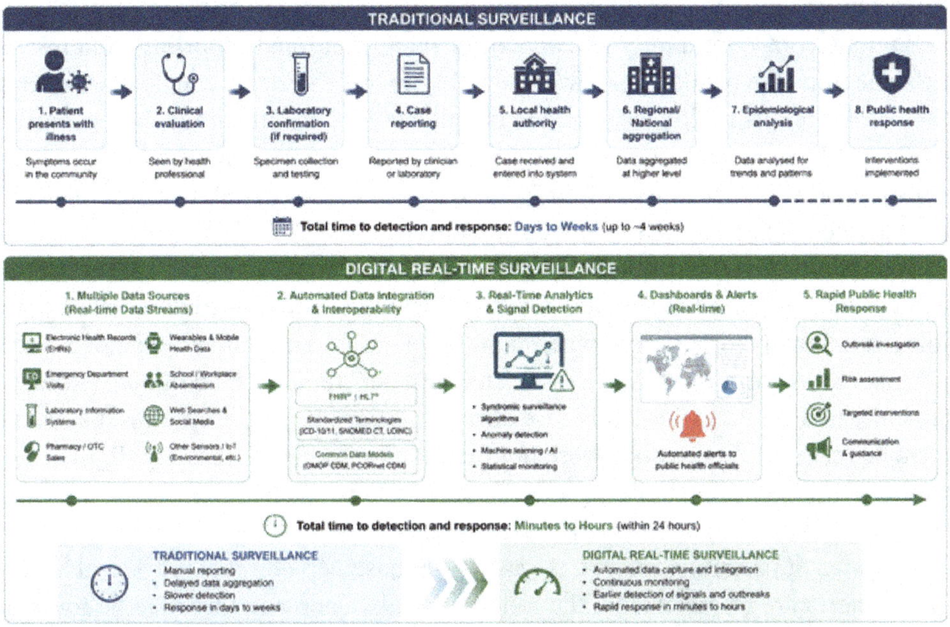

3.1 Outbreak Detection and Early Warning

One of the main challenges in real-time surveillance is separating meaningful signals from background noise. Health data are inherently variable. Seasonal patterns, holidays, shifts in healthcare-seeking behavior, and simple data entry errors can all create fluctuations that may appear significant but are not. To address this, a range of statistical approaches are used to detect unusual patterns while minimizing both false alarms and missed events. These include control charts, scan statistics, Bayesian methods, and machine learning techniques (Unkel et al., 2012).

In oral health, the use of real-time surveillance is still limited, but the potential applications are clear. For instance, a sudden increase in severe dental infections presenting at emergency departments could indicate a broader issue with access to care in a community. Spikes in dental trauma cases might point to specific incidents such as sports injuries or disaster events. Changes in antibiotic prescribing patterns within dental practices could also serve as early signals of emerging antimicrobial resistance. Bringing dental data into existing surveillance systems could therefore add an important layer of insight, particularly in understanding how oral and systemic health patterns intersect (Atchison et al., 2019).

The COVID 19 pandemic offered both a powerful demonstration and an important reality check for digital outbreak detection. In several settings, tools such as wastewater monitoring, mobility data, and social media analysis were able to pick up signs of community spread earlier than traditional reporting systems. At the same time, the pandemic showed how fragile these systems can be when underlying assumptions no longer hold. As people avoided healthcare facilities, shifted to telehealth, and changed their daily behaviors, the patterns captured in electronic health records also changed, often in ways that disrupted established models and reduced their reliability (Buehler et al., 2003).

For oral health, the pandemic exposed a different kind of vulnerability. Dental services were among the first to shut down, which meant that routine data collection was interrupted at a time when population stress and unmet care needs were increasing. Conditions such as stress related bruxism, temporomandibular disorders, and untreated dental caries likely rose during this period, yet the systems that would normally capture these trends were not functioning as usual. This highlights a key challenge for the future: building surveillance systems that can continue to generate meaningful data even when routine care is disrupted.

One area of particular interest is wastewater based epidemiology for oral health. Oral bacteria are released from the mouth via saliva and can therefore be found in wastewater systems. Community level monitoring of the presence and concentration of periodontal and/or cariogenic organisms could theoretically give a general overview of oral health trends without having to visit patients. This could be particularly useful in areas in which there is limited dental care access and limited routine surveillance data.

New studies seem to indicate that this is a potential. In recent pilot studies, it has been found that oral pathogens, such as *Porphyromonas gingivalis*, *Tannerella forsythia*, and *Treponema denticola*, can be detected in municipal wastewater samples using quantitative PCR (qPCR) and metagenomic sequencing (Johnson et al., 2025; Abe et al., 2024). A pilot study in three cities in Europe showed that the wastewater level of P. gingivalis was associated with the regional prevalence estimates of periodontal disease that had been determined using traditional survey methods ($r = 0.82$, $p < 0.001$), indicating that wastewater monitoring may be a useful complementary surveillance method (Schmidt et al., 2023). Likewise, the use of wastewater to detect *Streptococcus mutans* has been suggested as a proxy to assess sugar consumption habits and caries risk at the population level, especially in contexts with limited clinical surveillance, such as low-resource areas (García-Cruz et al., 2024).

Though these methods are still in the infancy stage, they have a number of constraints. These include standardization of sampling protocols, development of robust assays for oral specific pathogens in complex wastewater matrices and the need for correlation studies between wastewater concentrations and clinical disease burden (Simpson et al., 2025). Despite its limitations, however, the wastewater-based epidemiology is a novel and innovative extension of digital epidemiology, which may prove to be a notable contribution to dental health monitoring in areas lacking dental registries.

Although still at an early stage, this idea reflects the kind of creative thinking needed to expand digital epidemiology. It moves beyond traditional data sources and explores how existing infrastructure can be used in new ways to better understand population health, which is central to the broader vision of EpiDentomics.

3.2 Trend Monitoring and Situational Awareness

Real-time surveillance isn't just useful for outbreak detection. It also facilitates ongoing surveillance of long term trends, which is also important for planning. Rather than relying on periodic surveys to estimate the prevalence of conditions like periodontitis and dental caries, real-time electronic systems can provide regular updates. This can be done at sub group level, such as by geographical area, age, socioeconomic status and other health conditions and can be updated periodically (Brownstein et al., 2009).

This is a new opportunity for integrated oral and general health. It is possible to monitor the co-occurrence of conditions like periodontitis and diabetes in the population in close to real-time. Public health policy makers could map where these conditions are co-occurring, track the evolution of these patterns and measure the effect of interventions as they are introduced. This sort of real-time feedback is more responsive than static surveillance.

3.3 Resource Allocation and Decision Support

The availability of real-time data not only enhances surveillance. It affects resource allocation and decision making. For example, if new information shows that some communities are experiencing a greater unmet need, mobile clinics can be targeted accordingly. Health promotion strategies can be targeted at communities where risk is on the rise, rather than more generalized approaches. Even staffing levels in integrated oral and primary health centers can be adjusted, based on predictive models that estimate future demand based on current population trends (Khoury et al., 2016). This is a significant advance for the use of epidemiological knowledge. Rather than staying as reports and historical studies, it is used as part of routine health systems decision-making. In this way, digital epidemiology helps with clinical decision making by providing relevant, up to date evidence to those who need it (whether it is clinicians, service planners or policy makers).

Let's be a little more specific about how real-time decision support might work in integrated oral and general health services. For example, a regional health service might have a cloud-based dashboard that integrates data from dental and medical services and keeps it up to date. This type of system might show the concentration of conditions such as periodontitis and uncontrolled diabetes in particular communities, along with access to, and utilization of, services.

This type of information could help public health agencies. They could use mobile clinics to target areas of greatest need, prioritize community health workers in areas of risk and track over time whether integrated care strategies are making a difference. The tools to do so are already available. The barriers instead are related to the design, funding, and governance of the system - not to mention the legal issues around sharing data.

This is a more evolved way of thinking about population health, from separate, intermittent reporting to more ongoing connectedness. This could have a significant impact on communities that already have challenges accessing dental and medical care.

However, there is still little evidence on what type of integrated care works best. This is partly because the ability to do so has only recently emerged. Real-time surveillance systems can do more than monitor. They also enable us to learn from change itself. If a new care model is implemented in one jurisdiction but not another, these systems can monitor the changing picture in different populations over time to reveal how and why it works or fails. Such evidence can be developed more rapidly and at larger scales than is possible in clinical trials (Foláyan and Starr, 2024).

4. CLOUD COMPUTING AND THE INTERNET OF THINGS

The data sources and surveillance systems outlined above don't just collect data. They require a team to manage, analyses and connect big and varied data. An essential component of this infrastructure is cloud computing and the Internet of Things (IoT), which enables the storage, analysis and linking of today's big, fast and diverse health data.

4.1 Cloud-Based Health Data

Cloud computing is the provision of computing resources (storage, processing, networking and software) via the internet. There are several advantages for health research. It allows storage to scale as needed with relatively low up-front capital expenditure, provides opportunities for data analytics and machine learning, and makes it possible to back up and restore data. It can also enable multiple sites to collaborate without needing to build the same infrastructure (Dash et al., 2019).

The big cloud companies such as Amazon Web Services (AWS), Microsoft Azure and Google Cloud Platform offer healthcare solutions. They are compliant with laws like the Health Insurance Portability and Accountability Act (HIPAA) in the United States and the General Data Protection Regulation (GDPR) in Europe, and have capabilities to manage big health data, conduct genetic analysis, and to perform queries across multiple data sources (Kruse et al., 2016).

Cloud services are especially important for oral-general health studies. They enable integration of health data from multiple institutions and health areas. Providing appropriate security such as standardized information, de identification and governance, they can facilitate large studies which would not be possible within one institution.

4.2 Cloud Enabled Analytics and Collaboration

Cloud computing not only alters data storage. It also changes the way analyses are conducted and communicated. The steps in analyses can be recorded, documented and replicated more efficiently through code sharing and the use of cloud computing platforms for running analyses. This allows for result transparency and verification. Containerization technologies can package and share entire analytical environments, avoiding inconsistencies. Workflow managers can automate complex analyses, making them more scalable and reusable as new data are collected (Schatz, 2015). Another key trend is federated learning. Rather than sharing data across sites into a central location, models can be developed at each institution, and the results pooled. This approach can help resolve issues such as privacy, ownership and governance (Rieke et al., 2020). For instance, a model to predict the association between periodontal disease and systemic health could be trained across different countries without sharing individual patient data.

Federated learning is increasingly being put into practice in the fields of oral and systemic health research. Recent research from multi institutional dental informatics programs in the US and Europe demonstrate federated methods can be applied in practice. These systems involve a central team distributing an analysis plan for each institution to run locally (Gummin et al., 2023). Rather than transferring patient data, only aggregate data is sent back. This approach has been shown to yield estimates of prevalence of oral diseases and patterns of co-morbidity similar to what would be found from a fully centralised data set, without transferring patient-level information across institutional borders (Garza et al., 2016). This has profound implications for worldwide EpiDentomics. This means that in theory, a researcher could build a model for the risk of periodontitis using data from different countries simultaneously (such as dental clinics in Brazil, community health clinics in Kenya and hospital networks in Germany) without ever having to move patient level data from one place to another (Maiti et al., 2025). But there are a few requirements. Data models across participating institutions must be consistent and institutions must have sufficient computing power to do the analysis. This is not currently the case in every institution but is increasingly becoming an option with the growth of cloud-based resources. An alternative strategy that is emerging is synthetic data. This is where researchers train generative models on real clinical data and then generate new data that preserves the statistical properties but isn't related to individuals (Patel et al., 2022). This allows researchers to use a dataset that retains the same relationships but does not contain individual patient data. This might be highly beneficial in oral health. Synthetic data sets that retain the associations between oral health, systemic disease, socioeconomic status and clinical outcomes could be used for initial exploration, method development and training. This would allow researchers and institutions to undertake data driven research, particularly in situations where real patient data are not accessible due to legal or ethical considerations. Figure 4 illustrates cloud-enabled analytics and federated learning framework for oral–systemic epidemiology.

Figure 4. Cloud-enabled analytics and federated learning framework for oral–systemic epidemiology.

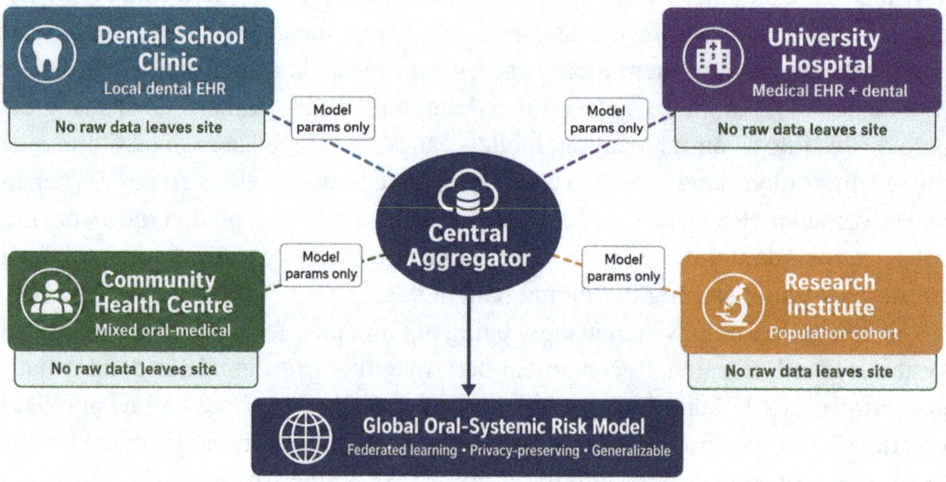

4.3 The Internet of Things in Healthcare

The Internet of Things (IoT) represents a rapidly expanding network of physical objects that have sensors, software and network connectivity, enabling them to gather and exchange data. In the health sector, this encompasses everything from medical devices (including implantable cardiac monitors and connected infusion pumps) to consumer devices (such as smart watches, continuous glucose monitors and even smart toothbrushes). It also includes environmental monitoring of variables such as air and water quality, temperature and humidity in health care facilities (Farahani et al., 2018).

From an epidemiologist's point of view, these devices are broadening the possibilities of measuring health and behaviors. For one thing, they allow data to be collected in real world situations. Rather than relying on self-reported data or recall, researchers can track behaviors as they happen in the real world. A second major benefit is the high resolution of these devices. Now, researchers can collect data at a very detailed time scale, for example, minute to minute physical activity, hourly variability in glucose, or moment to moment exposure to the environment. This fine level of detail allows one to more accurately link exposures and outcomes over time.

For oral health, these advances hold some exciting opportunities. For instance, smart toothbrushes can collect objective data on tooth brushing including time, method and coverage. This is significant as self-reported measures of oral health behavior are often unreliable and overestimate good behavior (Scheerman et al., 2018). When linked with clinical measures of oral disease, such as periodontal disease and dental caries, these measures would provide more insight into oral health behaviors.

IoT environmental sensors can provide an additional layer of data to complement oral health information, with epidemiological implications. Air quality sensors, such as particulate matter, ozone, and heavy metals, can be combined with oral health data to understand the impact of environmental exposures on oral health. This includes periodontal disease, risk of oral cancer, and abnormalities in children's teeth. Similarly, monitoring water quality can help detect populations exposed to low fluoride or other contaminants (such as heavy metals) where public health interventions can be targeted to prevent clinical problems from occurring. This is particularly important in low income urban areas, where the environment may pose greater risks and access to dental care is scarce, and where clinical surveillance may not pick up early signs of problems.

In addition to environmental monitoring, smart dental clinic systems are also revolutionizing data collection. Networked devices that automatically record procedure information in electronic health records; digital check in that records patient attendance; and chairside diagnostic technology that automatically uploads data to cloud storage, can all minimize the need for manual data entry, and increase the accuracy and timeliness of clinical data.

When these technologies are deployed, data from routine dental care are no longer archived away, but are part of a stream of epidemiological data. Even the most basic IoT technologies, such as sensors that count the use of dental hand pieces (as a proxy measure for procedures) can offer insights at the clinic level on service delivery and capacity. Such data are usually not included in billing systems, but can provide an overall sense of how services are being delivered and used.

4.4 Telehealth, Monitoring of Chronic Disease, and Quick Reporting

Telehealth has grown rapidly in recent years due to the use of IoT and cloud computing technologies. Telepatient monitoring helps to track health data continuously from the home and transfer it to health care professionals. This allows early signs of problems to be identified, unnecessary visits to the clinic to be avoided, and patients with chronic conditions to take more control of their own health.

In dentistry, teledentistry platforms provide new opportunities for delivering care outside of clinics. They can increase access to care in disadvantaged communities, enable the integration of oral health into primary health care, and, when linked to other medical systems, can help to provide a more comprehensive picture of patient health (Alabdullah and Daniel, 2018).

Such innovations are especially important in low and middle-income countries. Many areas have poor access to dental services, but high mobile phone and internet penetration. In these settings, IoT-based monitoring and teledentistry with AI-based diagnosis can help extend access to care. At the same time, such systems can collect useful population data, providing information about population-level health where conventional sources of data are sparse or non-existent.

5. ETHICS, PRIVACY AND GOVERNANCE IN DIGITAL EPIDEMIOLOGY

The technologies outlined above are impressive. But with them come challenges of privacy, equity, trust, and validity of epidemiological studies. We cannot delay their consideration or relegate them to a secondary task. For digital epidemiology to progress, these issues need to be confronted now, rather than being left for regulators to address after the fact (Arshed, Kazi, Kiran, et al., 2025).

5.1 Informed Consent and Re-Use

Research ethics are often premised on a clear and specific informed consent, generally acquired before a research project. This model is not well suited to digital epidemiology. Many of the data currently used for research are collected for clinical, administrative or commercial purposes. Secondary use of these data for research raises ethical and legal considerations which vary between jurisdictions (Dove et al., 2015).

To address this, several alternative models have been proposed. Broad consent allows individuals to agree, at the time of care, to the use of their de identified data for future research in general. This approach is commonly used in biobanking (Kaye et al., 2015). Dynamic consent goes a step further by using digital platforms that allow individuals to update their preferences over time, choosing which types of research they wish to support or decline (Steinsbekk et al., 2013). In the context of routine public health surveillance, many systems permit the use of data without explicit consent, provided that appropriate oversight and data protection measures are in place.

When it comes to integrating oral and general health data, it is important not to underestimate the sensitivity of dental information. Oral health patterns can reflect socioeconomic status, cultural practices, access to care, and conditions that may carry stigma. Individuals should have a clear understanding of how their dental and medical data might be linked and used for research or public health purposes.

The challenge of consent in integrated oral and general health research becomes even more complex when data are drawn from multiple institutions and sectors. A single patient's dental record from a private clinic, their electronic health record from a public hospital, and behavioral data from a wearable device owned by a commercial company may each be governed by entirely different consent arrangements. In some cases, one or more of these data sources may not involve explicit consent for research use at all. As a result, individuals may have agreed to secondary use of their hospital data without being aware that it could be linked with dental or consumer-generated data — or even that such linkage is technically possible (Dove et al., 2015). This creates what can be understood as a consent gap: the analytical value of integrated datasets depends on combining information across systems whose ethical and legal permissions are not naturally aligned. Addressing this requires deliberate coordination across institutions rather than assuming compatibility between governance frameworks.

This makes community engagement central to any viable consent model, particularly in settings where trust in health and research institutions has been historically undermined. Indigenous communities, ethnic minority groups, and populations with limited access to healthcare often carry legitimate concerns rooted in past experiences of exclusion or extractive research practices. Participation in digital health research is unlikely to be sustainable unless these groups are meaningfully involved in decisions about how data are collected, how they are used, and what benefits are returned to them (Nuzzo, 2020). For EpiDentomics to generate representative and credible evidence, such communities cannot be treated as passive data sources; they must be active participants in shaping the system.

5.2 Privacy, Anonymization, and Re Identification Risk

Protecting privacy in health research has traditionally relied on de identification, where direct identifiers such as names, dates of birth, and addresses are removed. However, when multiple datasets are combined, the risk of re identification increases significantly. Even without obvious identifiers, combinations of demographic details, clinical codes, location data, and timing information can make it possible to identify individuals within large datasets (Narayanan and Shmatikoff, 2008).

This challenge becomes even more pronounced when dental and medical data are linked. Dental records often include highly specific procedural and clinical details, which, when combined with other data sources, create more distinctive individual profiles. To manage these risks, several safeguards are used. These include limiting data collection to what is strictly necessary, restricting how data can be used, applying pseudonymization techniques, and using advanced approaches such as differential privacy to protect aggregate outputs. Secure data environments that prevent direct access to raw data are also increasingly important (Dwork and Roth, 2014).

5.3 Data Ownership, Control, and Equity

Ownership and use of health data and the distribution of benefits have become a salient concern. In many cases, health care organizations hold data about patients, and patients have access to their information, with the right to request data corrections, but they do not own their data. This means that large organizations, such as technology firms and research centers, can use data collected from patients to generate value, without sharing the rewards (Prainsack & Buyx, 2017).

Equality is another concern. Sub-populations under-represented in digital health data, such as those with lower access to technology, fewer interactions with the health system, or who are not involved in research are often excluded from analysis. This can mean models developed using these data do not work well for them and may even perpetuate inequitable allocation of resources. This can be remedied by efforts to include these groups, testing models for fairness, and designing governance structures to ensure equitable allocation (Obermeyer et al., 2019).

5.4 Bias, Fairness and Accountability

With the increasing use of machine learning in epidemiology, issues of bias and fairness have come to the fore. If models are developed using data that do not represent all relevant groups, they can perpetuate and even worsen existing disparities. For instance, a model predicting heart disease risk from dental data may not work as well for certain demographic subgroups if those groups are not well represented in the data used to train the model (Rajkomar et al., 2018).

Biases may creep in at various points such as data selection, variable selection, model design and evaluation. This needs to be done through transparency. Data sources, processing, assumptions and model testing and evaluation need to be transparently outlined (Lee et al., 2024). After models are deployed, it is important to monitor how they perform, especially to ensure they remain equitable. Methods from explainable AI that seek to explain model behaviour are particularly useful in health, where accountability is paramount (Doshi Velez and Kim, 2017).

Oral health analytics are especially susceptible to bias because dental data are poorly represented in most health data. Most predictive models are developed using data from groups who are insured, urban, and regularly access the formal dental system (Yarlagadda et al., 2025). These results in a systematic blind spot: individuals from groups with the greatest burden of oral disease - rural, uninsured and care-avoiding groups - tend to be less represented, and risk is misestimated (Obermeyer et al., 2019). When these models are applied to planning or allocation, there is a risk that programs may be targeted at the population that is overrepresented instead of the population most in need.

To address this issue, efforts should be made at the time of data collection rather than during statistical analysis. This includes deliberate oversampling of overlooked groups, broadening data collection beyond clinic settings (such as home or mobile data collection) and moving surveillance systems beyond the clinic (Arshed et al., 2025). Although post-hoc fairness corrections to models are still valuable, they can't address underrepresented or biased data (Arshed et al., 2024). Regulation is starting to catch up, with new guidelines for clinical AI models emphasizing diversity in training data and the need to monitor for performance differences across subgroups (Rajkomar et al., 2018). Figure 5 shows the lifecycle of algorithmic bias and fairness in artificial intelligence for oral health epidemiology.

Figure 5. Lifecycle of algorithmic bias and fairness in artificial intelligence for oral health epidemiology.

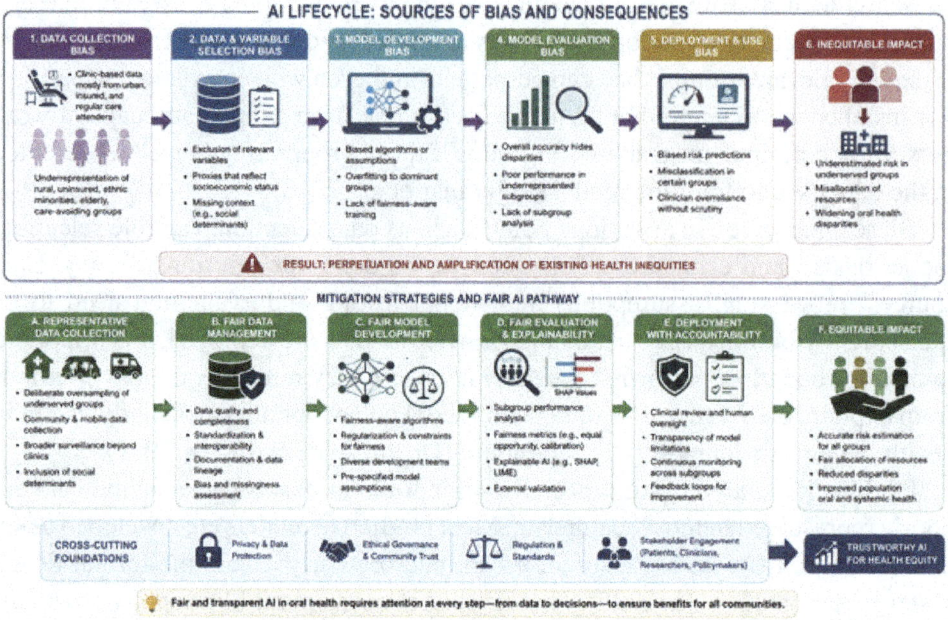

5.5 Regulation and Governance

Regulation in the form of laws like GDPR (Europe), HIPAA (US) and PIPEDA (Canada) are important frameworks for the collection, storage and use of health data. But laws aren't enough. Legislation can be slow to adapt to the pace of technological advances and simply complying with the law does not necessarily ensure ethical behaviour (Mittelstadt and Floridi, 2016).

Governance needs to be more holistic and proactive. This means putting in place data governance bodies that include a diversity of stakeholders, such as patients, community leaders, clinicians, researchers and data scientists. It also requires transparency, either through ensuring open data access, sharing analysis techniques, or reporting findings in a way that recognizes population variation.

Finally, there are mechanisms for accountability. These could be independent audits, processes to respond to data misuse or breaches, and mechanisms to mitigate harm. These measures help to maximize the potential of digital epidemiology while maintaining trust, equity and ethical considerations (Floridi et al., 2018). Table 4 ethical frameworks and governance mechanisms in digital health

Table 4. Ethical frameworks and governance mechanisms in digital health

Ethical Issue	Mechanism / Approach	Example Implementation	Key Limitations
Informed Consent	Broad consent frameworks; dynamic digital consent platforms	Biobank enrolment consent; digital portals allowing patients to adjust data-sharing preferences over time	Patients may not anticipate future linkage of their dental and medical data; consent fatigue in repeat encounters
De-identification & Privacy	Pseudonymisation; differential privacy; secure computation environments	NHS data anonymisation protocols; US Census differential privacy releases	Linkage of multiple individually de-identified datasets can still re-identify individuals in integrated systems
Data Ownership & Equity	Community data trusts; Indigenous data sovereignty frameworks; patient advisory boards	Maori Data Sovereignty Network; First Nations data governance principles in Canada and Australia	Power imbalances persist; commercial entities frequently control key data infrastructure and benefit from research outputs
Algorithmic Bias	Diverse training data requirements; equity audits; standardized model documentation	FDA AI/ML software as a medical device framework; EU AI Act transparency requirements	Bias correction after the fact is less reliable than ensuring representative data collection from the outset
Regulatory Compliance	GDPR (EU); HIPAA (US); PIPEDA (Canada); national data protection authorities	Institutional data governance committees; mandatory data protection impact assessments for new research uses	Regulations consistently lag behind technological capability; legal compliance alone does not guarantee ethical practice
Community Governance	Participatory design processes; community advisory boards; public deliberation on data use policies	Patient and public involvement (PPI) panels in UK health research; community health advisory boards	Risk of tokenistic engagement where communities are consulted but hold no real decision-making power

Ethical issues, governance mechanisms, implementation examples and limitations in digital health epidemiology. GDPR = General Data Protection Regulation; HIPAA = Health Insurance Portability and Accountability Act; PPI = patient and public involvement.

6. CONSEQUENCES FOR INTEGRATED ORAL-GENERAL HEALTH EPIDEMIOLOGY

The technologies we've discussed so far aren't just technological innovations. They have implications for the way we research, track, and address the links between oral and general health at the population level. What was previously hard to quantify is now more accessible, with new possibilities for research and public health initiatives.

6.1 Large-Scale Linkage of Dental and Medical Records

Perhaps the most obvious opportunity in EpiDentomics is to combine dental and medical records to understand the associations between oral and systemic health. We already know that these relationships are significant, such as the association between periodontitis and type 2 diabetes (Chapple et al., 2022), oral infections and heart disease (Sanz et al., 2020), poor dentition and nutritional deficiencies (Sahyoun et al., 2003), and maternal periodontitis and preterm birth (Offenbacher et al., 1996). But many of these studies have small sample sizes, making it difficult to control for potential biases.

Longitudinal data on a large scale holds the key. Linking dental and medical records across time, as is done with national registries in Nordic countries, provides the statistical power to identify more nuanced associations, causal links and the impacts of dental interventions on health (Sandlund et al., 2021). Large-scale research programs such as the United Kingdom Biobank and the All of Us Research Program in the US are starting to show how this can be realized, especially when clinical data are integrated with genomic and other biological data (Bycroft et al., 2018; All of Us Research Program Investigators, 2019). Figure 6 shows integrated EpiDentomics framework for longitudinal linkage of oral and general health data.

Figure 6. Integrated EpiDentomics framework for longitudinal linkage of oral and general health data.

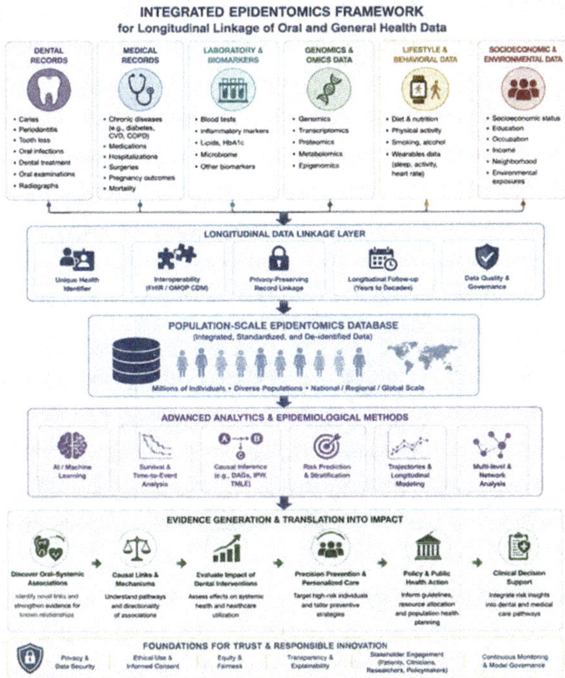

Table 3 illustrates how integrated longitudinal data can strengthen causal inference, improve risk prediction, and support precision prevention.

Table 3. Selected oral-Systemic associations in the evidence base epidemiology

Oral Condition	Systemic Condition	Association Direction	Key Evidence	Study Scale	Digital Data Potential
Periodontitis	Type 2 Diabetes	Bidirectional — each condition worsens the other	Chapple et al. (2022); Chang et al. (2020)	Thousands to hundreds of thousands	High — linked EHRs can track glycaemic control alongside periodontal staging over time
Periodontitis	Cardiovascular Disease	Periodontitis increases cardiovascular risk independently	Sanz et al. (2020); Rydén et al. (2016)	10,000 to 400,000+	High — large EHR linkage needed to distinguish causation from shared risk factors
Maternal Periodontal Disease	Preterm Birth / Low Birth Weight	Periodontal disease associated with adverse pregnancy outcomes	Offenbacher et al. (1996)	Hundreds to thousands	Medium — obstetric and dental records rarely linked; major gap for EpiDentomics
Poor Dentition / Tooth Loss	Malnutrition & Dietary Quality	Tooth loss limits dietary choices and nutrient intake	Sahyoun et al. (2003)	Community surveys	Medium — dietary app data combined with dental records could clarify dose-response
Oral Infection (*Streptococcus mutans*)	Infective Endocarditis	Oral bacteria can seed and colonise cardiac valves	Nomura et al. (2020)	Case series and registries	High — dental procedure records combined with hospital cardiac data could quantify population risk

Key oral-systemic epidemiologic associations, evidence sources, and potential contribution of digital health data. EHR = electronic health record.

6.1 Oral Health Indicators in Population Health Analytics

Digital health systems also make it possible to include oral health measures more routinely in population-level analysis. Indicators such as the DMFT index, periodontal staging and grading, and patient reported measures like the Oral Health Impact Profile can be incorporated into electronic systems and linked with other health data. This allows for more complete health profiles that reflect both oral and systemic conditions.

This shift is important because oral diseases are often overlooked in broader health assessments. Despite affecting more than 3.5 billion people globally, oral conditions remain underrepresented in major burden of disease estimates and are often given less priority in health policy and resource allocation (Kassebaum et al., 2017). Integrating oral health indicators into routine data systems is a key step toward addressing this gap and ensuring that oral health is considered alongside other major health concerns.

The WHO's Global Oral Health Status Report (2022) marked a major step forward by providing comparable country-level oral health profiles across all member states. However, it also made clear how dependent global oral health monitoring still is on survey-based and modelled estimates rather than continuous clinical data. In most countries, routine digital surveillance of oral conditions simply does not exist, meaning that population-level understanding of oral health remains episodic and incomplete.

A shift toward continuous digital monitoring would not only improve accuracy but fundamentally change what can be observed. It would allow health systems to track oral disease burden as it evolves over time, rather than relying on periodic snapshots. Importantly, it would also make it possible to monitor inequality directly. Instead of focusing only on average prevalence, systems could track how oral health outcomes differ across income groups, geographic regions, and demographic categories in near real-time. Foláyan and Starr (2024) argue that embedding equity tracking into surveillance systems is essential if oral health data are to support meaningful policy action rather than simply describing disease patterns.

6.2 Precision Public Health for Oral Systemic Conditions

The growing availability of detailed health data also supports the move toward precision public health. Instead of applying the same intervention strategies to entire populations, this approach focuses on tailoring prevention and care based on specific risk profiles within communities (Khoury et al., 2016).

In the context of oral and general health, this means identifying populations based on combined risks, including clinical conditions, behaviors, socioeconomic factors, and environmental exposures. For example, a community with high levels of both periodontitis and diabetes may require integrated clinical and preventive strategies, while another community might need interventions focused more on improving access to care or addressing dietary patterns.

By bringing together data from multiple sources, including clinical records, behavioral monitoring, and environmental indicators, it becomes possible to identify these patterns more clearly and respond in a more targeted way. This allows public health strategies to evolve continuously, rather than relying on fixed approaches that may not reflect local realities.

6.3 Learning Health Systems and Cross Disciplinary Collaboration

Integrated digital systems also support the development of learning health systems, where data from routine care are continuously used to improve practice. In this model, research and clinical care are not separate activities but part of an ongoing cycle of learning and improvement (Friedman et al., 2010). For oral and general health integration, this would involve closer collaboration between dental and medical professionals, supported by shared data systems. Clinicians could access more complete patient information, including relevant findings from both dental and medical care, and use this to inform decision making.

There are already examples of how this could work in practice. Clinical decision support tools could alert physicians when patients with chronic conditions, such as diabetes, have not received recent dental care. Similarly, dentists could be notified when changes in a patient's oral health may be linked to worsening systemic indicators such as glycemic control.

The main challenges here are not technical but organizational. Effective integration requires shared standards, aligned professional practices, and governance structures that support collaboration across disciplines. Without these, even the most advanced data systems will struggle to deliver their full potential.

7. FUTURE DIRECTIONS

Table 5. Future Directions: Technologies, Applications, and Prerequisites

Technology / Approach	Oral-Systemic Application	Readiness	Key Prerequisites
Federated Learning	Train periodontal risk models across dental and medical institutions without sharing raw patient records	High	Compatible data models at each participating site; local computing capacity; multi-institutional governance agreements
FHIR / OMOP Dental Extensions	Enable dental data to flow into multi-institutional research networks alongside medical records	Medium	Completion of OMOP dental module; vendor adoption incentives from professional and regulatory bodies
AI Diagnostic Imaging	Automated extraction of periodontal and caries findings from dental radiographs for population-level analysis	Medium	Diverse and representative training datasets; regulatory validation pathways; ongoing equity performance audits

continued on following page

Table 5. Continued

Technology / Approach	Oral-Systemic Application	Readiness	Key Prerequisites
Synthetic Data Generation	Release privacy-safe synthetic dental datasets that enable open research and student education without patient risk	Emerging	Generative AI trained on sufficiently large real-world dental datasets; validation frameworks to ensure data fidelity
Wastewater Epidemiology	Monitor community-level oral pathogen burden without requiring individual clinical contact — useful in underserved areas	Emerging	Oral pathogen assay development and standardisation; integration with existing wastewater surveillance infrastructure
Cross-Sector Dashboards	Real-time policy intelligence combining periodontitis prevalence, diabetes rates, dental access and socioeconomic indicators	Feasible now	Political will to integrate oral health into national monitoring systems; shared governance between dental and health authorities
IoT Oral Health Sensors	Connected toothbrushes and dental devices generating objective oral hygiene behavioural data for epidemiology	Feasible now	Consumer adoption beyond affluent populations; privacy frameworks for continuous device-generated personal data

Future directions in EpiDentomics: technologies, applications, readiness levels, and prerequisites for implementation. Readiness: Teal = feasible now; Orange = medium-term; Purple = emerging.

7.1 Interoperable Health Ecosystems

Achieving the goals of integrated oral and general health research will be largely dependent on the interoperability of health systems. Interoperability goes beyond technical standards. It also requires institutional partnerships, governance and incentives for collaboration in sharing data and partnerships over time.

Greater uptake of standards like FHIR in medical and dental systems will help. Simultaneously, adapting common data models such as OMOP to suit dental data, and creating federated research networks connecting multi-disciplinary institutions, will be crucial to moving this area forward. We can look to existing international initiatives such as the European Health Data Space and the Global Alliance for Genomics and Health as models (European Commission, 2022).

7.2 Privacy Preserving and Federated Learning

Federated learning is likely to be pivotal to the future of oral systemic epidemiology. Rather than data having to be combined in a central location, it enables models to be trained across multiple data sets while maintaining the physical location of the data. This overcomes many of the privacy, legal and logistical barriers currently preventing collaboration between institutions and countries (Rieke et al., 2020).

Approaches like secure multiparty computation, holomorphic encryption and synthetic data also add to the range of possibilities while ensuring data protection. Yet to see these methods used more widely, there will need to be more consistency in health systems so these methods can go from the niche to the mainstream.

7.3 Artificial Intelligence and Explainable Decision Support

Artificial intelligence (AI) is already having an impact on many aspects of health research and practice, such as imaging, prediction and clinical notes. When it comes to oral and general health, AI could uncover information that is otherwise hard to detect. For instance, it can be applied to extract more information about periodontal health from dental X-rays, or to predict the likelihood of a systemic disease when using oral health data, or to identify people who might need more integrated care (Lee et al., 2018).

But the success of these interventions depends on their development and implementation. Data sets used to train these models should be varied and representative, and the models should be validated in the target populations. They also need to be continually evaluated to prevent perpetuation of inequality. Explain ability is also crucial. Health practitioners and policymakers need to know how and why a model makes its predictions, both to increase trust in the model and to understand when it may not do well (Doshi Velez and Kim, 2017).

7.4 Building Capability in Low Resource Settings

But there is also a danger that digital innovation could increase global health disparities if it remains focused in high resource settings. A large burden of oral disease is found in low and middle income countries, but these countries are frequently overlooked in digital health research and development.

To tackle this, we need to invest in low cost and flexible digital technologies and training programs to build capacity in data science, epidemiology and digital health. It also requires collaborative and reciprocal research relationships that ensure the benefits and knowledge are shared. Without such initiatives, integrated oral-general health research will not benefit all (Naicker et al., 2009).

7.5 Ethics and Democratic Governance

Perhaps the most important area of future research is social. Data systems are not standalone and require trust to be successful. That means that the communities that provide data need to be involved in the design and governance of such systems.

Methods like participatory design, community advisory boards and public consultations around data use can ensure that these systems align with community values and priorities. Robust accountability measures are also needed to prevent or mitigate misuse and harm.

In the case of integrated oral and general health, this is critical for groups historically under-serviced by the dental system. Involving these communities in the development of data systems can help ensure that the resulting systems address their needs. Trust will be a key factor in the long term success of digital epidemiology (Nuzzo, 2020).

7.6 Cross Sector Oral Systemic Dashboards and Policy Intelligence

One of the most practical next steps for EpiDentomics is the development of real-time dashboards that bring together oral and general health data in a way that is easy to understand and use. Unlike research databases, which are often complex and designed for detailed analysis by specialists, these dashboards are meant for decision makers such as policymakers, healthcare planners, and clinical leaders. The goal is to present clear, actionable insights about population health without requiring advanced technical expertise.

A well designed national or regional dashboard could provide a continuously updated view of key indicators. This might include the geographic distribution of combined burdens such as periodontitis and diabetes, patterns of dental service use across different socioeconomic groups, antibiotic prescribing trends in dental care, rates of emergency visits related to oral conditions, and progress toward defined oral health targets. While similar tools already exist for some general health indicators in higher income settings, incorporating oral health into these systems would significantly improve its visibility and importance in policy discussions.

However, developing these dashboards is not only a technical task. It also involves changing how oral health is viewed within the broader health system. For a long time, oral health has been treated as separate from general healthcare, often receiving less attention and fewer resources. Shifting this perspective requires engagement with health ministries, insurance systems, and professional bodies to recognize oral health as an essential part of overall health.

The World Health Organization's Global Oral Health Status Report in 2022 marked an important step in this direction. By providing country-level evidence on the burden of oral disease and calling for its integration into primary care and universal health coverage, it strengthened the case for change (World Health Organization, 2022).

Digital epidemiology can support this shift by providing timely and locally relevant data that policymakers can act on. Instead of relying only on broad or outdated estimates, decision makers can use real-time information to understand current needs within their populations (Arshed, Kazi, Ashraf, et al., 2025). In this way, the argument for integrating oral and general health moves from theory to practice grounded in evidence that is directly relevant to the communities being served.

7.7 Future Direction

Several policy developments are now pushing oral health into the mainstream of digital health infrastructure. Within Europe, recent frameworks for cross-border health data exchange have begun to require that dental records be compatible with other clinical information systems. This marks a notable shift from earlier approaches, where oral health data were often excluded from broader health informatics planning or treated as an afterthought in interoperability discussions. The inclusion of dentistry in these regulatory instruments signals growing recognition that oral health is not a separate domain but an integral component of comprehensive health records.

On the global stage, the World Health Organization has launched an initiative aimed at establishing standardized digital surveillance protocols for oral health across dozens of low- and middle-income countries. This effort responds to the historical underrepresentation of oral conditions in routine disease monitoring systems, which has limited the visibility of dental diseases in global health priority-setting. Crucially, the initiative connects digital data collection directly to health equity goals, requiring that surveillance methods be designed to capture information from marginalized and underserved communities so that resource allocation can be guided by the needs of those who are most affected by oral diseases yet least visible in existing data systems.

Alongside these governmental and intergovernmental efforts, professional organizations have produced guidance for the ethical deployment of artificial intelligence in dental practice. These recommendations address the full lifecycle of AI tools, from their development through to clinical implementation. Key areas covered include the assessment of algorithmic bias, transparent reporting of model performance across different patient populations, adequate training for clinicians who will use these systems, and meaningful engagement with patient communities. A consistent theme across these professional guidelines is that AI should augment rather than supersede clinical expertise, and that patients retain the right to know when automated systems are informing decisions about their care.

8. CONCLUSION

The digital transformation of epidemiology brings both excitement and responsibility. On one hand, it offers new ways to monitor population health almost in real-time, to bring together different types of data at a scale that was not possible before, and to design interventions that respond more closely to the needs of specific communities. On the other hand, these advances raise important questions about privacy, fairness, and trust. Making full use of digital health data requires careful attention to how these systems are built and how their benefits are shared.

In the context of oral and general health, these changes are particularly significant. The idea behind EpiDentomics, which treats oral and systemic health as part of a single, connected system, has long been supported by scientific evidence but has been difficult to implement in practice. Digital tools are beginning to change that. The ability to link dental and medical records, include oral health signals in real-time surveillance, and use shared data platforms and advanced analytics creates new opportunities to study and manage health in a more integrated way.

At the same time, these developments do not automatically lead to better outcomes. The direction they take depends on decisions made by researchers, institutions, policymakers, and communities. Choices about data use, governance, and inclusion will shape whether digital epidemiology reduces health gaps or reinforces them.

Moving forward, the challenge is not only to build better systems, but to build them responsibly. This means creating digital infrastructure that is technically strong, ethically sound, transparent in its governance, and inclusive in its reach. If these conditions are met, the integration of oral and general health will move from an aspirational idea to a practical reality that benefits populations more broadly.

REFERENCES

Abe, M.. (2024). Detection of periodontal pathogens in wastewater: A pilot study. *Water Research*, *230*, 119532.

Alabdullah, J. H., & Daniel, S. J. (2018). Evidence for teledentistry in orthodontics: A systematic review. *The Angle Orthodontist*, *88*(6), 802–810. DOI: 10.2319/012218-52.1

All of Us Research Program Investigators. (2019). The "All of Us" Research Program. *The New England Journal of Medicine*, *381*(7), 668–676. DOI: 10.1056/NEJMsr1809937 PMID: 31412182

Arshed, M., et al.. (2025). Prevalence and associated factors of adherence to antihypertensive medication: A nationwide cross-sectional study. BMC Public Health, 25(1), Article number. https://doi.org/DOI: 10.1186/s12889-025-21456-6

Arshed, M., Kazi, A. K., Ashraf, W., Kiran, M., Arshed, M., Kazi, A. K., Ashraf, W., & Kiran, M. (2025). *Universal Health Coverage: Progress Toward Achieving Universal Health Coverage and Lessons Learned* [Chapter]. Innovation and Transformation of Public Health. IGI Global Scientific Publishing. (universal-health-coverage). Https://Services.Igi-Global.Com/Resolvedoi/Resolve.Aspx?Doi=10.4018/979-8-3373-1992-6.Ch002. https://doi.org/DOI: 10.4018/979-8-3373-1992-6.ch002

Arshed, M., Kazi, A. K., Kiran, M., Ali, S. M. F., Arshed, M., Kazi, A. K., Kiran, M., & Ali, S. M. F. (2025). *Challenges in Health Equity: Balancing Innovation With Fairness and Addressing Algorithmic Biases* [Chapter]. Innovation and Transformation of Public Health. IGI Global Scientific Publishing. (challenges-in-health-equity). Https://Services.Igi-Global.Com/Resolvedoi/Resolve.Aspx?Doi=10.4018/979-8-3373-1992-6.Ch004. https://doi.org/DOI: 10.4018/979-8-3373-1992-6.ch004

Arshed, M., Mahmud, A. B., Umer, M. F., & Mashhadi, F. (2024). Study protocol for a randomized control trial investigating the effectiveness of a multifaceted mHealth approach on adherence to antihypertensive treatment among patients in Pakistan. *Pakistan Journal of Medical Sciences*, *41*(1), 22–28. DOI: 10.12669/pjms.41.1.9272 PMID: 39867791

Atchison, K. A., Rozier, R. G., & Weintraub, J. A. (2019). Integration of oral health and primary care: Communication, coordination and referral. NAM Perspectives. Discussion Paper. National Academy of Medicine. https://doi.org/DOI: 10.31478/201905a

Brownstein, J. S., Freifeld, C. C., & Madoff, L. C. (2009). Digital disease detection: Harnessing the Web for public health surveillance. *The New England Journal of Medicine, 360*(21), 2153–2157. DOI: 10.1056/NEJMp0900702 PMID: 19423867

Brownstein, J. S., Freifeld, C. C., Reis, B. Y., & Mandl, K. D. (2008). Surveillance sans frontieres: Internet-based emerging infectious disease intelligence and the HealthMap project. *PLoS Medicine, 5*(7), e151. DOI: 10.1371/journal.pmed.0050151 PMID: 18613747

Buehler, J. W., Hopkins, R. S., Overhage, J. M., Sosin, D. M., & Tong, V. (2003). Framework for evaluating public health surveillance systems for early detection of outbreaks. *MMWR. Recommendations and Reports, 53*(RR-5), 1–11. PMID: 15129191

Bycroft, C., Freeman, C., Petkova, D., Band, G., Elliott, L. T., Sharp, K., Motyer, A., Vukcevic, D., Delaneau, O., O'Connell, J., Cortes, A., Welsh, S., Young, A., Effingham, M., McVean, G., Leslie, S., Allen, N., Donnelly, P., & Marchini, J. (2018). The UK Biobank resource with deep phenotyping and genomic data. *Nature, 562*(7726), 203–209. DOI: 10.1038/s41586-018-0579-z PMID: 30305743

Chang, Y., Lee, J. S., Lee, K.-J., Woo, H. G., & Song, T.-J. (2020). Improved oral hygiene is associated with decreased risk of new-onset diabetes: A nationwide population-based cohort study. *Diabetologia, 63*(5), 924–933. DOI: 10.1007/s00125-020-05112-9 PMID: 32128623

Chapple, I. L. C., & Genco, R. J. (2022). Diabetes and periodontal diseases: Consensus report of the Joint EFP/AAP Workshop on Periodontitis and Systemic Diseases. *Journal of Clinical Periodontology, 40*(s14, S14), S106–S112. DOI: 10.1111/jcpe.12077 PMID: 23627322

Christen, P. (2012). A survey of indexing techniques for scalable record linkage and deduplication. *IEEE Transactions on Knowledge and Data Engineering, 24*(9), 1537–1555. DOI: 10.1109/TKDE.2011.127

Cowie, M. R., Blomster, J. I., Curtis, L. H., Duclaux, S., Ford, I., Fritz, F., & Zalewski, A. (2017). Electronic health records to facilitate clinical research. *Clinical Research in Cardiology : Official Journal of the German Cardiac Society, 106*(1), 1–9. DOI: 10.1007/s00392-016-1025-6 PMID: 27557678

Dash, S., Shakyawar, S. K., Sharma, M., & Kaushik, S. (2019). Big data in healthcare: Management, analysis and future prospects. *Journal of Big Data, 6*(1), 1–25. DOI: 10.1186/s40537-019-0217-0

Doshi-Velez, F., & Kim, B. (2017). Towards a rigorous science of interpretable machine learning. arXiv preprint arXiv:1702.08608.

Dove, E. S., Knoppers, B. M., & Zawati, M. H. (2015). An ethics safe harbor for international genomics research? *Genome Medicine*, *7*(1), 1–4. DOI: 10.1186/s13073-015-0204-4 PMID: 25606059

Dwork, C., & Roth, A. (2014). The algorithmic foundations of differential privacy. *Foundations and Trends in Theoretical Computer Science*, *9*(3-4), 211–407. DOI: 10.1561/0400000042

European Commission. (2022). *European Health Data Space. Proposal for a Regulation of the European Parliament and of the Council (COM/2022/197 final)*. Publications Office of the European Union.

Eysenbach, G. (2009). Infodemiology and infoveillance: Framework for an emerging set of public health informatics methods to analyze search, communication and publication behavior on the internet. *Journal of Medical Internet Research*, *11*(1), e11. DOI: 10.2196/jmir.1157 PMID: 19329408

Farahani, B., Firouzi, F., Chang, V., Badaroglu, M., Constant, N., & Mankodiya, K. (2018). Towards fog-driven IoT eHealth: Promises and challenges of IoT in medicine and healthcare. *Future Generation Computer Systems*, *78*, 659–676. DOI: 10.1016/j.future.2017.04.036

Floridi, L., Cowls, J., Beltrametti, M., Chatila, R., Chazerand, P., Dignum, V., Luetge, C., Madelin, R., Pagallo, U., Rossi, F., Schafer, B., Valcke, P., & Vayena, E. (2018). An ethical framework for a good AI society: Opportunities, risks, principles, and recommendations. *Minds and Machines*, *28*(4), 689–707. DOI: 10.1007/s11023-018-9482-5 PMID: 30930541

Foláyan, M. O., & Starr, J. R. (2024). Grand challenges and future oral epidemiology research. *Frontiers in Oral Health*, *4*, 1349252. DOI: 10.3389/froh.2023.1349252 PMID: 38268765

Friedman, C. P., Wong, A. K., & Blumenthal, D. (2010). Achieving a nationwide learning health system. *Science Translational Medicine*, *2*(57), 57cm29. Advance online publication. DOI: 10.1126/scitranslmed.3001456 PMID: 21068440

García-Cruz, I.. (2024). Wastewater surveillance for sugar consumption and caries risk assessment. *Environmental Science & Technology Letters*, *11*(3), 215–221.

Garza, M., Del Fiol, G., Tenenbaum, J., Walden, A., & Zozus, M. N. (2016). Evaluating common data models for use with a longitudinal community registry. *Journal of Biomedical Informatics*, *64*, 333–341. DOI: 10.1016/j.jbi.2016.10.016 PMID: 27989817

Gualtero, D. F., Contreras, A., Lafaurie, G. I., Castillo, D. M., Zúñiga-Rincón, L., Trujillo, T. G., & Blanco, S. D. (2023). Oral microbiome mediated inflammation, a potential inductor of vascular diseases: A comprehensive review. *Frontiers in Cardiovascular Medicine*, *10*, 1250263. DOI: 10.3389/fcvm.2023.1250263 PMID: 37711554

Gummin, D. D., Mowry, J. B., Beuhler, M. C., Spyker, D. A., Rivers, L. J., Feldman, R., Brown, K., Pham, N. P. T., Bronstein, A. C., & DesLauriers, C. (2023). 2022 Annual report of the national poison data system®(NPDS) from America's Poison Centers®: 40th annual report. *Clinical Toxicology : The Official Journal of the American Academy of Clinical Toxicology and European Association of Poisons Centres and Clinical Toxicologists*, *61*(10), 717–939. DOI: 10.1080/15563650.2023.2268981 PMID: 38084513

Hajishengallis, G. (2022). Interconnection of periodontal disease and comorbidities: Evidence, mechanisms, and implications. *Periodontology 2000*, *89*(1), 9–18. DOI: 10.1111/prd.12430 PMID: 35244969

Henning, K. J. (2004). Overview of syndromic surveillance: What is syndromic surveillance? MMWR Supplements, 53, 5-11.

Joda, T., & Spallek, H. (2023). Editorial: Precision dentistry and ehealth in oral healthcare. *Frontiers in Oral Health*, *4*, 1155166. DOI: 10.3389/froh.2023.1155166 PMID: 36960387

Johnson, P.. (2025). Metagenomic detection of oral pathogens in municipal wastewater: A feasibility study. *The Science of the Total Environment*, *850*, 157962.

Kahn, M. G., Callahan, T. J., Barnard, J., Bauck, A. E., Brown, J., Davidson, B. N., & Zozus, M. N. (2016). A harmonized data quality assessment terminology and framework for the secondary use of electronic health record data. *EGEMS (Washington, DC)*, *4*(1), 1244. DOI: 10.13063/2327-9214.1244 PMID: 27713905

Kassebaum, N. J., Smith, A. G. C., Bernabe, E., Fleming, T. D., Reynolds, A. E., Vos, T., & Marcenes, W. (2017). Global, regional, and national prevalence, incidence, and disability-adjusted life years for oral conditions for 195 countries, 1990-2015: A systematic analysis for the Global Burden of Diseases, Injuries, and Risk Factors. *Journal of Dental Research*, *96*(4), 380–387. DOI: 10.1177/0022034517693566 PMID: 28792274

Kaye, J., Whitley, E. A., Lund, D., Morrison, M., Teare, H., & Melham, K. (2015). Dynamic consent: A patient interface for twenty-first century research networks. *European Journal of Human Genetics : EJHG*, *23*(2), 141–146. DOI: 10.1038/ejhg.2014.71 PMID: 24801761

Khoury, M. J., Iademarco, M. F., & Riley, W. T. (2016). Precision public health for the era of precision medicine. *American Journal of Preventive Medicine*, *50*(3), 398–401. DOI: 10.1016/j.amepre.2015.08.031 PMID: 26547538

Kruse, C. S., Goswamy, R., Raval, Y. J., & Basha, S. (2016). Challenges and opportunities of big data in health care: A systematic review. *JMIR Medical Informatics*, *4*(4), e5359. DOI: 10.2196/medinform.5359 PMID: 27872036

Lazer, D., Kennedy, R., King, G., & Vespignani, A. (2014). The parable of Google Flu: Traps in big data analysis. *Science*, *343*(6176), 1203–1205. DOI: 10.1126/science.1248506 PMID: 24626916

Ledger, D., & McCaffrey, D. (2014). Inside wearables: How the science of human behavior change offers the secret to long-term engagement. *Endeavour Partners*, *200*(93), 1–17.

Lee, J. H., Kim, D. H., Jeong, S. N., & Choi, S. H. (2018). Detection and diagnosis of dental caries using a deep learning-based convolutional neural network algorithm. *Journal of Dentistry*, *77*, 106–111. DOI: 10.1016/j.jdent.2018.07.015 PMID: 30056118

Lee, J. H., Kim, Y. T., & Lee, J. B. (2024). Identification of dental implant systems from low-quality and distorted dental radiographs using AI trained on a large multicenter dataset. *Scientific Reports*, *14*(1), 12606. DOI: 10.1038/s41598-024-63422-z PMID: 38824187

Listl, S., Galloway, J., Mossey, P. A., & Marcenes, W. (2015). Global economic impact of dental diseases. *Journal of Dental Research*, *94*(10), 1355–1361. DOI: 10.1177/0022034515602879 PMID: 26318590

Maiti, N., Chawla, R., Toure, B., Agrawal, P., & Abba, S. H. (2025, November). Federated Learning for Collaborative Dental Diagnosis Across Hospitals Without Compromising Privacy. In *2025 Tenth International Conference on Science Technology Engineering and Mathematics (ICONSTEM)* (pp. 1-8). IEEE. DOI: 10.1109/ICONSTEM65670.2025.11374623

Mandl, K. D., Gottlieb, D., & Ellis, A. (2020). SMART on FHIR: A standards-based, interoperable apps platform for electronic health records. *Journal of the American Medical Informatics Association : JAMIA*, *23*(5), 899–908. DOI: 10.1093/jamia/ocv189 PMID: 26911829

Meskó, B., Drobni, Z., Benyei, E., Gergely, B., & Gyorffy, Z. (2017). Digital health is a cultural transformation of traditional healthcare. *mHealth*, *3*, 38. DOI: 10.21037/mhealth.2017.08.07 PMID: 29184890

Mittelstadt, B. D., & Floridi, L. (2016). The ethics of big data: Current and foreseeable issues in biomedical contexts. *Science and Engineering Ethics*, *22*(2), 303–341. DOI: 10.1007/s11948-015-9652-2 PMID: 26002496

Naicker, S., Plange-Rhule, J., Tutt, R. C., & Eastwood, J. B. (2009). Shortage of healthcare workers in developing countries: Africa. Ethnicity & Disease, 19(1 Suppl 1), S1-60-4.

Narayanan, A., & Shmatikoff, V. (2008). Robust de-anonymization of large sparse datasets. *2008 IEEE Symposium on Security and Privacy*, 111-125. https://doi.org/ DOI: 10.1109/SP.2008.33

Nuzzo, R. (2020). How participatory approaches can make epidemiology more equitable and ethical. *Nature Medicine*, *26*(11), 1669–1672. DOI: 10.1038/s41591-020-1145-1

Obermeyer, Z., Powers, B., Vogeli, C., & Mullainathan, S. (2019). Dissecting racial bias in an algorithm used to manage the health of populations. *Science*, *366*(6464), 447–453. DOI: 10.1126/science.aax2342 PMID: 31649194

Offenbacher, S., Katz, V., Fertik, G., Collins, J., Boyd, D., Maynor, G., McKaig, R., & Beck, J. (1996). Periodontal infection as a possible risk factor for preterm low birth weight. *Journal of Periodontology*, *67*(10, Suppl), 1103–1113. DOI: 10.1902/jop.1996.67.10.1103

Patel, V. A., Bhattacharya, P., Tanwar, S., Gupta, R., Sharma, G., Bokoro, P. N., & Sharma, R. (2022). Adoption of federated learning for healthcare informatics: Emerging applications and future directions. *IEEE Access : Practical Innovations, Open Solutions*, *10*, 90792–90826. DOI: 10.1109/ACCESS.2022.3201876

Paul, M. J., & Dredze, M. (2011). You are what you tweet: Analyzing Twitter for public health. *Proceedings of the Fifth International AAAI Conference on Weblogs and Social Media*, 265-272.

Prainsack, B., & Buyx, A. (2017). *Solidarity in biomedicine and beyond*. Cambridge University Press. DOI: 10.1017/9781139696593

Raghupathi, W., & Raghupathi, V. (2014). Big data analytics in healthcare: Promise and potential. *Health Information Science and Systems*, *2*(1), 1–10. DOI: 10.1186/2047-2501-2-3 PMID: 25825667

Rajkomar, A., Hardt, M., Howell, M. D., Corrado, G., & Chin, M. H. (2018). Ensuring fairness in machine learning to advance health equity. *Annals of Internal Medicine*, *169*(12), 866–872. DOI: 10.7326/M18-1990 PMID: 30508424

Redd, T. K., Campbell, J. P., Brown, J. M., Kim, S. J., Ostmo, S., Chan, R. V. P., & Kalpathy-Cramer, J. (2021). Prediction of referral-warranted retinopathy of prematurity using a deep learning model trained on wide-field retinal images. *Nature Communications*, *12*(1), 1–11. PMID: 33397941

Rieke, N., Hancox, J., Li, W., Milletari, F., Roth, H. R., Albarqouni, S., Bakas, S., Galtier, M. N., Landman, B. A., Maier-Hein, K., Ourselin, S., Sheller, M., Summers, R. M., Trask, A., Xu, D., Baust, M., & Cardoso, M. J. (2020). The future of digital health with federated learning. npj. *Digital Medicine*, *3*(1), 1–7. DOI: 10.1038/s41746-020-00323-1 PMID: 33015372

Romero-Laorden, J. I., Lorenzo, F., Solis, J. H., & Lopez-Berges, M. (2022). Integration of dental and medical electronic health records: A systematic review of the evidence and challenges. *The Journal of the American Dental Association*, *153*(8), 741–753.

Rydén, L., Buhlin, K., Ekstrand, E., de Faire, U., Gustafsson, A., Holmer, J., Kjellström, B., Lindahl, B., Norhammar, A., Nygren, Å., Näsman, P., Rathnayake, N., Svenungsson, E., & Klinge, B. (2016). Periodontitis increases the risk of a first myocardial infarction: A report from the PAROKRANK study. *Circulation*, *133*(6), 576–583. DOI: 10.1161/CIRCULATIONAHA.115.020324 PMID: 26762521

Sahyoun, N. R., Krall, E., & Russell, R. M. (2003). Poor dentition in community-dwelling elderly was associated with malnutrition but not with a specific nutritional deficiency. *The American Journal of Clinical Nutrition*, *77*(2), 411–416. PMID: 12540402

Salathe, M., Bengtsson, L., Bodnar, T. J., Brewer, D. D., Brownstein, J. S., Buckee, C., Campbell, E. M., Cattuto, C., Khandelwal, S., Mabry, P. L., & Vespignani, A. (2012). Digital epidemiology. *PLoS Computational Biology*, *8*(7), e1002616. DOI: 10.1371/journal.pcbi.1002616 PMID: 22844241

Sandlund, M., Huss, L., & Theorell-Haglow, J. (2021). Nordic register-based research in dentistry: A systematic review of study designs and applications. *Acta Odontologica Scandinavica*, *79*(1), 1–10. PMID: 32401086

Sanz, M., Marco del Castillo, A., Jepsen, S., Gonzalez-Juanatey, J. R., D'Aiuto, F., Bouchard, P., Chapple, I., Dietrich, T., Gotsman, I., Graziani, F., Herrera, D., Loos, B., Madianos, P., Michel, J.-B., Perel, P., Pieske, B., Shapira, L., Shechter, M., Tonetti, M., & Wimmer, G. (2020). Periodontitis and cardiovascular diseases: Consensus report. *Journal of Clinical Periodontology*, *47*(3), 268–288. DOI: 10.1111/jcpe.13189 PMID: 32011025

Schatz, M. C. (2015). Biological data sciences in genome research. *Genome Research, 25*(10), 1417–1422. DOI: 10.1101/gr.191684.115 PMID: 26430150

Scheerman, J. F. M., van Loveren, C., van Meijel, B., Dusseldorp, E., Wartewig, E., Verrips, G. H. W., & van Empelen, P. (2018). Psychosocial correlates of oral hygiene behaviour in people aged 9-19: A systematic review with meta-analysis. *Community Dentistry and Oral Epidemiology, 46*(1), 43–55. DOI: 10.1111/cdoe.12325

Schmidt, A.. (2023). Community-level periodontal disease monitoring using wastewater-based epidemiology. *Environmental Research, 220*, 115164.

Simpson, A.. (2025). Wastewater-based epidemiology: Methodological considerations for pathogen surveillance. *Current Opinion in Environmental Science & Health, 33*, 100432.

Stankevic, E., Bjørnland, T., Kunzmann, A. T., Jansonius, N. M., & Magnusson, P. K. E. (2024). Genome-wide association study identifies host genetic variants influencing oral microbiota diversity and metabolic health. *Scientific Reports, 14*(1), 14738. DOI: 10.1038/s41598-024-65538-8 PMID: 38926497

Steinsbekk, K. S., Kare Myskja, B., & Solberg, B. (2013). Broad consent versus dynamic consent in biobank research: Is passive participation an ethical problem? *European Journal of Human Genetics : EJHG, 21*(9), 897–902. DOI: 10.1038/ejhg.2012.282 PMID: 23299918

Tran, N. H., Zhang, X., Li, M., & Shan, B. (2021). Deep learning in cancer diagnosis, prognosis and treatment selection. *Genome Medicine, 13*(1), 152. DOI: 10.1186/s13073-021-00968-x PMID: 34579788

Unkel, S., Farrington, C. P., Garthwaite, P. H., Robertson, C., & Andrews, N. (2012). Statistical methods for the prospective detection of infectious disease outbreaks: A review. *Journal of the Royal Statistical Society. Series A, (Statistics in Society), 175*(1), 49–82. DOI: 10.1111/j.1467-985X.2011.00714.x

World Health Organization. (2022). *Global oral health status report: Towards universal health coverage for oral health by 2030*. World Health Organization. https://www.who.int/publications/i/item/9789240061484

Yarlagadda, S. K., Samavati, N., Ghorbanifarajzadeh, M., Levinta, V., Sojoudi, A., Inam, W., & Dolan, T. A. (2025). Development and validation of an AI-enabled oral score using large-scale dental data. *Scientific Reports, 15*(1), 20398. DOI: 10.1038/s41598-025-07484-7 PMID: 40593131

Zimmerman, B., Tsoi, S., Khosrowpour, B., & Ghazali, M. (2022). The state of dental electronic health records and opportunities for FHIR integration. *Journal of the American Medical Informatics Association : JAMIA*, *29*(4), 703–710. DOI: 10.1093/jamia/ocab282

Chapter 6
The EpiDentomic Paradigm:
Reimagining Epidemiology at the Oral Systemic Digital Interface

L. B. Muralidhar
http://orcid.org/0000-0003-3453-613X
Jain (Deemed to be) University, India

ABSTRACT

Contemporary epidemiology is increasingly challenged by multimorbidity, population ageing, and the rapid expansion of digital health infrastructures, yet oral health remains marginalised within mainstream population health frameworks. This book chapter proposes EpiDentomics as a novel integrative paradigm that reimagines epidemiology at the oral–systemic–digital interface. Drawing on classical and systems epidemiology, digital epidemiology, artificial intelligence, and global health policy. It critically engages with methodological, ethical, and governance debates, including data interoperability, causal inference, and equity concerns. An integrative Oral Systemic Digital Epidemiology Nexus framework is advanced to connect biology, behaviour, environment, and data across clinical, population, and policy levels. By bridging dentistry, public health, and digital intelligence, the chapter positions EpiDentomics as a foundation for precision population health, inclusive surveillance systems, and future-oriented epidemiological research and practice.

DOI: 10.4018/979-8-3373-8402-3.ch006

INTRODUCTION: WHY EPIDEMIOLOGY NEEDS AN EPIDENTOMIC TURN

EpiDentomics brings the disciplines of oral, systemic, and digital epidemiology together to redefine oral health by placing it in the population-health landscape. It is based on three pillars: precision public health, causal inference, and complex systems thinking, and it explores the interconnections of biological processes, social gradients, behaviors, and data infrastructures in their joint contributions to risk and policy relevance (Khoury et al., 2016; Pearl et al., 2016; Rutter et al., 2017). This chapter critically reviews the concept of oral-health marginalization, reviews methodological progress in integrated data, and outlines the theoretical and policy significance of the paradigm. Therefore, EpiDentomics can be used as an analytical tool and for surveillance, research, and governance to support oral health priorities (World Health Organization, 2022).

EpiDentomics is not equal to, but builds on, precision public health, digital epidemiology, precision dentistry, oral systems medicine, learning health systems or population health informatics. Precision public health is largely about leveraging increasingly detailed information at finer resolution to better target, time, and assess population-level interventions (Khoury et al., 2016; Kearns et al., 2021). Digital epidemiology enhances the sources of observations of population health, their speed, and their reach or scale by leveraging electronic records, online information environments, sensors, and other digitally generated traces (Eysenbach, 2009; Salathé, 2018). The focus of precision dentistry is usually on individual diagnosis, risk prediction, prognosis, and choice of treatment, while oral systems medicine focuses on the interdependent nature of oral and systemic health. Learning health systems are concerned with continual improvement—they transform the routine collection of clinical data into evidence and then use that evidence to feed into health care.

EpiDentomics, however, differs from prevailing approaches, as shown in Table 1, because it considers the oral–systemic–digital relationship the primary epidemiological subject for analysis. It's a combination of four requirements that are not usually formalized together – the biological pathways are considered in addition to social, environmental, commercial, and health-system determinants; the oral conditions are analyzed as components and indicators of the broader processes of population health, not as discrete outcomes; digital infrastructures are discussed not only as tools for collecting information, but also as entities that shape measurement, inclusion, classification, and intervention; and the predictive findings are assessed using causal, equity, transportability, and governance criteria before being translated to policy or clinical action.

The value of EpiDentomics lies not in its being an overlooked aspect of oral–systemic relations or in digital technology being a novel epidemiology, but in the ways it can enhance both. It aims to define how oral-health evidence, systemic outcomes, structural determinants, clinical processes, and digital data architectures can be studied within a single multilevel causal and implementation framework. This also defines the edge of the investigation as EpiDentomic if it is based solely on dental data, AI, or precision targeting. It should explicitly link oral and systemic health determinants to observed health outcomes to recognize the social and institutional production of this data and to assess the potential of the resulting knowledge to inform equitable and accountable intervention.

These five related gaps are subsequently left in the literature. First, conventional oral epidemiology has established the burden and inequality, but in many instances, it has been separated from general health surveillance within an institutional setting. Second, the biological plausibility and consistent relationships found in oral–systemic research have been established, but residual confounding, reverse causation, and variability in case definitions and clinical samples limit causal inference. Third, digital epidemiology and dental AI increase observability and predictability but often fail to theorize about different types of use and need. Fourth, precision approaches enhance stratification but might also obscure risks arising from commercial, social, financial, and geographic factors. Fifth, routine data can be used to generate feedback on care, but people without access to dental services could be left out of the learning cycle. EpiDentomics addresses these gaps in a unique way by integrating causal explanation, measurement critique, multilevel determinants, digital infrastructures, implementation pathways, and governance into a single oral–systemic population-health framework.

Table 1. Distinguishing EpiDentomics from Related Frameworks

Framework	Primary object	Main unit of analysis	Typical data or methods	Primary objective	Limitation addressed by EpiDentomics
Traditional oral epidemiology	Distribution and determinants of oral diseases	Individuals and populations	Surveys, clinical indices, administrative data	Measure burden, risk factors, and inequalities	Often treats oral outcomes separately from systemic disease and digital infrastructure.
Oral systems medicine	Biological relationships between oral and systemic conditions	Patient and biological system	Biomarkers, clinical studies, and mechanistic research	Explain oral–systemic biological interdependence	May under-specify population heterogeneity, social causation, and data governance
Precision dentistry	Individual diagnosis, prognosis, and treatment	Individual patient	Genomics, imaging, biomarkers, predictive models	Personalize dental prevention and treatment	May individualize structurally produced risk and emphasize prediction over population causation
Digital epidemiology	Digitally generated population-health signals	Digital populations and data streams	EHRs, sensors, platforms, online data	Improve the timeliness and scale of surveillance	Does not necessarily center oral health or integrate oral–systemic mechanisms
Precision public health	Stratified population intervention	Population subgroups	Geospatial, genomic, and risk-stratification tools	Target interventions more accurately	It may not specify how oral health, dental care, and dental data should be integrated.
Learning health systems	Continuous evidence-to-practice cycle	Healthcare organization or network	Routine clinical data, feedback systems	Improve care through continuous learning	Often depends on clinically observed populations and may not capture unrecorded oral health needs.

continued on following page

Table 1. Continued

Framework	Primary object	Main unit of analysis	Typical data or methods	Primary objective	Limitation addressed by EpiDentomics
Population health informatics	Information infrastructure for population-health management	Health systems and populations	Linked records, dashboards, and decision support	Support surveillance and management	May remain technically oriented without an explicit oral–systemic causal theory
EpiDentomics	Oral–systemic population-health processes as observed and acted upon through digital infrastructures	Individuals, populations, places, institutions, and data systems	Multilevel data linkage, causal inference, spatial analysis, AI, implementation evaluation	Explain and intervene in oral–systemic inequalities through causally valid, equitable and governed population intelligence	Integrates oral–systemic biology, structural determinants, digital measurement, causal reasoning and policy feedback in one framework

The chapter is designed for researchers, postgraduate students, dental public health professionals, epidemiologists, health informaticians, health system leaders, and health policymakers who are interested in and concerned with how oral health evidence can be linked to systems health surveillance, digital infrastructures, causal analysis, and equitable implementation.

CONCEPTUAL FOUNDATIONS OF EPIDENTOMICS: INTEGRATING DISCIPLINARY SILOS

EpiDentomics involves not only a new focus for oral health research on the multiple intellectual traditions of epidemiology, but also a new integration of the traditions with the complexity of the modern world, digitization, and the oral-systemic link. The oral-systemic health continuum is a central theme in this extension; it provides biological plausibility and a leverage point for integration. The role of dysbiosis and immunosuppression in local microenvironments and the subsequent systemic inflammatory consequences has been a useful model for illustrating pathways underlying the epidemiological associations of periodontitis that go beyond mere mechanisms (Hajishengallis, 2015; Kinane et al., 2017).

There are bidirectional and syndemic relationships; for example, there is clinical and consensus evidence indicating that diabetes and cardiovascular disease have a relationship, and that periodontal conditions are related to diabetes and cardiovascular disease; population heterogeneity needs to be recognized, and causal interpretations made with caution (Chapple et al., 2013; Sanz et al., 2020). The next is digital epidemiology and population intelligence, which further deepens and expands observation, linkage, and action, based on 'infodemiology', electronic health records, and multi-institutional repositories, provided that interoperability, governance, and analytic validity are appropriately addressed (Eysenbach, 2009; Kalenderian et al., 2013).

Machine learning has revolutionized dental diagnosis for dentists and facilitated risk stratification, but it remains vulnerable to machine learning biases, lack of transparency, and inequitable use of models, thus necessitating explainable and ethical machine learning models (Brall et al., 2019; Schwendicke et al., 2021). Combining all these factors, EpiDentomics proposes that oral health is an early indicator of systemic dysregulation and an amplifier of the chronic disease burden, both of which depend on context, access, and social patterning. This non-deterministic framing is difficult to tackle with a single method and calls for a hybrid approach to causal inference, systems thinking, and digital population intelligence for value-oriented public health that is sensitive to equity (Listl et al., 2019; Kearns et al., 2021; World Health Organization, 2021).

THE ORAL SYSTEMIC DISEASE INTERFACE: EVIDENCE, MECHANISMS, AND DEBATES

A few of the many well-studied relationships include the bidirectional relationship between periodontal disease and diabetes. Consensus reports, based on the synthesis of clinical, epidemiological, and mechanistic evidence, suggest that poor glycaemic control is associated with increased periodontal inflammation, and periodontal infection is associated with worsening insulin resistance and metabolic control (Chapple et al., 2013; Nazir, 2017).

This interaction could be described as an example of a syndemic relationship, meaning that there is an increased risk of a biological susceptibility compounded by a shared behavioral and social risk factor, in this instance, cigarette smoking, diet, and limited access to preventive services. Cardiovascular disease is the second biggest area of research. An association between periodontitis and atherosclerotic events, such as myocardial infarction and stroke, has been reported in large observational studies and expert consensus documents, although the magnitude of the association varies by population and study design (Linden et al., 2013; Sanz et al., 2020). Maternal periodontal disease also has been correlated with low birth weight and preterm birth. But there is systematic review evidence suggesting heterogeneity and contextual effects (baseline risk, access to health services, and quality of measurement) (Ide & Papapanou, 2013).

These associations have been greatly supported by biological plausibility in the past decade. The oral microbiome is recognized as a dynamic ecological community, and inflamed periodontal tissues are recognized as potential sources of microbial products and inflammatory mediators that can enter the circulation, as revealed by mechanistic studies. Pathogenic bacteria and inflammatory mediators can enter the bloodstream from the oral cavity during periodontal dysbiosis, leading to the activation of endothelial dysfunction, inflammatory responses, and metabolic dysfunction (Hajishengallis, 2015; Kinane et al., 2017). It has been proposed that immune dysregulation, or exaggerated or maladaptive immune host responses, is a unifying pathway between host responses to periodontal inflammation and systemic sequelae. Understands how these responses relate to metabolism and circulation in the body, and explains how these metabolic and vascular processes generate epidemiological patterns of diabetes and cardiovascular disease (CVD) incidence and mortality (Sanz et al., 2020). Importantly, these pathways do not work independently of one another but are shaped by and linked to the interplay among psychosocial stress, environmental exposures, and lifetime disadvantage, thus reinforcing the biopsychosocial models of disease causation (Diez Roux, 2012; Marmot, 2017).

In EpiDentomics, the oral–systemic evidence is not considered to be proof of a universal causal relationship. Rather than that, the longevity of associations and the fact that this evidence is incomplete and/or there is some residual confounding, variability in measures, and population variability indicate a need for a more explicit analytical framework. There are four different possible explanations that need to be distinguished in order to justify EpiDentomics, namely a direct effect of an oral condition on a systemic outcome, reverse causation from a systemic disease to oral deterioration, common causation through behavioral or structural determinants, and selection (or measurement) processes triggered by access to healthcare and to clinical documentation. All are questions that can be answered by existing oral epidemiology. But these questions are not typically incorporated into a single design for digital data provenance, algorithmic classification, health system feedback, and equity impacts. EpiDentomics does not claim to establish a causal relationship between debated oral–systemic associations, but rather is intended to organize this integration.

GLOBAL BURDEN AND INEQUALITIES IN ORAL SYSTEMIC DISEASES: A POPULATION-LEVEL PERSPECTIVE

The evidence from GBD indicates that most oral diseases remain common and that progress towards an epidemiological transition has been minimal since 1990 (Bernabe et al., 2020; Kassebaum et al., 2017). This persistence is important within

EpiDentomics, since oral-systemic associations are not uncommon, but rather common population-wide exposures, with the exception of very rare clinical associations (Backstrom et al., 2015). Given their high prevalence, the potential public-health significance of causal contributions to cardiometabolic, vascular, or inflammatory outcomes (Chapple et al., 2013; Lamster, 2022; Sanz et al., 2020) is high. Dental coverage is not part of broad-based public coverage, meaning that out-of-pocket spending is a key measure of risk that should be disaggregated by year and by regional and/or income group.

But the populations most affected, both orally and systemically, are the ones least reached by integrated care and thus face a structural disparity between knowledge and implementation of biomedical care, with the greatest inequity (Marmot, 2017; Diez Roux, 2012). From a methodological point of view, the observed associations could be due to shared risk factors, residual confounding, or different disease definitions (Baelum & Lopez, 2013; Faggion et al., 2017). The policy question is then which interventions (what counterfactuals) change systemic outcomes for which people and under what circumstances (Hernan & Robins, 2020; Pearl et al., 2016). This changes the way that oral disease is perceived as being part of multimorbidity and inequality.

DIGITAL TRANSFORMATION OF EPIDEMIOLOGY: FROM SURVEILLANCE TO PREDICTION

Digital transformation in epidemiology involves paradigm shifts in the standards for evidence, visibility of the population, and authority within surveillance and intervention. In classical systems, inferences are drawn from retrospective surveys, sentinel sites, or administrative reports, whereas digital infrastructure enables continuous, high-dimensional inference but also raises issues of validity, accountability, and equity (Salathé, 2018; Brall et al., 2019). The evidence base incorporates a variety of sources, including electronic health records, practice systems, claims, repositories, imaging archives, wearables, and Internet of Things (IoT) devices, all with varying structures, temporal resolution, and population coverage. Observational research, quality monitoring, learning health systems (Kalenderian et al, 2013), and other types of research rely on cross-institutional dental data, which platforms like BigMouth demonstrate is possible.

These benefits are, however, dependent on interoperability, standardization and governance – which is uneven and can foster distinctions between dental and medical data systems (Mertz et al., 2017). AI takes this transformation further through diagnostic, predictive, and decision-support tools, such as imaging and orthodontic analysis (Schwendicke et al., 2019; Khanagar et al., 2021; Wirtz et al., 2023). This change is beneficial to precision public health efforts, however, accuracy does not imply causation. Thus, digital epidemiology should view models as tools for decision-making with respect to their causal interpretation, representativeness, and attention to upstream structural determinants (Khoury et al., 2016; Hernán & Robins, 2020).

ARTIFICIAL INTELLIGENCE IN EPIDENTOMIC INTELLIGENCE: OPPORTUNITIES AND LIMITATIONS

While machine learning has many potential applications in precision public health, EpiDentomics applications require more than predictive accuracy (Khoury et al., 2016; Kearns et al., 2021). Reviews show that the use of reviews to diagnose and treat caries and to make periodontal prognoses has expanded, as well as in the interpretation of images and planning of treatment, both using clinical, behavioral, imaging, and sociodemographic data with limited evidence of external validity and population benefit (Khanagar et al., 2021; Wirtz et al., 2023; Nassar et al., 2024). In dental radiology, deep learning has shown promising results in detecting and identifying lesions and landmarks. Transfer is limited to routine care. However, due to the homogeneous nature of the training data and controlled acquisition setting, devices, protocols, operators, comorbidities, and image quality vary (Schwendicke et al., 2019; Ni et al., 2022).

Therefore, interpretability needs to be coupled with external validation, calibration, distribution-shift testing, and independent audit, not just visualization (Schwendicke et al., 2021). Causal reasoning is always important as advanced models can yield accurate but policy-inaccurate connections (Faggion et al., 2017; Hernan & Robins, 2020). Stewardship, accountability, and equity-focused governance are needed in tandem with continuous monitoring to achieve generalisability, as this is a socio-technical process besides being statistical (Ahmed et al., 2021; AlHumaid et al., 2020; Brall et al., 2019).

The model of an evaluation pathway ought to be separable into technical, clinical, implementation, and population impact. The technical assessment should report discrimination, calibration in the large, calibration slope, clinically meaningful decision thresholds, uncertainty, and failure patterns. Modeling is an especially critical part of the process, since a model might identify the correct rank of individuals but yield an incorrect absolute risk estimate, which may result in inappropriate referrals or resource allocation. Validation of the evaluation should be conducted at external, geographic, demographic, institutional, and temporal levels, in addition to internal random splits.

The algorithmic auditing should take place prior to deployment and at predetermined time points after deployment. The following are intended areas for audit: Data provenance, intended use, excluded populations, missingness, subgroup performance, threshold effects, security, clinician override, patient complaints, evidence of data drift, and concept drift. The results of the audit should be subject to monitoring by an accountable, multidisciplinary body with the authority to adjust, limit, or remove the system. In addition, human–AI interaction, flow impact, safety and real-world clinical performance should be evaluated in early clinical studies, following the DECIDE-AI approach, rather than evaluating accuracy in a retrospective fashion.

Institutions might be able to work together without creating a central repository of all person-level data through other privacy-preserving approaches, such as federated learning. However, federated analysis can't guarantee that re-identification, model leakage, institutional bias, or differences in data-generating processes will not occur. Yet data governance agreements, local validation and monitoring of institutional contributions and performance remain required, along with secure aggregation and, when appropriate, differential privacy.

In addition, foundation and generative models pose further challenges due to the difficulty of examining their training data, representations, and behavior, as well as their downstream applications. They are not intended to be a stand-alone diagnostic or policy decision maker in oral-health applications. They produce outputs that need to be validated according to the task, traced back to their sources, checked by humans, communicated with uncertainty, and limited in secondary use. WHO recommendations also emphasize autonomy, safety, transparency, accountability, inclusiveness, equity, responsiveness and sustainability as key principles of governance for health-AI.

The regulatory status of a system needs to be determined by what the system does and its risk, and not by how it is described on the market. Even if not offered as a diagnostic instrument, an EpiDentomic system could have material consequences for screening, referral, insurance, or public resource allocation. Governance should therefore include evidence before deployment, tracking of evidence after deployment, evidence for incidents, change control, recording of evidence of changes to the model, human accountability, and mechanisms to allow those potentially affected to challenge consequences of classifications.

SPATIOTEMPORAL AND ENVIRONMENTAL EPIDEMIOLOGY: MAPPING RISK IN CONTEXT

However, the results of GIS-based clustering analyses were always consistent, and it was found that the burden of oral disease was not randomly distributed but concentrated at known 'hotspots', where the various interacting elements of socioeconomic deprivation, commercial exposures, and poor access to services combined. The analysis of the urban GIS reveals evident spatial trends in dental caries gradients that are similar to deprivation at the neighborhood level, indicating that place structure shapes oral morbidity in ways not explained by individuals' characteristics (Matsuo et al., 2021). The present results support the multilevel findings that neighborhood income has a "contextual" effect on caries, in addition to the effect of individual SES, and illustrate the value of neighborhood context not only in influencing individual exposure patterns but also in influencing individual response capacity (Celeste et al., 2011).

Of particular importance, spatial clustering is analytical, generative, and descriptive – it helps strengthen and increase the plausibility of a geographically patterned oral-systemic comorbidity (Lamster, 2022; Peres et al., 2019). These are not biologic in nature but are rather related to environmental and occupational exposures, and are epidemiologically important. Based on the systematic review, occupational stress and environmental pollutants are shown to affect periodontal outcomes more than known behavioral risk factors, though the results are inconsistent and measurement methods often vary (Shrestha et al., 2022).

This is a methodological frontier in this context, where spatial information and artificial intelligence models are combined. Geocoded clinical data, deprivation indices, environmental exposures and service access can be fused together in multiple ways to enhance risk stratification and facilitate place-based prevention, in keeping with precision public health (Khoury et al., 2016; Kearns et al., 2021). Yet, beyond the potential for structural disadvantages, spatial proxies can be used as tools for inequity rather than equity and can reinforce inequity when not used with ethical safeguards (Brall et al., 2019; AlHumaid et al., 2020). Explainable AI is thus essential for identifying environmental conditions that can be changed, from proxies for institutionalized inequalities (Schwendicke et al., 2021). The operationalization of inequality is possible using spatiotemporal epidemiology, both as a measure of a geography of preventable risk in terms of micro-spatial heterogeneity and as a measure of lack of service availability, with EpiDentomics also aligned with upstream systems-based intervention strategies, rather than with individual behavior-focused approaches (Frieden, 2010; Watt et al., 2019).

TRANSLATIONAL AND PRECISION PUBLIC HEALTH APPLICATIONS: FROM INSIGHT TO INTERVENTION

The success of EpiDentomics is measured by its contributions to oral-systemic epidemiology and digital epidemiology, improving the state of the art in population health. Because oral diseases continue to be prevalent and they show social and geographical gradients, precision public health, which focuses on directing prevention at an individual level, is well-adapted to oral diseases (Khoury et al., 2016; Kassebaum et al., 2017; Bernabe et al., 2020; Peres et al., 2019). The key focus is on transforming analytic knowledge to ensure its application is equitable, while avoiding the risk that stratification tools are exploited by predominantly already-visible populations. A risk stratification approach can be used in dentistry to guide recall frequency, prevention, and referral, but it can be confusing when applied at the individual level rather than as part of a structural approach to disease production (Divaris, 2019; Riley et al., 2017). Therefore, in assessing risk, EpiDentomics takes a multi-level approach that includes biological susceptibility, clinical history, neighborhood deprivation, access to services, and behavioral conditions (Diezroux, 2012; Celeste et al., 2011).

If structural determinants are driving risk, then fluoridation is not the answer to targeting downstream, nor is sugar regulation, nor is tobacco control, nor is universal coverage, nor is primary care that's accessible (Frieden, 2010; Watt et al., 2019). Oral-systemic predictive prevention models and digital twins could aid in counterfactual assessment of oral-systemic trajectories, although the validity of these models relies on explicit causal assumptions, specified interventions, transparent model validation and model transportability (Faggion et al., 2017; Hernán & Robins, 2020; Pearl et al., 2016). Clinical decision support can help with improving imaging, diagnosis, referral, care coordination, and more. But for benefits to be realized, there needs to be interoperable records, integrated workflows, communicated uncertainty, accountability, ongoing funding, and monitoring of unequal uptake, benefits, and harms (Schwendicke et al., 2019, 2021; Mertz et al., 2017).

POLICY, GOVERNANCE, AND GLOBAL HEALTH PERSPECTIVES: INSTITUTIONALIZING THE EPIDENTOMIC PARADIGM

National exchange architectures need to include oral-health information and not create an independent information domain for dentistry to enable the implementation of digital health reform for EpiDentomics. Multiple longitudinal records of individuals are necessary for analyzing shared risk factors, multimorbidity, and temporality in oral-systemic pathways (Hernan & Robins, 2020; Pearl et al., 2016). Ayushman Bharat Digital Mission (ABDM) in India, the TEFCA in the USA, and the European Health Data Space provide examples of different infrastructures of identity, exchange, trust, primary use, and secondary research.

Their significance depends on the encoding of dental diagnoses, periodontal measures, tooth loss, imaging metadata, preventive attendance, treatment histories, and referral outcomes within interoperable standards and their integration with medical records. Otherwise, technologically advanced medical exchange systems could still allow the exclusion of the oral-health benefit. Such endeavors should, therefore, be viewed as facilitators rather than signifiers of integration. They need to be judged on their utility using the available dental data, the mapping of terminology, the interoperability of images, the coverage of providers, the patient's rights, and follow-up across sectors. Interoperability is also epistemological due to the influence of standards on the codability, comparability, and usability of concepts for causal inference (Faggion et al., 2017).

Some countries continue to use different diagnostic thresholds and different practices for recording diagnoses, making it difficult to compare them nationally and internationally, and making it challenging to transport the model or models (Baelum & Lopez, 2013; Divaris, 2019). There is also variation by setting: high-income settings may have vendors and workforces, lower-resource settings may have workforce coverage, reimbursement, coding standards, and routine dental data, but may not have vendors or workforces (Petersen, 2014). Therefore, to ensure effective integration of EpiDentomics, funding for preventive care, inclusion of core oral health indicators in the monitoring of non-communicable diseases, harmonization of data models and validation of measures, as well as ethical oversight of cross-domain analytics are needed (Frieden, 2010; Watt & Sheiham, 2012; Listl et al., 2019). It needs to communicate technically about connectivity into actionable, accountable initiatives. Interoperable infrastructure will thus be an essential tool, but not the solution, for equity-oriented public health governance (World Health Organization, 2022; Lamster, 2022).

ETHICAL, EQUITY, AND SOCIETAL IMPLICATIONS: WHO BENEFITS FROM EPIDENTOMICS

EpiDentomics brings together oral epidemiology, digital systems, big data, and AI, but must be seen as legitimate if the sharing of the benefits and burdens of population intelligence is equitable. Due to the high prevalence and social patterning of oral diseases, incomplete or biased data can lead to the creation of predictive systems that replicate gradients in oral disease such as caries, periodontal disease, and tooth loss (Peres et al., 2019; Bernabe et al., 2020; Bernabe & Marcenes, 2011; Celeste et al., 2011). But the ethical challenge is not just one of privacy; it is also one of justice as a public health concern and of how data-intensive dentistry fits into that (Marmot, 2017; Patrick et al., 2006). Another danger of technocratic modeling is the tendency to supplant the decisions of who caused what, what to value, and who is responsible for what. Apparent neutrality of risk scores can result in the risk score reflecting historical practice patterns rather than underlying disease (Baelum & Lopez, 2013; Faggion et al., 2017; Hernan & Robins, 2020; Pearl et al., 2016).

In addition to its technical faults, imaging also carries extra hazards, such as "overfitting" and "data drift," which can create a lack of performance in low-resource contexts and raise equity issues, rather than just technical problems, in this capacity (Schwendicke et al., 2019; Khanagar et al., 2021). As such, EpiDentomics must involve the participation of all stakeholders in the data collection process, and involve regular subgroup validation and calibration, established stewardship and audit mechanisms, and community engagement in challenging harmful classifications. It has six interrelated areas, namely: oral health, systemic health, structural determinants, clinical and behavioral factors, digital infrastructure, and governance. It also distinguishes between the causal process and the measurement process because the disease that is recorded is dependent on access, threshold diagnosis, coding, and linkage processes, and is not necessarily a reflection of the prevalence of the disease in the population.

Four assumptions are made: oral-systemic relations are heterogeneous; individual risk is socially nested; data infrastructures are non-neutral; and prediction is not enough without a specified intervention, a causal estimand, a target population, a pathway of implementation, and a governance structure. They prevent digital observation from being confused with epidemiological representation and/or causality. These principles relate analytical accuracy to responsible and equitable action.

These assumptions generate testable propositions:

Proposition 1: The association between oral conditions and systemic outcomes will vary across populations according to shared determinants, baseline risk, healthcare access, and measurement practices.

Proposition 2: Models integrating oral, systemic, social, and service-access information will improve risk characterization over oral-clinical data alone, but apparent improvement will not necessarily imply causal validity or equitable benefit.

Proposition 3: Differences in dental-service utilization and diagnostic coding will mediate or distort the relationship between underlying oral-health need and digitally observed disease.

Proposition 4: External validation across institutions and demographic subgroups will reveal performance and calibration differences that are obscured by internal validation.

Proposition 5: Linking risk stratification to preventive care, referral, and upstream resource allocation will generate greater population benefit than using prediction without an implementation pathway.

Proposition 6: Governance arrangements that include transparent documentation, subgroup auditing, community participation, and mechanisms for appeal will improve legitimacy and reduce the risk of discriminatory deployment.

These propositions make EpiDentomics empirically examinable. They allow the framework to be evaluated, modified, or rejected, rather than serving only as a broad metaphor for interdisciplinary integration.

AN INTEGRATIVE FRAMEWORK FOR EPIDENTOMICS: THE EPIDENTOMIC CAUSAL-MEASUREMENT-IMPLEMENTATION FRAMEWORK

Figure 1. The EpiDentomic Causal-Measurement-Implementation Framework

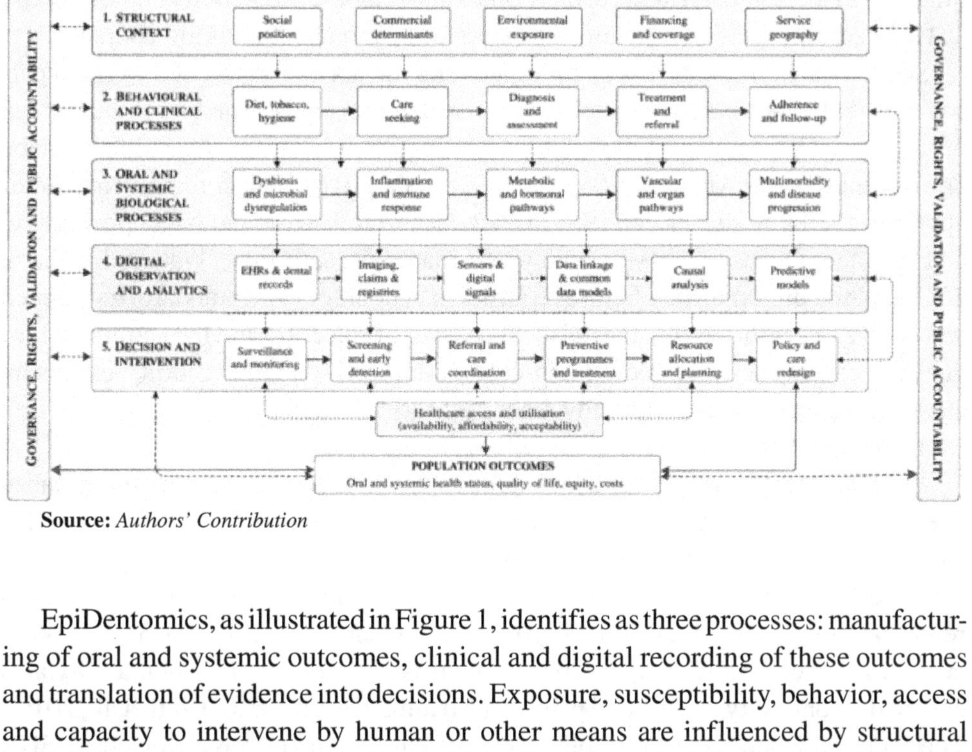

Source: *Authors' Contribution*

EpiDentomics, as illustrated in Figure 1, identifies as three processes: manufacturing of oral and systemic outcomes, clinical and digital recording of these outcomes and translation of evidence into decisions. Exposure, susceptibility, behavior, access and capacity to intervene by human or other means are influenced by structural conditions, and biological and clinical processes lead to disease. Outcomes are only visible as data when they are used in healthcare, are understood as conventions/diagnostic rules, coded, linked, and processed by algorithms. Later disease trends, services used and data available are then altered by analytical outputs, which affect screening, referral, financing, and resource allocation and policy. Governance, validation and rights are therefore throughout the process as other decisions may compound early mistakes.

Mechanistic pathways, population heterogeneity, structural determinants and digital infrastructures are all conceptually part of the causal interpretation as active components of synthetic epistemology, meaning EpiDentomics (Hajishengallis, 2015; Lamster, 2022; Marmot, 2017). Biological plausibility includes dysbiotic biofilms, immune dysfunction and chronic inflammation which are pertinent to cardiometabolic and inflammatory pathways (Hajishengallis, 2015; Kinane et al., 2017). But the framework is not biological reductionist as all the factors related to oral and systemic risk (diet, tobacco, hygiene, care seeking, economic structures and cultural norms) work together (Watt & Sheiham, 2012; Kranz et al., 2019). All aspects of clinical management are also a method of measurement: case definitions, imaging procedures, treatment choices and coding practices define the way in which illness is made an analyzable record (Baelum & Lopez, 2013; Schwendicke et al., 2019). Recorded profiles are thus a mixture of health and institution contact.

Social context is another way of broadening the definition of risk beyond a person's attributes. Attention to patterned oral-systemic inequities and what they reveal of why precision cannot be molecular stratification (Celeste et al., 2011; Bernabe & Marcenes, 2011; Marmot, 2017; Khoury et al., 2016). The common-risk-factor approach therefore makes connections between oral disease and NCD prevention, and maintains focus on power, policy and material conditions (Watt & Sheiham, 2012). While digital infrastructures transform encounters into standardized, linked and analyzable information, they also add a layer of selection and measurement bias due to inconsistencies in coding and case definitions—interoperability is thus an epidemiological capacity, not only a connectivity (Kalenderian et al., 2013; Mertz et al., 2017).

Feedback occurs as clinical data become the basis for surveillance, surveillance goes into policy, and policy shifts access, care, data and disease (Frieden, 2010; Rutter et al., 2017). AI shortens this cycle, but needs to be tested for transportability, assessed for fairness, and managed with accountability due to the issue of underrepresentation and the lack of data provenance which impacts performance (Wirtz et al., 2023; Schwendicke et al., 2020). The trust, consent, and accountability also ensure the continuity of data and privacy (AlHumaid et al., 2020; Brall et al., 2019). The framework needs to be flexible across resource contexts, relying on dense EHR systems where possible, and, where they do not, on surveys and sentinel systems, mobile tools, and/or integration within primary care (Petersen, 2014; World Health Organization, 2022). Theoretically it seeks to disaggregate the processes of causation, measurement, and incentives for the system, while its agenda on the applied side is to ensure interoperable standards, fair and transparent validation of AI, and interventions that bridge the gap between surveillance and prevention and redesigning care.

This co-optimization helps to place oral health in the suite of NCD and universal coverage strategies, and changes digital observation into actionable, accountable, and equitable population action (Lamster & Meyerowitz, 2021).

An EpiDentomic system in operation can be broken down into six phases: question specification, data acquisition, harmonization and linkage, causal or predictive analysis, implementation and continuous evaluation. The process starts off with a decision about a population health need, not a data set. This can be done when adults with diabetes are identified who would benefit from a periodontal examination; when the location of preventive dental care services can be assessed; and to study the effectiveness of integrated dental–medical referral in the reduction of avoidable disease burden.

A minimum dataset should contain five variable groups:

1. **Oral-health variables:** caries status, periodontal measures or validated case classification, tooth loss, oral pain, functional limitation, oral cancer indicators, preventive attendance, treatment history, and date of assessment.
2. **Systemic-health variables:** diabetes diagnosis and glycaemic indicators, cardiovascular diagnoses and risk factors, pregnancy status and outcomes where relevant, inflammatory comorbidities, prescribed medication, body mass index, tobacco exposure, and relevant laboratory measures.
3. **Social and environmental variables:** age, sex or gender where analytically justified, socioeconomic position, insurance or coverage status, geographical location at an appropriately privacy-protective level, service accessibility, food and tobacco environments, and indicators of deprivation.
4. **Data-quality and provenance variables:** source institution, date and method of collection, coding system, device or imaging protocol, missingness indicators, diagnostic criteria, and linkage quality.
5. **Governance and implementation variables:** legal basis for processing, consent or authorized secondary-use mechanism, permitted users, audit history, referral completion, intervention uptake, clinician override, and reported adverse or inequitable outcomes.

Data should be linked to its origin and should be converted to a harmonised common model using the use of validated terminology mapping. Data should be separated from analytical data sources, access should be controlled based on roles, data should be encrypted, access should be logged, data should be kept for a specific period of time as per the rule and governance should be undertaken by an independent body. In the case that it is not suitable to transfer data centrally or is not allowed by law, federated approaches can allow for the local training or analysis of a model while sharing some parameters or summarizing results. These arrangements are not necessarily inherently secure or fair, nor are they necessarily private, and as such need to be tested, governed and evaluated for institutional heterogeneity.

There should be distinction between the analytical pathway for descriptive surveillance, prediction, causal estimation and implementation evaluation. Burden and inequality are given through descriptive analyses. Future risk estimates are made using predictive models which need to be calibrated, discriminated, evaluated for groups of patients, and validated. Causal analyses include a set of assumptions, time horizon, estimand, comparator, an intervention, and a population to be targeted. Implementation analyses examine the acceptability, feasibility, adoption, fidelity, sustainability and impacts of model-supported decisions.

Evaluation should extend beyond overall accuracy. Recommended indicators include:

- completeness and representativeness of linked data;
- linkage error and missingness by subgroup;
- discrimination and calibration;
- sensitivity and specificity at clinically meaningful thresholds;
- false-positive and false-negative rates across relevant groups;
- external validity and temporal stability;
- referral completion and preventive-service uptake;
- changes in oral and systemic outcomes;
- patient-reported experience and burden;
- resource use and cost;
- clinician override and automation-bias events;
- differential benefit or harm by socioeconomic, geographic, and demographic group; and
- evidence of model or data drift.

The operational unit is therefore not the algorithm alone but the complete pathway from data generation to decision, intervention, outcome, audit, and system adaptation.

To illustrate a primary-care network looking to enhance periodontal assessment in adult patients with poorly controlled type 2 diabetes. The target population would be adults who are being treated for diabetes in the network (with and without dental attendance recorded). Medical records would provide glycaemic data, comorbidities, medication intake, smoking and primary-care data. Periodontal measures, tooth loss, preventive attendance, radiographic information and treatment history would be provided in dental records. The deprivation and travel time to dental services, and availability of local workforce could be described at the area level.

The first step in the system would be to determine if there are sufficient linked records for the target population. People who don't have a dental record would not be considered "periodontally healthy" because no dental data would be observed; absence of dental data would be modeled as an access and utilization related observation process. Predictive portion might be able to forecast the likelihood of clinically important periodontal disease. However, if there was to be a referral threshold this would indicate the threshold based on a transparent, systematic consideration of expected benefit, service capacity, and consequences of not detecting the disease and of unnecessary service.

A comparison of an integrated referral approach to usual care would be used in the causal evaluation. The main estimand could be the difference in the percentage of adults that have completed a periodontal assessment at 12 months, between the two groups. Secondary outcomes might be uptake of periodontal treatment, changes in glycaemic control, uprise in oral health related quality of life, cost and differential uptake by deprivation and rurality. Implementation outcomes would be acceptance of referrals, referral completion, referral waiting time, clinician override, burden on the patient, disruption of the clinician's workflow and sustainability.

Involvement in governance would be from dentistry, primary care, epidemiology, information governance, community groups and patient groups. The model would be tested externally prior to expansion, adjusted should there be a change in case mix or changed clinical practices and would be halted should there be data in the subgroup monitoring process that showed that harm to the model was materially unequal. As the example shows, EpiDentomics is not a dental risk score, but a fully connected cycle connecting measurement, causal assessment, service redesign, equity assessment and governance.

LIMITATIONS, CHALLENGES, AND UNRESOLVED TENSIONS

The EpiDentomic paradigm is attractive because it offers the potential to integrate oral-systemic biology in a scalable, timely and predictive way with digital population analytics. But, it has not yet come together as a scientific and policy programme due to a range of epistemic, methodological, institutional and governance tensions. Such restrictions are not flaws in the temporary implementation of these algorithms, but indicators of what is considered evidence, whose conditions come to light, and whose institutions are tasked to act upon algorithmic knowledge. First constraint is data quality. Case definitions, clinical thresholds and practices of measuring these diseases are still not uniform, even among dental epidemiologists (Baelum & Lopez, 2013), particularly in the case of periodontal monitoring, where the patterns of periodontal disease observed depend partly on the diagnostic conventions used(Baelum & Lopez, 2013). .

These issues can be exacerbated by the use of electronic dental records, as missingness is indicative of inequity of access, differences in coding style between providers, and more likely to be captured for procedures than unmet need for the condition, which gives service users an advantage over unserved need users (Mertz et al., 2017; Kranz et al., 2019). Standardisation is not therefore only 'technical'. The choices made in terms of what to classify, how fine to be precise and for what purpose share the authority of classification and specify which inequities are measurable (Kalenderian et al., 2013). As data becomes more complex with the addition of radiomics, utilization and data from wearable devices, methodological risk rises. Convenience sampling and clinical cohorts are already easily subject to overinterpretation, and the high dimensional adjustment can create mediators or colliders which can yield precise but causally misleading estimates (Faggion et al., 2017; Hernán & Robins, 2020). The tension is important as data can provide better stratification and hide social forces and contextual causation (Diez Roux, 2012; Marmot, 2017).

Additionally, scaling up is a constraint in low resource areas. Increased ambition of platforms does not necessarily lead to greater funding for interoperable systems, and a lack of available personnel, a fragmented care continuum, weak information systems, and inadequate maintenance capacity can also hinder ambitious platforms (World Health Organization, 2021, 2022; Lamster & Meyerowitz, 2021; Petersen, 2014). The spread of digitalisation can also further inequalities if populations living in urban areas and covered by insurance and those with internet access are over-represented in national statistics, while those living in rural areas and who provide informal care are systematically under-represented (Patrick et al., 2006; Watt et al., 2019). Surveillance, however, needs to be proportional to institutional capacity, community trust, access to services, and continued funding, not replace the need for universal access (Frieden, 2010; Petersen, 2014). These issues are exacerbated by the disciplinary silos as dentistry and medicine have distinct cultures, funding solutions, referrals, and records (Peres et al., 2019; Lamster, 2021). These divisions contribute to differentials in standards of evidence, and to under-investment and poor accountability for prevention (Listl et al., 2019; Rutter et al., 2017; Watt et al., 2019).

These findings should contribute to shaping a minimum interoperable dataset and reconciling the tension between prediction and causal interpretation, as well as to the establishment of rights-based stewardship and testing of combinations of surveillance, prevention, referral, and care redesign to reduce oral-systemic burden instead of simply improving measurement (AlHumaid et al., 2020; Brall et al., 2019; Kearns et al., 2021; Wirtz et al., 2023; Schwendicke et al., 2020, 2021). These priorities are linking technical development with value, and avoid the slippery slope of measurement becoming policy. If predictive precision is privileged over causal validity, if multiple ways of representing oral-health inequality are not provided for, if there is no institutional accountability and if no action is taken on the social conditions that create oral-health inequality, then EpiDentomics remains uncredible (Watt & Sheiham, 2012; Khoury et al., 2016).

IMPLICATIONS AND FUTURE RESEARCH DIRECTIONS: ADVANCING THEORY, PRACTICE, AND POLICY

While oral disease is highly prevalent and has high disability burden and has been distributed in a patterned way across society, oral conditions are still poorly represented in many national surveillance systems and accountability frameworks for NCDs. The institutional impact of this under-measurement is that things that are not well recorded are not given the priority in prioritising, funding, planning the workforce, and prevention. EpiDentomics thus views invisibility as a challenge to explain and suggests that oral health measures should only be included in the population health intelligence when there is a connection between measurement and services, prevention and equity. While this role is within the framework of digital epidemiology which relies on electronic records and communication traces as well as on sensor-enabled environments, it also challenges the thesis that more data equals more population knowledge (Eysenbach, 2009; Salathé, 2018; Mertz et al., 2017). Therefore it makes sense to redefine epidemiology to incorporate oral-health intelligence, as an adjunct to the traditional oral/ systemic dichotomy.

The curricula should include counter-factual reasoning, causal diagrams and identification logic, as well as unstable case definitions and diagnostic variation and treatment-related outcome distortion (Pearl et al., 2016; Hernán & Robins, 2020; Faggion et al., 2017; Baelum & Lopez, 2013). Data literacy should include information on the provenance of the eHR, coding incentives, missingness, harmonisation across sites, and the privacy, benefit to society and ways in which algorithms can be biased, distributive effects, and accountability for risk-based decisions (Kalenderian et al., 2013; Brall et al., 2019; AlHumaid et al., 2020).

Interoperable dental-medical data should be considered as an important epidemiological infrastructure to be used in the policy development process. There needs to be standardized terminology, common definition of outcomes and rights-preserving linkage mechanisms to link oral status, systemic disease, and service use (Mertz et al., 2017). The WHO oral-health resolution and global strategy place oral indicators in the context of NCD monitoring and global control, but it will take a clear commitment to financing, accountability and a cross-ministerial approach to ownership for implementation. (World Health Organization, 2021, 2022; Lamster & Meyerowitz 2021). A tiered approach to surveillance is a viable option: a basic set of data on basic oral outcomes, access, and shared risk factors should be obtained from all systems; a more complex set of data could be obtained from higher capacity systems, including imaging, biomarker proxies, longitudinal utilization, and wearable-derived behaviors. The latter tiering mitigates this risk of the displacement of analyticity by universal visibility, especially for people in rural areas or without access to costs (Kranz et al., 2019; Patrick et al., 2006).

To this end, the future research should be a synthesis of the longitudinal inference, biological integration and responsible artificial intelligence. Biological data should be integrated into biopsychosocial explanations, and not deterministic ones (Sanz et al., 2020; Diez Roux, 2012; Hajishengallis, 2015; Marmot, 2017), as should be the case with the other international longitudinal studies, which can help to clarify the temporality, shared risk, causal pathways, selection and attrition. Predictive accuracy is not the only aspect of AI evaluation that needs to be taken into account, as the other aspects such as transportability, calibration, interpretability, subgroup performance, fairness and data drift need to be considered as well (Schwendicke et al., 2020, 2021; Wirtz et al., 2023). Its main contribution is analytical—the relationship between choices of measurement and institutional power, as well as the need for evidence systems to be measured by those they represent and benefit and in practice. EpiDentomics can thus only enable precision population health when precision is more than just technical prediction, but also visibility in a sense of equality, stratification in a sense of accountability, care pathways and paths of integration, and system evaluation in a continuous sense (Khoury et al., 2016; Kearns et al., 2021; Watt et al., 2019).

REFERENCES

Ahmed, N., Abbasi, M. S., Zuberi, F., Qamar, W., Halim, M. S., Maqsood, A., & Khan, A. (2021). Artificial intelligence in dentistry: Unlocking new possibilities. *International Journal of Environmental Research and Public Health, 18*(6), 2711.

AlHumaid, J.. (2020). Ethical considerations of artificial intelligence in healthcare: A focus on dentistry. *BMC Medical Ethics, 21*, 1–9.

Baelum, V., & López, R. (2013). Periodontal disease epidemiology—Learn it, teach it, and use it. *Periodontology 2000, 62*(1), 7–15. DOI: 10.1111/j.1600-0757.2012.00449.x PMID: 23574461

Bernabe, E., & Marcenes, W. (2011). Income inequality and tooth loss in the United States. *Journal of Dental Research, 90*(6), 724–729. DOI: 10.1177/0022034511400081 PMID: 21508433

Bernabe, E., Marcenes, W., Hernandez, C. R., Bailey, J., Abreu, L. G., Alipour, V., Amini, S., Arabloo, J., Arefi, Z., Arora, A., Ayanore, M. A., Bärnighausen, T. W., Bijani, A., Cho, D. Y., Chu, D.-T., Fischer, F., Folayan, M. O., Futran, N. D., Haagsma, J. A., & Kassebaum, N. J. (2020). Global, regional, and national levels and trends in the burden of oral conditions, 1990–2017. *Journal of Dental Research, 99*(4), 362–373. PMID: 32122215

Brall, C., Berlin, C., & Schwappach, D. (2019). Ethics of artificial intelligence in public health: A conceptual framework. *BMC Medical Ethics, 20*, 1–14.

Celeste, R. K., Fernandes, I. B., & Nadanovsky, P. (2011). The contextual effect of neighborhood income on dental caries in adults: A multilevel analysis. *Community Dentistry and Oral Epidemiology, 39*(3), 193–201. PMID: 21070318

Chapple, I. L. C., & Genco, R. (2013). Diabetes and periodontal diseases: Consensus report. *Journal of Periodontology, 84*(4S, 4-s), S106–S112. DOI: 10.1902/jop.2013.1340011 PMID: 23631572

Diez Roux, A. V. (2012). Conceptual approaches to the study of health disparities. *Annual Review of Public Health, 33*(1), 41–58. DOI: 10.1146/annurev-publhealth-031811-124534 PMID: 22224879

Divaris, K. (2019). Predicting dental caries outcomes in children: A "risky" concept. *Journal of Dental Research, 98*(13), 1405–1406. PMID: 31746686

Eysenbach, G. (2009). Infodemiology and infoveillance: Framework for an emerging set of public health informatics methods to analyze search, communication, and publication behavior on the Internet. *Journal of Medical Internet Research, 11*(1), e11. DOI: 10.2196/jmir.1157 PMID: 19329408

Faggion, C. M.Jr. (2017). Methodological issues in periodontal research: Causal inference and evidence hierarchies. *Journal of Clinical Periodontology, 44*(9), 868–875.

Frieden, T. R. (2010). A framework for public health action: The health impact pyramid. *American Journal of Public Health, 100*(4), 590–595. DOI: 10.2105/AJPH.2009.185652 PMID: 20167880

Hajishengallis, G. (2015). Periodontitis: From microbial immune subversion to systemic inflammation. *Nature Reviews. Immunology, 15*(1), 30–44. DOI: 10.1038/nri3785 PMID: 25534621

Hernán, M. A., & Robins, J. M. (2020). *Causal inference: What if?* Chapman & Hall/CRC.

Ide, M., & Papapanou, P. N. (2013). Epidemiology of the association between maternal periodontal disease and adverse pregnancy outcomes—Systematic review. *Journal of Periodontology, 84*(4S, 4-s), S181–S194. DOI: 10.1902/jop.2013.134009 PMID: 23631578

Kalenderian, E.. (2013). BigMouth: A multi-institutional dental data repository. *The Journal of the American Dental Association, 144*(12), 144–153.

Kassebaum, N. J.. (2017). Global, regional, and national prevalence, incidence, and disability-adjusted life years for oral conditions, 1990–2015: A systematic analysis. *Journal of Dental Research, 96*(4), 380–387. DOI: 10.1177/0022034517693566 PMID: 28792274

Kearns, C., Peres, M. A., & Watt, R. G. (2021). The future of dental public health: Precision, prevention, and integration. *Community Dentistry and Oral Epidemiology, 49*(5), 369–375.

Khanagar, S. B., Al-Ehaideb, A., Maganur, P. C., Vishwanathaiah, S., Patil, S., & Naik, S. (2021). Developments, applications, and performance of artificial intelligence in dentistry – A systematic review. *Journal of Dental Sciences, 16*(1), 508–522. DOI: 10.1016/j.jds.2020.06.019 PMID: 33384840

Khoury, M. J., Iademarco, M. F., & Riley, W. T. (2016). Precision public health for the era of precision medicine. *American Journal of Preventive Medicine, 50*(3), 398–401. DOI: 10.1016/j.amepre.2015.08.031 PMID: 26547538

Kinane, D. F., Stathopoulou, P. G., & Papapanou, P. N. (2017). Periodontal diseases. *Nature Reviews. Disease Primers*, *3*(1), 17038. DOI: 10.1038/nrdp.2017.38 PMID: 28805207

Kranz, A. M., Gahlon, G., Dick, A. W., & Stein, B. D. (2019). Characteristics of US adults who delay dental care due to cost. *Journal of Public Health Dentistry*, *79*(4), 331–339. PMID: 31407343

Lamster, I. B. (2021). Oral health's inextricable connection to systemic health. *Periodontology 2000*, *87*(1), 11–16. PMID: 34463994

Lamster, I. B. (2022). The nexus of oral and general health: Review and future directions. *Periodontology 2000*, *89*(1), 9–15. PMID: 35244969

Lamster, I. B., & Meyerowitz, C. (2021). The 2021 WHO resolution on oral health: Implications for global oral health. *Journal of Public Health Dentistry*, *81*(3), 177–179.

Linden, G. J., & Herzberg, M. C., & Working Group 4 of the Joint EFP/AAP Workshop. (2013). Periodontitis and systemic diseases: Clinical evidence. *Journal of Clinical Periodontology*, *40*(s14), S20–S29. PMID: 23627330

Listl, S.. (2019). Value-based oral healthcare: Concepts and application. *Community Dentistry and Oral Epidemiology*, *47*(6), 515–523.

Marmot, M. (2017). Social justice, epidemiology, and health inequalities. *European Journal of Epidemiology*, *32*(7), 537–546. DOI: 10.1007/s10654-017-0286-3 PMID: 28776115

Matsuo, H.. (2021). Spatial distribution of dental caries and socioeconomic status in an urban setting: A GIS-based study. *Community Dental Health*, *38*(2), 101–107.

Mertz, E. A.. (2017). Data systems and oral health surveillance: Opportunities and challenges. *Journal of Public Health Dentistry*, *77*(S1), S59–S69.

Nassar, H. M.. (2024). A panorama of machine learning in dentistry. *Journal of Clinical and Translational Research*, *10*(4), 1–22.

Nazir, M. A. (2017). Prevalence of periodontal disease, its association with systemic diseases, and prevention. *International Journal of Health Sciences (Qassim)*, *11*(2), 72–80. PMID: 28539867

Ni, Y., Alwell, K., & Kravitz, N. D. (2022). Deep learning for cephalometric landmark detection in orthodontics: A systematic review. *The Angle Orthodontist*, *92*(5), 659–667.

Patrick, D. L., Lee, R. S. Y., Nucci, M., Grembowski, D., Jolles, C. Z., & Milgrom, P. (2006). Reducing oral health disparities: A focus on social and cultural determinants. *BMC Oral Health*, *6*(S1, Suppl 1), S4. DOI: 10.1186/1472-6831-6-S1-S4 PMID: 16934121

Pearl, J., Glymour, M., & Jewell, N. P. (2016). *Causal inference in statistics: A primer*. Wiley.

Peres, M. A., Macpherson, L. M. D., Weyant, R. J., Daly, B., Venturelli, R., Mathur, M. R., Listl, S., Celeste, R. K., Guarnizo-Herreño, C. C., Kearns, C., Benzian, H., Allison, P., & Watt, R. G. (2019). Oral diseases: A global public health challenge. *Lancet*, *394*(10194), 249–260. DOI: 10.1016/S0140-6736(19)31146-8 PMID: 31327369

Petersen, P. E. (2014). Strengthening of oral health systems: Oral health through primary health care. *Medical Principles and Practice : International Journal of the Kuwait University, Health Science Centre*, *23*(S1), 3–9. DOI: 10.1159/000356937 PMID: 24525450

Riley, P., Lamont, T., Worthington, H., Clarkson, J. E., & Beirne, P. (2017). Recall intervals for oral health in primary care patients. *Cochrane Database of Systematic Reviews*, *2017*(12), CD004346. PMID: 24353242

Rutter, H., Savona, N., Glonti, K., Bibby, J., Cummins, S., Finegood, D. T., Greaves, F., Harper, L., Hawe, P., Moore, L., Petticrew, M., Rehfuess, E., Shiell, A., Thomas, J., & White, M. (2017). The need for a complex systems model of evidence for public health. *Lancet*, *390*(10112), 2602–2604. DOI: 10.1016/S0140-6736(17)31267-9 PMID: 28622953

Salathé, M. (2018). Digital epidemiology: What is it, and where is it going? *Life Sciences, Society and Policy*, *14*(1), 1–5. DOI: 10.1186/s40504-017-0065-7 PMID: 29302758

Sanz, M., Marco Del Castillo, A., Jepsen, S., Gonzalez-Juanatey, J. R., D'Aiuto, F., Bouchard, P., Chapple, I. L. C., Dietrich, T., Gotsman, I., Graziani, F., Herrera, D., Loos, B. G., Madianos, P., Michel, J. B., Perel, P., Pieske, B., Shapira, L., Shechter, M., Tonetti, M. S., & Wimmer, G. (2020). Periodontitis and cardiovascular diseases: Consensus report. *Journal of Clinical Periodontology*, *47*(3), 268–288. DOI: 10.1111/jcpe.13189 PMID: 32011025

Schwendicke, F., Giannakakis, A., Parthasarathy, S., Krois, J., & Samek, W. (2021). Explainable artificial intelligence in dentistry. *Journal of Dental Research*, *100*(10), 1074–1081.

Schwendicke, F., Golla, T., Dreher, M., & Krois, J. (2019). Convolutional neural networks for dental image diagnostics: A scoping review. *Journal of Dentistry*, *91*, 103226. DOI: 10.1016/j.jdent.2019.103226 PMID: 31704386

Schwendicke, F., Samek, W., & Krois, J. (2020). Artificial intelligence in dentistry: Chances and challenges. *Journal of Dental Research*, *99*(7), 769–774. DOI: 10.1177/0022034520915714 PMID: 32315260

Shrestha, R. M.. (2022). Environmental and occupational determinants of periodontal disease: A systematic review. *International Journal of Environmental Research and Public Health*, *19*(4), 1938. PMID: 35206125

Watt, R. G., Daly, B., Allison, P., Macpherson, L. M. D., Venturelli, R., Listl, S., Weyant, R., Mathur, M. R., Guarnizo-Herreño, C. C., Celeste, R. K., Peres, M. A., Kearns, C., & Benzian, H. (2019). Ending the neglect of global oral health: Time for radical action. *Lancet*, *394*(10194), 261–272. DOI: 10.1016/S0140-6736(19)31133-X PMID: 31327370

Watt, R. G., & Sheiham, A. (2012). Integrating the common risk factor approach into a social determinants framework. *Community Dentistry and Oral Epidemiology*, *40*(4), 289–296. DOI: 10.1111/j.1600-0528.2012.00680.x PMID: 22429083

Wirtz, A.. (2023). Machine learning in dentistry: A scoping review. *Clinical Oral Investigations*, *27*(1), 45–63. PMID: 36459238

World Health Organisation. (2021). *Resolution WHA74.5: Oral health.* World Health Assembly.

World Health Organisation. (2022). *WHO global strategy on oral health.* World Health Organisation.

Chapter 7 Towards a Global EpiDentomic Observatory: Advancing AI-Driven Epidemiology and Educational Innovation

Pardeep Kumar
http://orcid.org/0000-0003-0308-7634
Lovely Professional University, India

Sanjeev Kumar
http://orcid.org/0000-0002-7375-7341
Lovely Professional University, India

ABSTRACT

The overlap of artificial intelligence (AI) and epidemiology has produced unprecedented opportunities to track, predict, and respond to the problems concerning the state of the health of the population, simultaneously enhancing the innovative quality of health education. An EpiDentomic Observatory is an international organization that is an interdisciplinary partnership to apply AI-driven data analysis, real-time surveillance of diseases, and knowledge exchange between institutions to improve epidemiological studies and education. Predictions about disease outbreaks and implementing intervention strategies based on the synthesis of large-scale health, demographic, and environmental data can enable further and more accurate, faster and efficient responses to the issue of public health due to the capabilities of the AI models to identify trends. Meanwhile, the observatory will also be an instrument

DOI: 10.4018/979-8-3373-8402-3.ch007

of educational innovation, which will enable learners, researchers and healthcare providers to access interactive and data-driven learning. Such integration promotes predictive modeling

INTRODUCTION

Conceptual Foundations of the EpiDentomic Observatory:

The observatory allows these factors to be synthesized into a single analytical framework, enabling timely, data-driven, context-driven interventions. EpiDentomics' conceptualization is also characterized by a two-fold focus on knowledge creation and educational interactions, ensuring that knowledge gained from complex data analyses is translated into operational skills and competencies for students, practitioners, and researchers (Gawande et al., 2025). Combining epidemiology, AI, and education within the observatory's framework is an intentional attempt to bridge the divide between theoretical understanding, analytical skills, and practice. Epidemiology provides the methodological basis, including the systematic study of disease occurrence, prevalence, and risk factors, as well as the evaluation of intervention effectiveness. Conventional epidemiological methods have always been based on observational research, clinical trials, and statistical inference to draw insights towards the informal public health policy and practice. Although the above methods are fundamental, the growing complexity of contemporary health issues has necessitated the adoption of novel computational methods capable of processing large volumes of multidimensional data (Epelde, 2024). The models are especially useful in complex and unpredictable situations, where rapid changes in disease patterns or population behavior require swift, evidence-based responses. Predictive modeling will improve decision-making at local health facilities and in national and international policy-making frameworks by simulating possible scenarios and projecting their probable consequences. In addition, predictive modeling serves as an interface between abstract data analysis and practical public health interventions; thus, complex calculations can be translated into insights that guide the design and execution of interventions. In the educational field, predictive models enable students and practitioners to interact with real data, develop critical analysis skills, and gain a more intuitive understanding of the cause-and-effect relationships among health and other systemic factors (Fatima et al., 2023).

The conceptual pillars of EpiDentomics also highlight the need for interdisciplinary collaboration and knowledge sharing. Health outcomes are rarely determined by a single factor, and solving complex population health problems requires integrating knowledge of epidemiology, data science, behavior, environmental factors, and health policy. Not only does this collaborative orientation improve the quality and relevance of epidemiological research, but it also supports educational objectives by introducing learners to a variety of viewpoints, analytical methods, and problem-solving approaches. The observatory also helps to create a talented, flexible, and internationally oriented population in terms of the workforce in the field of public health, as it leads to the creation of a culture of collaboration and life-long learning, which will enable the workforce to be adequately equipped to address the arising health challenges (Amarachukwu Bernaldine Isiaka et al., 2024). One important aspect of the EpiDentomic structure is data integration, driven by the need to combine information from heterogeneous sources to yield deep, practical insights. Health-specific data include clinical records, laboratory findings, environmental surveillance data, demographic surveys, social determinants of health, and more movement patterns, and most recently, unstructured data from social media and other internet resources.

TECHNOLOGICAL FRAMEWORK

The technological platform on which a Global EpiDentomic Observatory is based is central to the potential to transform epidemiological research and health education through artificial intelligence (AI) and advanced data analytics. The dynamism of the diseases in question, the high population mobility, and the complexity of interactions between the environment and the population, which are inherent to modern public health, demand a computational infrastructure capable of handling diverse, vast datasets in real time and inferring actionable information. This infrastructure is enabled by AI and machine learning models that offer analytical capabilities faster and more predictive than conventional statistical systems (Da Silva, 2024). Those technologies enable the identification of hidden patterns in epidemiological data, enabling predictions of disease outbreaks and optimal interventions at different spatial and temporal scales (Abdelouahed et al., 2025). Their use in the observatory system enables converting raw health data into practical knowledge, thereby improving the efficiency, precision, and responsiveness of public health systems. The technological framework of the Global EpiDentomic Observatory is shown in Table 1

Table 1. Technological Framework of the Global EpiDentomic Observatory; Source: Author Compilation

Component	Description	Purpose/Impact
AI and Machine Learning Models	Algorithms for pattern recognition, forecasting, and optimization	Identify trends, predict outbreaks, optimize interventions
Data Acquisition	Collection of health, demographic, and environmental datasets	Provide diverse, multi-source input for analysis
Real-Time Disease Surveillance Systems	Continuous monitoring of epidemiological and environmental data	Enable timely detection of emerging health threats
Data Integration and Management	Harmonization, storage, and preprocessing of heterogeneous data	Ensure accuracy, accessibility, and interoperability for analysis
Analytical Infrastructure	High-performance computing, cloud-based platforms, and visualization tools	Support large-scale processing, predictive modeling, and actionable insights
Knowledge Translation Tools	Dashboards, reports, and visualization interfaces	Convert complex data outputs into actionable information for decision-makers

Machine learning has a range of modeling methods, especially those that are better applicable in epidemiological settings. Random forests, support vector machines, and gradient boosting algorithms are supervised learning models that can be used to develop relationships between predictor variables and health outcomes, enabling powerful risk stratification and disease incidence models. Unsupervised learning methods, including clustering and dimensionality reduction, can reveal latent structure and patterns in complex data sets and uncover relations that might otherwise be hidden when using standard analysis tools (Varela et al., 2017). Deep learning models, such as convolutional and recurrent neural networks, can be extended to support large-scale, high-dimensional and frequently unstructured information, such as medical imaging, genomics and social media feeds. These AI-based models are trained on combined datasets in the observatory to capture spatial and temporal trends in disease and high-risk populations, and to generate probabilities used to inform targeted interventions. Notably, the observatory focuses on explainable AI strategies that ensure the outputs of models are understandable to the general public, health practitioners, and policymakers, thereby enhancing trust, transparency, and actionable decision-making (Martins et al., 2023).

Real-time surveillance not only enhances responsiveness to health emergencies within the population but also supports longitudinal research by ensuring datasets are continuously updated to reflect the evolving dynamics of the disease. The final aspect of the technological base is data integration, storage, and management, in which the different datasets are organized, accessible, and secure for analysis. The observatory has advanced data warehousing technologies, cloud-based data storage systems, and high-performance computing capabilities to manage the volume and density of epidemiological data (Lappalainen et al., 2025). They are employed to standardize, correlate, and format heterogeneous sources of data, such as structured and unstructured data, using data integration pipelines that normalize, relate variables, and format them as needed for subsequent analysis. To obtain reproducibility and regulatory compliance, which metadata management and data lineage tracking provide, the following types of processes are required: transparency, data provenance, quality, and transformation processes (Bruce et al., 2018). In addition to storage and integration, it has implemented effective data governance policies to ensure privacy, ethical use, and security against unauthorized access. The observatory infrastructure is encrypted, anonymized, and uses role-based access controls so that only researchers and educators can access sensitive health information, while allowing them access to the information they need to analyze and learn (Oyeyemi et al., 2024).

The technological infrastructure is designed to be dynamic and open-ended, enabling it to meet the evolving needs of public health systems and education programs. Modular design principles allow adding new streams of data, new computational devices, and algorithms to the existing ones, making the observatory responsive to new epidemiological patterns and technological advances. The AI models will be retrained and tested on new data, forming a dynamic learning model that will improve predictive accuracy over time. Cloud computing and distributed processing architectures enable the observatory to manage computational workloads, enabling it to process large datasets and run parallel analytical processes across different geographic locations. More importantly, visualization and dashboard applications will be integrated into the observatory, transforming complex analytical outputs into a convenient format that can be easily accessed by many stakeholders, including researchers, educators, policymakers, and practitioners in public health. Between high-performance computational analysis and actual use, they turn data discovery, scenario modelling, and decision-making into interactive processes (Ramirez Varela et al., 2018). In addition to its mission to conduct epidemiological research, the technological framework also supports the observatory's educational mission. Students, trainees, and practitioners are introduced to real-world datasets, analytical pipelines, and predictive models, and gain practical experience with the tools and methods of modern epidemiology. By incorporating AI-based analytical systems into the educational curriculum, computational literacy, critical thinking, and data-driven decision-making are promoted, and learners are trained to manage the challenges of modern public health practice. Experiential learning opportunities are offered through interactive simulation environments, scenario-based modeling exercises, and group-based data analysis projects to reinforce theoretical knowledge and develop practical skills. By integrating technological capacity with learning goals, the observatory can ensure that its analytical breakthroughs are directly translated into educational impact, creating a new generation of employees who can use AI to improve society's health. In addition to its mission to conduct epidemiological research, the technological framework also supports the observatory's educational mission. Students, trainees, and practitioners are introduced to real-world datasets, analytical pipelines, and predictive models, and gain practical experience with the tools and methods of modern epidemiology (Pratt et al., 2024). By incorporating AI-based analytical systems into the educational curriculum, computational literacy, critical thinking, and data-driven decision-making are promoted, and learners are trained to manage the challenges of modern public health practice. Experiential learning opportunities are offered through interactive simulation environments, scenario-based modeling exercises, and group-based data analysis projects to reinforce theoretical knowledge and develop practical skills. By integrating technological capacity with learning goals, the observatory can ensure that its analytical breakthroughs are directly translated into educational impact, creating a new generation of employees who can use AI to improve society's health (Ramírez Varela et al., 2023).

APPLICATIONS IN PUBLIC HEALTH

The clustering algorithms and anomaly detection models can identify areas with abnormal spikes in disease incidence, whereas temporal modeling methods forecast the direction of outbreaks based on historical trends, mobility data, and population density. With this kind of foresight, the observatory can increase preparedness locally and internationally, enabling the efficient and effective distribution of resources, human resources, and interventions (Brabham et al., 2014). Pattern identification and disease forecasting are most important for emerging or changing pathogens. The AI models trained on various datasets can identify associations between environmental factors, demographic features, and disease occurrence that might otherwise go unnoticed using traditional statistics. For example, climatic information can be used in predictive algorithms to forecast the outbreak of a species-carrying disease, e.g., dengue or malaria, by matching temperature, rainfall, and humidity patterns with the mosquito's breeding cycle (Fletcher-Lartey & Caprarelli, 2016). In a similar manner, movement and transportation data could be used to predict the geographic distribution of infectious diseases, enabling authorities to issue targeted travel warnings, screening measures, and localized containment measures. In addition to infectious diseases, predictive models are also used in managing chronic diseases, where population clusters at a high risk of developing a condition (diabetes, cardiovascular disease, and cancer) are identified. The observatory enables proactive disease management, shifting the population's approach to health security by transforming the response strategy from reactive to preventive when diseases are developing (Freeman, 2018).

Another important use of the observatory is to optimize intervention strategies, which is made easier by the ability to simulate various situations and measure the potential effects of different actions in public health. The process of intervention optimization involves determining the most efficient use of resources, the time and resource intensity of interventions, and the population most likely to respond. For example, vaccination campaigns can be prioritized based on predicted outbreak hotspots, demographic vulnerability, and population density to reach as many individuals as possible with minimal waste (Iwelunmor et al., 2014). On the same note, predictive models based on projected disease burden and geographic distribution can inform resource allocation for medical supplies, hospital capacity planning, and staffing. The observatory is also central to improving population health decision-making by providing policymakers, health administrators, and frontline practitioners with timely, evidence-based information. Scenario modeling interfaces, interactive dashboards, and data visualization tools can be used to convert complex information outputs from analytical processes into usable, actionable information (Tracy et al., 2018). Both predictive analytics and situational knowledge enable decision-makers to research different intervention strategies, evaluate potential outcomes, and choose courses of action. In addition, the observatory promotes lifelong learning and feedback, through which the consequences of applied interventions are fed back into the models to optimize future predictions and recommendations. This cyclic and dynamic methodology ensures that public health strategies are dynamic to changing conditions, citizen practices, and disease dynamics. This linking of predictive analytics to decision-support systems transforms the research-practice gap into an informed, accountable and open form of governance of public health (Menon & Koura, 2025).

Additional evidence of the practical effects of the EpiDentomic Observatory across various health settings is provided by case studies and examples of successful implementation worldwide. In recent outbreaks of infectious diseases, AI-based surveillance systems have been shown to predict the occurrence and distribution of pathogens over time and to inform population health-related decisions. The observatory's impact is realized not only in the immediate response to the outbreak but also in long-term planning and population health assessment. Predictive modeling will facilitate the strengthening of the health system by revealing gaps in infrastructure, workforce distribution, and service delivery (Nykiforuk & Flaman, 2011). The observatory can be used to identify areas of continuous vulnerability, support investments in healthcare facilities, and contribute to training and capacity-building by analyzing historical data and real-time surveillance. In addition, the observatory helps promote equity in health by identifying populations at disproportionate risk due to disease, environmental factors, or social determinants of health. This can then be used to formulate specific interventions to tackle these inequalities, ensuring that public health interventions are fair and inclusive. The observatory can be used to improve the effectiveness and ethical basis of public health practice, demonstrating that analytics developed with AI can support evidence-based, equitable, and socially responsible health governance (Khoury et al., 2018).

One of the key factors in successful implementation is the interoperability of data systems and the integration of multi-source information. Health data is naturally heterogeneous, encompassing structured clinical records, unstructured textual reports, image datasets, and environmental sensor readings. By linking local, national, and global actors, the observatory enhances the ability of health systems to act effectively on endemic and emerging health issues and also ensures global health security and resilience (Edo-Osagie et al., 2020). Besides, the observatory helps draft flexible policy frameworks that can adapt to rapidly evolving epidemiological conditions. Predictive modeling enables policymakers to see into the future of disease and assess the potential effects of the various policy alternatives. For example, the effects of social distancing, vaccination, or environmental interventions can be evaluated using models to provide evidence for legislative and administrative actions (Odone et al., 2019). This proactive policy evaluation capability ensures that public health actions are grounded in empirical evidence and are more efficient and accountable. In addition, the observatory enables ongoing monitoring and assessment, allowing policies to be improved in response to new information, emerging threats, or unintended consequences. The observatory creates a feedback mechanism by connecting predictive analytics to policy development, enhancing alignment among research, operational planning, and governance. Other uses of the EpiDentomic Observatory in public health also include global health security and emergency preparedness. Scenario planning, predictive modeling and integrated surveillance allow authorities to mitigate the impact of environmental crises, natural disasters, and pandemics. The observatory can enhance situational awareness and coordinated action across different areas and states by providing a centralized platform for gathering and analyzing a wide range of data. Such integrated platforms have been used to facilitate quick, evidence-based, and coordinated responses to Ebola outbreaks in West Africa and to influenza surveillance across multiple continents, providing evidence of their importance. These cases remind the observatory of the potential to serve as a model of what global public health infrastructure can be by integrating technological advances with strategic coordination to safeguard populations worldwide.

The uses of the Global EpiDentomic Observatory in public health include identifying disease patterns, forecasting outbreaks, optimizing interventions, supporting decision-making, building educational capacity, and implementing interventions internationally. The observatory offers practical insights based on AI-supported predictive modeling, coupled with an array of health data and real-time surveillance, to support effective responses to and preparedness for prolonged risk and to promote better health equity among populations. Key Applications of the Global EpiDentomic Observatory are shown in Table 2.

Table 2. Key Applications of the Global EpiDentomic Observatory; Source: Author Compilation

Application	Methods/Tools	Impact
Disease Pattern Identification & Forecasting	Machine learning, predictive modeling	Early outbreak detection, high-risk population identification
Optimizing Interventions	AI simulations, reinforcement learning	Efficient resource allocation, targeted public health strategies
Decision Support	Dashboards, scenario modeling	Evidence-based policymaking, adaptive response
Data Integration & Surveillance	Real-time pipelines, cloud storage	Holistic understanding of health trends, timely alerts
Education & Capacity Building	Interactive simulations, predictive models	Enhanced analytical skills, experiential learning

EDUCATIONAL INNOVATION AND CAPACITY BUILDING

The participants will gain practical experience working with multi-source datasets, learning to preprocess, integrate, and analyze information from clinical records, environmental sensors, demographic surveys, and social determinants of health. It also focuses on model interpretability, reproducibility, and ethical concerns, so that learners can not only learn how to produce predictions, but also how to critically assess their assumptions, limitations, and implications for society. The observatory integrates predictive analytics training into an operational epidemiological platform and equips learners with the analytical skills they will apply to tackle real-life public health issues, fostering a culture of lifelong learning and methodological rigor. The inter-institutional and interdisciplinary work is another feature of the observatory's educational policy, which corresponds to the nature of the constantly interconnected modern health problems. Public health is not limited to a single field and therefore involves biological, environmental, social, and behavioral determinants that demand contributions from various disciplines (Lazaro-Mojica & Fernandez, 2021). The observatory supports collaborative learning and research by providing joint platforms for accessing data, using analytical tools, and solving problems, enabling members of various institutions and geographic areas to collaborate on complex health scenarios. Epidemiologists, data scientists, environmental health experts, clinicians, policy analysts, and educators might work collaboratively to develop interdisciplinary understanding, share knowledge, and drive innovation. The observatory trains learners in teamwork, communication, and cross-disciplinary reasoning by involving them in problem-solving and data-driven research, equipping them with the skills to work in collaborative public health settings (Ramirez-Montoya, 2020). This method will improve learning quality and support the overall goal of global health capacity building: establishing networks of professionals who can respond to cross-border problems. The development of evidence-based decision-making skills is a crucial outcome of the observatory's educational activities. It is common for public health professionals to make decisions in an uncertain environment, with limited resources, competing priorities, and changing information.

Moreover, the observatory's digital infrastructure enables ongoing evaluation and feedback, helping learners track their progress, identify knowledge gaps, and deepen their understanding through repeated practice. The observatory provides an interactive, enjoyable learning experience integrated with digital technology that meets the requirements of the modern health professional. Ethical, equitable, and socially responsible practice is also highlighted in the observatory's capacity-building. One of the training modules covers data privacy, algorithmic bias, fair resource distribution, and the social consequences of predictive modeling. Students are also given the opportunity to critically examine the assumptions underlying AI models, assess the potential implications of interventions across diverse groups, and focus on fairness and inclusivity in decision-making (Gil et al., 2018). Incorporating ethical considerations into experiential learning can ensure that future public health professionals not only become competent in their fields but also develop a responsible attitude toward their roles in society. Such congruence between the development of analytical skills and their moral sensitivity contributes to the strengthening of the credibility, trustworthiness, and influence of the field of public health practice in a globally interconnected environment.

In addition to personal competencies, the observatory supports capacity building within the organization and its systems. Those institutions that are members of the observatory have access to common data resources, analytical platforms, and collaborative networks, enabling local expertise, research projects, and course development. Faculty and trainers are assisted in incorporating AI-based analytics into curricula, creating interactive study modules, and advising students in applied epidemiological research (Zhuang & Liu, 2022). The cross-institutional collaboration will enable sharing of best practices, methodological innovations, and research outcomes and enhance the overall power of the health education ecosystem. The development of human and institutional capacity facilitates the sustainability, scalability, and long-term impact of global health education and practice through the observatory. The two-fold priority of research and education at the observatory is also designed to ensure that technological progress in predictive analytics and data integration is directly translated into learning outcomes. By involving learners in real-world applications, the observatory helps close the gap between theoretical knowledge and practical skills; thus, they emerge as professionals who have mastered analytical methods and, at the same time, are practical in decision-making (Riccomini et al., 2021).

CHALLENGES AND CONSIDERATIONS

Although AI and machine learning can be powerful tools for analyzing complex data and generating predictive insights, their effectiveness depends on the quality, completeness, and representativeness of the input data. Flaws such as data gaps, measurement errors, inconsistent reporting, and time lags may undermine the model's precision and decrease the forecast's credibility. Another limitation of models is computational, including processing capacity and memory, as well as the ability to scale algorithms to high-dimensional problems or even real-time datasets. In addition, AI models can be viewed as simplifications of complex biological and social processes, and their forecasts are subject to uncertainty due to missing variables, stochastic dynamics, or changing environmental conditions. Strict model validation, quantification of uncertainty, and clear communication of limitations to stakeholders to avoid misunderstandings or reliance on predictive outputs are therefore necessary. Constant improvement of the model, retraining using new data and testing the scenarios are required in order to keep the model accurate and relevant in the fast-changing epidemiological environment. A third key consideration for the observatory is equity and accessibility in global implementation. The distribution of health issues and technological assets is uneven across countries and regions, casting doubt on the inclusiveness, scalability, and sustainability of AI-based public health interventions. Knowledge transfer, technical support, and locally specific model and intervention development could be supported through collaborative relationships between high- and low-resource institutions. Moreover, one should focus on the linguistic, cultural, and contextual factors that affect data interpretation, model applicability, and educational interactions to ensure the observatory can be used to promote inclusivity and relevance in an international context. Agreements on data sharing, intellectual property, and cross-border regulatory compliance underscore the need for careful negotiation to avoid delays, conflicts, and legal risks. The need to sustain the flow of data, real-time processing, and high system availability requires strong IT infrastructure, human resources and long-term funding, which may not be evenly distributed among the participating organizations. The institution's commitment, and the organization's governance and working procedures, are thus essential to ensuring that the observatory operates reliably, effectively, and fairly in the long run.

The interpretation and communication of AI-driven insights creates another difficulty. Predictive models are analytically complex, but their outputs are counter-intuitive, complex, and probabilistic. To translate insights into practical public health responses, one needs knowledge of epidemiology, statistics, and decision science, as well as the ability to communicate effectively with policymakers, practitioners, and the general public. Incorrect interpretation of model results, overconfidence in predictions, or a lack of transparency can undermine confidence and reduce the effectiveness of interventions. The observatory focuses on explainable AI, user-friendly dashboards, scenario-driven visualization, and training programs to counter this risk by promoting data literacy among the various stakeholders. These steps are used to ensure AI insights are utilized in a responsible and effective way by developing awareness and trust in model results.

Social and cultural issues involve the ethical, technical, and operational factors that determine the observatory's implementation success. Relevance, trust and sustainability require engagement with local communities, stakeholder involvement and sensitivity to local health needs. To address this, sustainable financial models, institutional partnerships, and strategic planning are necessary. Developing local expertise and encouraging cross-institutional cooperation, along with the development of an open-source solution, will make the observatory less dependent on external support and, eventually, more resilient, enabling it to deliver consistent value over time.

The rapid development of AI and epidemiological research aggravates the problem of data privacy, security, technical accuracy, equity, and sustainability. The capabilities and complexity of the observatory continue to increase with advances in machine learning, data integration, and computational infrastructure, with opportunities and threats. Proactive governance, responsive policies, and continuous stakeholder involvement are also necessary to keep up with technological changes, comply with regulations, and align ethical goals with the organization. Risk management systems, scenario planning, and ethical oversight committees are hence important for anticipating, mitigating, and responding to emerging challenges and for maximizing the benefits of the observatory.

The observatory has to navigate the tension between global standardization and local acculturation. Although standardized data formats, data analytical pipeline, and operational protocols enable comparability, interoperability, and cross-border cooperation, they might not sufficiently reflect local epidemiological peculiarities, cultural practices, and resource limitations. It is necessary to balance global consistency and local relevance by adopting context-sensitive modeling, flexible frameworks, and participatory methods that empower local stakeholders to adapt tools and interventions to their specific needs. Through standardization and flexibility, the observatory can achieve the highest scientific rigor and usefulness, enabling world-class insights to be applied across diverse local environments. Altogether, ethical, technical, operational, and social issues and considerations of the Global EpiDentomic Observatory are numerous. The privacy of data, its security, and ethical regulation must be ensured and transparent, whereas technical constraints and the quality of the model must be rigorously validated, improved, and understood. It is important that equity, access, and sustainability be put in place in order to make the world more inclusive, relevant, and impactful in the long term. To address these issues, the planning process requires inter-institutional cooperation, interventions that promote participation, and flexible governance systems that incorporate aspects of technology innovation, ethics, and social and practical issues.

FUTURE DIRECTIONS

Federated learning enables models to be trained on decentralized data without sensitive patient data being transmitted, allowing institutions to collaboratively design models without violating data privacy. Transfer learning enables predictive models to be used in new geographic areas, populations, or disease profiles, thereby increasing their scalability and applicability. These developments, in combination with improved computational infrastructure, cloud computing platforms, and high-performance analytics, will enable observatories to deliver more accurate, timely, and actionable insights to support evidence-based decision-making and proactive public health interventions. Another important area of future development is the integration of emerging educational technologies. Immersion and experience: Digital learning environments, augmented reality (AR), virtual reality (VR), and interactive simulators can offer immersive, experiential training for students, practitioners, and policymakers. Using such platforms, incorporating real-time epidemiological data and AI-based predictive models, learners will have the opportunity to interact with dynamic scenarios, experiment with intervention strategies, and see the outcomes of their decisions in simulated conditions. AI-based adaptive learning technologies have the potential to customize instructional content and its complexity to the individual learner's progress and capabilities, increasing engagement, retention, and skill development. The inclusion of gamification elements, problem-solving through scenarios, and online collaboration sites also promotes active engagement, multidisciplinary cooperation, and critical thinking. The educational aspect of the observatory could therefore become a technology-enriched, globally networked learning system that can create data-literate, analytical, and adaptable public health professionals prepared to solve the complex problems of the twenty-first century.

Policy and strategic implications are necessary for the observatory's future path. As observatories expand and their analytical capabilities improve, it is necessary to reflect on how these insights can be incorporated into local, national, and international decision-making systems. The outputs generated by AI-based observatories can inform health resource distribution, epidemic preparedness, vaccination, environmental health policy, and health equity interventions. The implementation of outputs from observatories requires sound governance systems, ethical considerations, and their institutionalization, ensuring that policies are evidence-based, fair, and contextual. Moreover, as observatories span international boundaries, it is necessary to coordinate regulatory systems, data-sharing policies, and networks that enable cross-country research, knowledge sharing, and a coordinated response to international health threats. By strategically planning policies that enable technological innovation to follow specific trends, observatories can do the most to improve health outcomes and ensure responsible, transparent, and sustainable governance. One aspect of further evolution is the convergence of various and new streams of data to increase predictability and context. In addition to the conventional clinical, demographic, and environmental data, observatories may include new sources such as genomic sequences, wastewater surveillance, mobile health (mHealth) data, social media analytics, and wearable device outputs.

Global observatories can also serve as data-sharing platforms, sites of methodological innovation, and places for capacity building to create transnational networks of researchers, educators, and practitioners. This type of collaboration increases the strength, applicability and utility of predictive models and facilitates harmonization of surveillance practices, ethical principles and best practices. Coordination across borders is especially important for addressing pandemics, vector-borne diseases, environmental health hazards, and other issues that cross national borders. The joint research and comparative studies, as well as common educational material, can also be supported by collaborative platforms and enhance preparedness to act globally, disseminate knowledge, and coordinate actions. Adaptive governance and policy innovation are also a priority emerging trend. The more complex insights generated by observatories, the more decision-makers need to devise ways to translate predictive analytics into operational policy without compromising ethical principles, transparency, and stakeholder trust. The use of scenario-based planning, repeated policy analysis and feedback loops between model outputs and policy outcomes are bound to be the main elements of observatory-based governance. It might also be necessary for the policy to address cross-sectoral issues, such as environmental health, urban planning, social determinants of health, and global mobility, given the interrelationships among modern public health hazards. Anticipatory policymaking, proactive resource deployment, and the design of effective and equitable interventions can be facilitated by strategic foresight informed by simulations conducted with AI and predictive modeling.

Another important aspect of further development is international cooperation. Global observatories can also serve as data-sharing platforms, sites of methodological innovation, and places for capacity building to create transnational networks of researchers, educators, and practitioners. This type of collaboration increases the strength, applicability and utility of predictive models and facilitates harmonization of surveillance practices, ethical principles and best practices. Coordination across borders is especially important for addressing pandemics, vector-borne diseases, environmental health hazards, and other issues that cross national borders. The joint research and comparative studies, as well as common educational material, can also be supported by collaborative platforms and enhance preparedness to act globally, disseminate knowledge, and coordinate actions.

CONCLUSION

The Global EpiDentomic Observatory is one of the first interdisciplinary models combining artificial intelligence, epidemiology, and education and can help revolutionize research, decision-making, and capacity-building in public health. Across the different dimensions discussed in this paper, several major findings emerge, underscoring the opportunities for observation that the observatory will provide in redefining the scientific and educational environment of global health. To begin with, predictive modeling based on AI, combined with multi-source datasets including clinical, demographic, environmental, and behavioral data, will enable the visualization of disease dynamics, population susceptibility, and intervention efficacy at a granular level. Such capabilities are important not only for responding to outbreaks of infectious diseases but also for addressing chronic diseases, environmental health hazards, and emerging threats to people's health. Another advantage of global collaboration is that the observatory fosters cross-institutional and cross-national data sharing, enabling comparative research and helping coordinate emergency responses to health issues. The observatory helps achieve better population health outcomes, resilience, and preparedness for future challenges by advancing data-driven, evidence-based solutions. Moreover, incorporating ethical and equitable concerns makes the interventions inclusive, socially responsible, and considerate of the needs of vulnerable groups.

The observatory can serve as an example in experiential, technology-based education that aligns with current requirements in public health education. Growth and consolidation of observatory platforms, along with their maintenance, are, in the future, a data-driven vision for global health. The growth of observatories to other nations, institutions, and information will result in more reliable predictions, more analysis areas, and more convenient coordination of responses on a worldwide scale. Better AI solutions, cloud computing, and data integration will enable more sophisticated simulations and real-time analytics, along with adaptive interventions; future educational technologies, including virtual and augmented reality and gamified learning engines, will transform training experiences to an even higher level. The coordination of policies and strategies will also play a significant role in operationalizing predictive insights into actionable interventions, ensuring that resource allocation, health governance, and emergency preparedness are data-driven.

REFERENCES

Abdelouahed, M., Yateem, D., Amzil, C., Aribi, I., Abdelwahed, E. H., & Fredericks, S. (2025). Integrating artificial intelligence into public health education and healthcare: Insights from the COVID-19 and monkeypox crises for future pandemic readiness. *Frontiers in Education*, *10*, 1518909. DOI: 10.3389/feduc.2025.1518909

Brabham, D. C., Ribisl, K. M., Kirchner, T. R., & Bernhardt, J. M. (2014). Crowdsourcing Applications for Public Health. *American Journal of Preventive Medicine*, *46*(2), 179–187. DOI: 10.1016/j.amepre.2013.10.016 PMID: 24439353

Bruce, L. C., Frassl, M. A., Arhonditsis, G. B., Gal, G., Hamilton, D. P., Hanson, P. C., Hetherington, A. L., Melack, J. M., Read, J. S., Rinke, K., Rigosi, A., Trolle, D., Winslow, L., Adrian, R., Ayala, A. I., Bocaniov, S. A., Boehrer, B., Boon, C., Brookes, J. D., & Hipsey, M. R. (2018). A multi-lake comparative analysis of the General Lake Model (GLM): Stress-testing across a global observatory network. *Environmental Modelling & Software*, *102*, 274–291. DOI: 10.1016/j.envsoft.2017.11.016

Da Silva, R. G. L. (2024). The advancement of artificial intelligence in biomedical research and health innovation: Challenges and opportunities in emerging economies. *Globalization and Health*, *20*(1), 44. DOI: 10.1186/s12992-024-01049-5 PMID: 38773458

Edo-Osagie, O., De La Iglesia, B., Lake, I., & Edeghere, O. (2020). A scoping review of the use of Twitter for public health research. *Computers in Biology and Medicine*, *122*, 103770. DOI: 10.1016/j.compbiomed.2020.103770 PMID: 32502758

Epelde, F. (2024). How AI Could Help Us in the Epidemiology and Diagnosis of Acute Respiratory Infections? *Pathogens (Basel, Switzerland)*, *13*(11), 940. DOI: 10.3390/pathogens13110940 PMID: 39599493

fatima, G., Allami, R. H., & Yousif, M. G. (2023). *Integrative AI-Driven Strategies for Advancing Precision Medicine in Infectious Diseases and Beyond: A Novel Multidisciplinary Approach* (Version 1). arXiv. DOI: 10.48550/ARXIV.2307.15228

Fletcher-Lartey, S. M., & Caprarelli, G. (2016). Application of GIS technology in public health: Successes and challenges. *Parasitology*, *143*(4), 401–415. DOI: 10.1017/S0031182015001869 PMID: 26831619

Freeman, M. (Ed.). (2018). *The Ethics of Public Health* (1st ed.). Routledge., DOI: 10.4324/9781315239927

Gawande, M. S., Zade, N., Kumar, P., Gundewar, S., Weerarathna, I. N., & Verma, P. (2025). The role of artificial intelligence in pandemic responses: From epidemiological modeling to vaccine development. *Molecular Biomedicine*, *6*(1), 1. DOI: 10.1186/s43556-024-00238-3 PMID: 39747786

Gil, A. J., Rodrigo-Moya, B., & Morcillo-Bellido, J. (2018). The effect of leadership in the development of innovation capacity: A learning organization perspective. *Leadership and Organization Development Journal*, *39*(6), 694–711. DOI: 10.1108/LODJ-12-2017-0399

Isiaka, A. B., Anakwenze, V. N., Ilodinso, C. R., Anaukwu, C. G., Ezeokoli, C. M.-V., Noi, S. M., Agboola, G. O., & Adonu, R. M.Amarachukwu Bernaldine IsiakaVivian Nonyelum AnakwenzeChiamaka Rosemary IlodinsoChikodili Gladys AnaukwuChukwuebuka Mary-Vin EzeokoliSamuel Mensah NoiGazali Oluwasegun AgboolaRichard Mensah Adonu. (2024). Harnessing Artificial Intelligence for Early Detection and Management of Infectious Disease Outbreaks. *International Journal of Innovative Research and Development*. Advance online publication. DOI: 10.24940/ijird/2024/v13/i2/FEB24016

Iwelunmor, J., Newsome, V., & Airhihenbuwa, C. O. (2014). Framing the impact of culture on health: A systematic review of the PEN-3 cultural model and its application in public health research and interventions. *Ethnicity & Health*, *19*(1), 20–46. DOI: 10.1080/13557858.2013.857768 PMID: 24266638

Khoury, M. J., Bowen, M. S., Clyne, M., Dotson, W. D., Gwinn, M. L., Green, R. F., Kolor, K., Rodriguez, J. L., Wulf, A., & Yu, W. (2018). From public health genomics to precision public health: A 20-year journey. *Genetics in Medicine : Official Journal of the American College of Medical Genetics*, *20*(6), 574–582. DOI: 10.1038/gim.2017.211 PMID: 29240076

Lappalainen, H. K., Baklanov, A., Bäck, J., Arvanitidis, C., Basart, S., Bernier, N., Berod, D., Bornman, T., Buttigieg, P. L., Carmichael, G., Dañobeitia, J., De Roeck, Y.-H., Dey, S., Gerasopoulos, E., Feig, G., Gani, S., Glaves, H., Häme, S., Juurola, E., & Kulmala, M. (2025). Towards a Global Ground-Based Earth Observatory (GG-BEO): Leveraging existing systems and networks. *Big Earth Data*, *9*(4), 615–650. DOI: 10.1080/20964471.2025.2574174

Lazaro-Mojica, J., & Fernandez, R. (2021). Review paper on the future of the food sector through education, capacity building, knowledge translation and open innovation. *Current Opinion in Food Science*, *38*, 162–167. DOI: 10.1016/j.cofs.2020.11.009

Martins, J., Onofre, M., & Hallal, P. C. (2023). Launch of the Global Observatory for Physical Education (GoPE!). *Journal of Physical Activity & Health, 20*(7), 573–574. DOI: 10.1123/jpah.2023-0099 PMID: 37130590

Menon, S., & Koura, K. G. (2025). Artificial intelligence for tuberculosis control: A scoping review of applications in public health. *Journal of Global Health, 15*, 04192. DOI: 10.7189/jogh.15.04192 PMID: 40709592

Nykiforuk, C. I. J., & Flaman, L. M. (2011). Geographic Information Systems (GIS) for Health Promotion and Public Health: A Review. *Health Promotion Practice, 12*(1), 63–73. DOI: 10.1177/1524839909334624 PMID: 19546198

Odone, A., Buttigieg, S., Ricciardi, W., Azzopardi-Muscat, N., & Staines, A. (2019). Public health digitalization in Europe. *European Journal of Public Health, 29*(Supplement_3), 28–35. DOI: 10.1093/eurpub/ckz161 PMID: 31738441

Oyeyemi, A. L., Ramirez Varela, A., Lambert, E. V., Kohn, E. R., Hallal, P. C., & Pratt, M. (2024). An Overview of Physical Activity Research Evolution in Africa: The Global Observatory for Physical Activity—GoPA! *Journal of Physical Activity & Health, 21*(5), 434–444. DOI: 10.1123/jpah.2023-0455 PMID: 38412851

Pratt, M., Ramírez Varela, A., & Hallal, P. C. (2024). Celebrating 10 Years of the Global Observatory for Physical Activity—GoPA! *Journal of Physical Activity & Health, 21*(5), 423–424. DOI: 10.1123/jpah.2024-0233 PMID: 38621673

Ramirez-Montoya, M. S. (2020). Challenges for Open Education with Educational Innovation: A Systematic Literature Review. *Sustainability (Basel), 12*(17), 7053. DOI: 10.3390/su12177053

Ramírez Varela, A., Hallal, P. C., Mejía Grueso, J., Pedišić, Ž., Salvo, D., Nguyen, A., Klepac, B., Bauman, A., Siefken, K., Hinckson, E., Oyeyemi, A. L., Richards, J., Salih Khidir, E. D., Inoue, S., Amagasa, S., Jauregui, A., Da Silva, M. C., Lee, I.-M., Ding, M., & Pratt, M. (2023). Status and Trends of Physical Activity Surveillance, Policy, and Research in 164 Countries: Findings From the Global Observatory for Physical Activity—GoPA! 2015 and 2020 Surveys. *Journal of Physical Activity & Health, 20*(2), 112–128. DOI: 10.1123/jpah.2022-0464 PMID: 36535269

Ramirez Varela, A., Salvo, D., Pratt, M., Milton, K., Siefken, K., Bauman, A., Kohl, H. W.III, Lee, I.-M., Heath, G., Foster, C., Powell, K., & Hallal, P. C. (2018). Worldwide use of the first set of physical activity Country Cards: The Global Observatory for Physical Activity - GoPA! *The International Journal of Behavioral Nutrition and Physical Activity, 15*(1), 29. DOI: 10.1186/s12966-018-0663-7 PMID: 29587783

Riccomini, F. E., Cirani, C. B. S., Carvalho, C. C. D., & Storopoli, J. E. (2021). Educational innovation: Trends for higher education in Brazil. *International Journal of Educational Management*, *35*(3), 564–578. DOI: 10.1108/IJEM-07-2019-0245

Tracy, M., Cerdá, M., & Keyes, K. M. (2018). Agent-Based Modeling in Public Health: Current Applications and Future Directions. *Annual Review of Public Health*, *39*(1), 77–94. DOI: 10.1146/annurev-publhealth-040617-014317 PMID: 29328870

Varela, A. R., Pratt, M., Powell, K., Lee, I.-M., Bauman, A., Heath, G., Martins, R. C., Kohl, H., & Hallal, P. C. (2017). Worldwide Surveillance, Policy, and Research on Physical Activity and Health: The Global Observatory for Physical Activity. *Journal of Physical Activity & Health*, *14*(9), 701–709. DOI: 10.1123/jpah.2016-0626 PMID: 28513338

Zhuang, T., & Liu, B. (2022). Sustaining Higher Education Quality by Building an Educational Innovation Ecosystem in China—Policies, Implementations and Effects. *Sustainability (Basel)*, *14*(13), 7568. DOI: 10.3390/su14137568

Chapter 8

Tech-Driven Health Communication and Nudging in Oral-Systemic Care: The EpiDentomics Model

Jyotsna Slesha Sudharsan K.
http://orcid.org/0009-0008-5322-192X
Saveetha Dental College and Hospitals, India & SIMATS School of Management, Saveetha Institute of Medical and Technical Sciences (SIMATS), Saveetha University, Chennai, India

K. C. Raja Shree
http://orcid.org/0009-0009-1029-910X
Saveetha School of Management, Saveetha Institute of Medical and Technical Sciences, India

P. Praveen Kumar
http://orcid.org/0000-0002-0707-039X
SRM Institute of Science and Technology, Vadapalani, India

ABSTRACT

This chapter explores digital Public Health Campaigns, social media epidemiology and nudging for oral and systemic health promotion and also demonstrates the rise of "digital persuasion ecosystems", public health environments driven by social media data, real-time surveillance, AI-enabled communication, and behavioural science models. As global health systems move toward precision public health and data-informed decision-making, digital campaigns have grown more impactful,

DOI: 10.4018/979-8-3373-8402-3.ch008

reshaping how health education is created, delivered, and consumed. Within the broader EpiDentomics framework, digital public health becomes a central pillar for preventing both oral diseases and systemic conditions connected to oral health.

INTRODUCTION

One of the tribulations in the entire world is dental problems, which pose a burden on the health of both poor and rich countries. According to the World Health Organization and the Global Burden of Disease Study, 3.5 billion individuals in the globe have dental issues. These issues actually impact the lives of people due to such reasons as tooth decay, loss of teeth, and mouth cancer due to gum disease. Such kinds of dental problems make people find it difficult to live. The World Health Organization and the Global Burden of Disease Study are discussing such problems as dental caries, periodontitis, and teeth and oral malignancy loss (Sanz et al., 2020). Despite the fact that severe periodontitis disables the functional ability of hundreds of millions of the world's population, with a strong tendency of poor quality-of-life changes and socioeconomic costs, the most widespread health issue in the world is dental caries in permanent teeth. Dental conditions are preventable conditions, which remain common in the lifespan of an individual and induce a lot of inequality since they are known to cause disparities in health, mostly between the socio-economically vulnerable social groupings.

The point is, medical services and oral health remain objects. They are isolated despite the fact that we are increasingly aware of the ways in which issues with our teeth and mouth can impact our body. We are discussing such things as diabetes and heart disease and pregnancy problems and breathing infections and muscle problems. Dental health and healthcare are discrete, although we possess much evidence that they are interrelated. This happens in the case of healthcare and dental health. Systemic inflammatory processes in general have been shown to be influenced by oral inflammatory processes, whereas the connection between oral and systemic disease has been emphasized by common risk factors such as tobacco use, poor dietary habits, stress, and poor hygienic practices (Tu et al., 2023). Oral health goals are also not factored into national surveillance systems or objectives of universal health coverage.

Conventional promotion programs on oral health have been based virtually solely on an informational approach to education with the supposition that increased knowledge will inevitably translate to healthier behaviour. School-based lectures, brochures, posters, and ad hoc awareness campaigns are still widespread as methods in public health. However, decades of behavioural science have determined that knowledge is an insufficient basis for maintaining behaviour change (Oyekunle et al., 2024). Oral health behaviours are strongly affected by habits, social rules, emotional incentives, accessibility, and environmental prompts, including the frequency of brushing teeth, sugar consumption, cessation of smoking, and use of dental care. The ongoing disparity between promise and delivery of oral health promotion relying on education highlights the ineffectiveness of one-way models of communication that do not consider the contextual constraints or cognitive biases and motivational deficits. Consequently, the majority of the oral health education initiatives are more likely to increase the awareness in the short term but have minimal long-term effects on preventing diseases.

The digital transformation is currently the paradigm shift in the sphere of public health as it influences the creation, distribution, and consumption of health-related information

(Keesara et al., 2020). The AI-related products of AI, big data analytics systems, mHealth solutions, and social network platforms provide various AI-related technologies like real-time communications, customized therapies, and mass surveillance to a degree that never existed before over the past century. Social networking sites like Instagram, YouTube, and TikTok, and social network platforms like X and previous sites like Twitter platforms, e.g., have become ecosystems where different myths and ideals related to health are exchanged and presented at any given time. The technologies that are based on AI processes can process massive amounts of information to find trends and anticipate threats, and take actions in accordance with the generated identity in both individual and social dimensions.

The COVID-19 pandemic has made the application of telehealth and digital health communication faster globally. Lockdowns, inability to reach dental practices, and health issues in general make communities and health professionals have no alternative but to rely on digital platforms widely to obtain health information. Teleconsultation services, mobile apps, chatbots, health-related education campaigns on the web, and the spread of algorithmic content have become invaluable to the continuity of health and involvement in communities. It is interesting to note that one of the relevant lessons of the COVID-19 pandemic is the positives and negatives of digital health to be readily influenced or poorly influenced regarding health behaviours and health outcomes. The necessity of evidence-based and ethical approaches in digital health during that time has been emphasized (Salathe al., 2012).

Considering this evolving landscape, there seems to be an increasing awareness of the fact that fluid risky behaviours, incessant living circumstances, and dynamism in the motivations of people cannot and ought not to be dealt with by the implementation of generic health communications where their focus is on only some of the episodes and behaviours, and with their objectives being only short-term objectives. Behavioural nudges and behavioural insights that influence individuals to make healthy decisions without employing forceful interventions are slowly becoming crucial aspects in contemporary health systems and interventions.

It is against this backdrop that the idea of EpiDentomics is an integrative concept in the spirit of systemic and dental health promotion. Epidemiology, dentomics the combination of clinical, biological, and behavioural oral health data, artificial intelligence, and digital nudging have come together to constitute EpiDentomics. EpiDentomics is geared towards closing the gap in oral and general health systems over the years in terms of population-level surveillance and individual-level behavioural intelligence. This approach involves clinical-source-in-real-time, social media, and digital health data in order to assist in the creation of accurate public health measures in an equitable, adaptable, and scalable way.

The EpiDentomics model of dental disease prevention is one that acknowledges that dental disease prevention is a dynamic environment. The initial point of initiation begins with the constant flow of data that is handled through artificial intelligence analysis methods, like digital behaviour patterns and oral-related information collection and analysis. The information system is digital, and it offers the channel of delivery of interventions and communication products that are required to deliver to the community (Michie et al., 2011). The purpose of feedback processes in this chapter is to enable and to solicit reactions to emerging disease threats and behavioural patterns, through the synthesis of oral disease prevention and the creation of full digital public health systems and research through the EpiDentomics approach, which is the third objective. Secondly, exploring what seems to be a radical change in the sphere of oral health promotion due to the knowledge and innovations linked to the digital technologies, as well as the new ideas of AI and social media, and their usages in and to the new post-COVID reality formed by the population, and influencing human behaviours (Fathima & Sakthi, 2023). Thirdly, the chapter acts as a platform and conceptual entry point to our EpiDentomics integrative framework, a proposed conceptual framework indicating a vision of accuracy, stakeholder involvement, and a future-oriented and values-driven approach and perspective to the promotion of dental and systemic health.

This monograph and this introductory first chapter are split into three sections: First, this chapter presents and discusses a theoretical base and framework concerning digital public health and its innovations; secondly, this chapter also presents and discusses a detailed framework of EpiDentomics and its related specific definition; and thirdly, this monograph ends with a conclusion and future research and application suggestions.

THEORETICAL FOUNDATIONS

The EpiDentomics paradigm is based on several interconnected fields of theorizing that collectively account for the development, maintenance, and treatment response of oral health outcomes. The various viewpoints introducing the dynamics of oral and systemic health in the digital age are facilitated by the above frameworks that cross-cut across disciplines, including the biological and behavioural, to the digital.

Oral–Systemic Health Theory: The characteristic feature of the concept of oral-systemic health is a strengthened connection between oral health and systemic health. It claims that oral disease is a clinical and physiological health issue that does not differ from systemic health. Actually, the co-relationship between periodontitis and diabetes mellitus is the most investigated example of the association relationships between oral disease and systemic health. Periodontitis, which is an incurable bacterial infection of dental biofilms leading to an inflammatory condition, has been revealed to influence diabetes regulation in diabetic patients. The causes of insulin resistance are pro-inflammatory mediators released as a consequence of the inflammation of the periodontal tissues (C-reactive protein, interleukin-6, and tumour necrosis factor-alpha) released into the bloodstream. (Taylor & Borgnakke, 2008) Diabetes causes high blood sugar that may lead to the aggravation of gum disease. It interferes with the process of fighting infection in your body, and you become more likely to be infected and lose tissue in your gums. It is a two-way road: any issues with the metabolism of your body may lead to problems with your mouth, and vice versa. In addition to diabetes, the concept of oral health and overall health association means that the distribution of bacteria and chronic inflammation are the mechanisms through which dental complications are associated with respiratory infections, brain problems, heart diseases, and pregnancy issues (Baima et al., 2025). Infection in the gums and the bad stuff that they produce can be transferred to the blood by the sores in your gums. This may result in the condition of your blood vessels and cause plaque formation. In addition, the inhalation of oral germs has also been associated with lung infection, predominantly in elderly individuals and those already ill. The Oral-Systemic Health Theory dwells upon the significance of perceiving pastoral disease prevention as a systemic health effect rather than a dental problem. The early detection and management of the general health care issues related to oral health care can guarantee the improved quality of life, cut down the fringe health care expenses, and save the general health care without any problems. EpiDentomics is guided by the oral-systemic health theory in its approach in general.

Shared Risk Factor Approach (SRFA): The Shared Risk Factor Approach is a population-level theoretical paradigm that describes the factor that explains why oral disorders appear to co-occur with other NCDs. It considers the combination of behavioural, social, and environmental factors, which each contribute to the occurrence of many health outcomes simultaneously, instead of addressing a disease individually, and prioritizes all the conditions under investigation equally (Sheiham & Watt, 2000). The major common risk factors are tobacco use, high sugar and excessive alcohol use, chronic stress, inactivity, and poor hygiene practices. As an example, tobacco smoking is a significant risk factor for heart disease, chronic respiratory disease, oral cancer, and periodontal disease. On the same note, high sugar consumption leads to metabolic syndrome, type 2 diabetes, obesity, and caries. Psychosocial stress has influence on oral parafunctional habits, immunological functionality, food choices, and compliance to health behaviour. SRFA is actually vital in areas where resources are limited, as treatment of certain diseases may be prohibitively costly or difficult to access by all persons. Health promotion can make a greater impact on a wider range of diseases by addressing the factors that bring the health issues in the first place. Delivering campaigns using digital platforms is very rational since the issues of several risky behaviours can be addressed simultaneously with uniform messages and change-supporting options. The digital medium can provide integrated campaigns that promote reduction of stress, good hygiene, healthy eating, and smoking cessation in a single communication system. To illustrate, when a digital program assists in reducing the amount of sugar consumed by people, it would prevent diabetes, obesity, and cavities simultaneously. EpiDentomics framework applies SRFA to ensure that the promotion of oral health is not an independent operation as a prevention measure of non-communicable diseases but rather a component of the overall plan.

Behavioural Science and Nudging: The findings in the study of behaviour have questioned people acting rationally in making personal health-related choices. Although the real-world actions are not necessarily in the standards of rationality due to cognitive limitations, feelings, and other environmental cues, the undeterred view of health education presupposes that human beings evaluate their health hazards and advantages in a rational manner. Dual-process theories of cognition identify two styles of thinking. This comprises System 1, which happens to be fast-paced and automatic and is characterized by the use of habits and routines, and System 2, which happens to be systematic and slow and is characterized by the use of reasoning and thinking. The automatic processing System 1 rules most of our daily habits pertaining to our health and hygiene, including brushing your teeth, enjoying some snacks, smoking, and even paying visits to the dental office, all of which are dominated by the automatic processing of System 1. According to Thaler and Sunstein (2008), nudging is a concept in behavioural economics that entails changes to the environment, which are small. Such changes make us choose better habits, but we are free to make our own choices. Nudges can be used to assist with health by appealing to our healthier instincts through such means as standard options, reminders, feedback, and what is seen as normal in society. As an illustration, in oral health, you can come across messages on how other people are maintaining their hygiene in their mouths. Or, you might have the automatic brush or floss reminders. The other concept is having signs leading to sugar-free alternatives or even having dental check-ups as the default one. They have the potential to enhance the effectiveness of nudges because we can easily access information in a short amount of time and manipulate it to suit us through the use of digital tools. The action section of the EpiDentomics concept is behavioural science and nudging, to transform our daily information into the ability to change what we are doing. EpiDentomics is not just a matter of sharing information but is extended to long-term behavioural change because therapies are compared to the real human decision-making processes.

Digital Epidemiology and Infodemiology: Digital epidemiology can, using the tools of digital data flows, such as social media messages, search engine queries, mobile application data, and online forums, offer surveillance of population health in near real time and thereby expand the traditional surveillance tools (Salathé, et al., 2018). The reason behind this is that, unlike the traditional surveys or medical care, digital data is reflective of spontaneous reporting of symptoms, behaviour, opinions, and the emotional state. Social media platforms are like health barometers of the people, and they provide a pointer of new trends towards popular opinion, health-seeking behaviours, and perceptions of diseases. Using different analytics methods, like sentiment analysis and topic modelling, researchers can track the dissemination of false information and define the increasing number of people worried about the issue and reactions to health interventions. One more area to be considered is infodemiology, which examines the dissemination of health-related information (true and false) through the Internet and how it works. Poor information spreads like a wildfire in times of health crisis, damaging the prevention efforts. Myths on dental work, home remedies, and fluoride are common in oral health on the Internet (Abidin, 2018). They can alter the decision-making process of the people in relation to obtaining treatment, as well as the level of trust they have in dentists. Digital epidemiology is relevant to the issue of oral health since it is able to identify premature conditions in the behaviours of people prior to visiting a dentist. To give an example, the number of individuals who would begin discussing toothaches, bleeding gums, or fear of the dentist could increase. This information will assist in determining where to invest resources, risk discussions, and the online projects to concentrate on. Imagine that digital epidemiology is the brains of the EpiDentomics system. It allows you to monitor things, make a plan in seconds and create oral health campaigns that are improved by what you learn.

Integrative Role in the EpiDentomics Model: These theoretical underpinnings combined together support the multi-layered nature of the EpiDentomics model. Biological rationale of integration is determined by oral-systemic health theory; population-level prevention rationale is ensured by SRFA; the design of successful intervention is informed by behavioural science and nudgifor; and real-time intelligence is ensured by digital epidemiology. Their combination allows promoting oral and systemic health in a precision-oriented, behaviour-oriented, digitally responsive way.

RESEARCH GAP

There are lack of existing frameworks that amalgamates the oral-systemic health with technology and behavioural dimensions. Also, existing studies highly focus on surveys and fragmented interventions. We can witness the confined integration of social media data, electronic health records and behavioural inputs. Therefore, the proposed model namely EpiDentomics framework would address the gap and assist in implementing digital public health network.

Table 1. Positioning EpiDentomics within Existing Frameworks

Framework	Focus	Limitation	EpiDentomics Contribution
Precision Public Health	Population prediction	Limited oral health focus	Integrates oral-systemic health
Learning Health Systems	Continuous learning	Limited behavioural nudging	Includes AI nudges
Precision Dentistry	Clinical oral care	Limited population perspective	Population + individual focus
Digital Epidemiology	Surveillance	Limited intervention design	Surveillance + intervention
AI Health Ecosystems	Prediction	Limited oral integration	Oral-systemic integration

The EpiDentomics Conceptual Model

The EpiDentomics conceptual model is presented as a digital-enabled, integrative model that is expected to overcome the historical limitations of promoting oral health and preventing illness. The model provides a theoretical framework for understanding the dynamics of oral-systemic health coupled with an operational infrastructure of implementing behaviour-focused, precision-oriented, and public health interventions by integrating epidemiology, dentomics, artificial intelligence, and behavioural science.

Figure 1. Epidentomics

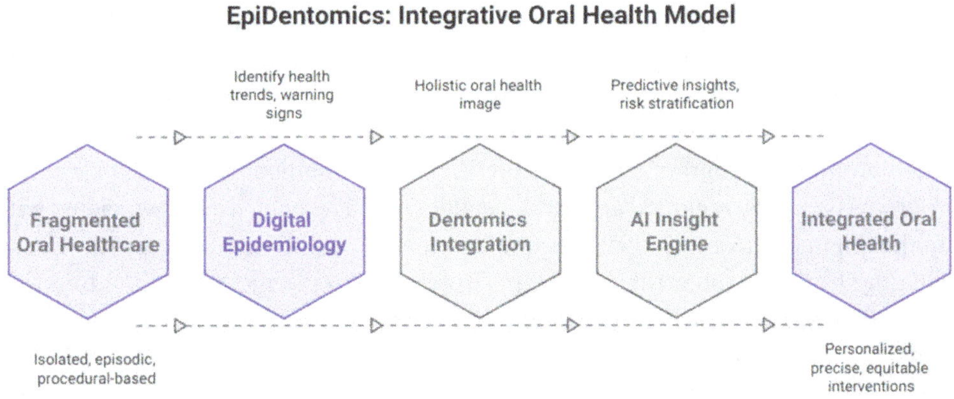

Source: *(Primary)*

There is the fragmentation of the demographic, healthcare, and behavioural spheres in the contemporary oral healthcare. Clinical dentistry has failed to transition to a more episodic and procedural-based system within a closed system which does not have any connection with the public health infrastructure, and surveillance trends are being collected on a demographic basis in a routine that is not very relevant to healthcare. As far as the behavioural approaches are concerned, they are often short-term and generic with respect to healthcare. Due to this sub-specialty, there is a lack of space in addressing the more associated causes of oral sickness, a healthcare interruption, or timely diagnosis of the condition. The health promotion programs involving oral health continue to operate in isolation even though they share similar risk factors with respect to the biological links. The related oral health practices in this age of modern technology still portray severely changing trends or erroneous forces and sociocultural tendencies, which the existing healthcare networks are not addressing effectively. The EpiDentomics model assists in integrating various things in two significant aspects. First, it uses data on a large number of individuals to identify health trends in time. Second, it links data of your mouth to your health condition. Third, it applies what it learns to assist people to make long-term and healthy changes. The fact that this model is practical is what matters. It provides us with a means to intervene, obtain feedback, and improve on matters with time. It is also able to interpret much complex information. This makes it a thing of learning and improving, rather than a fixed, independent activity, to take care of your mouth.

Digital Epidemiology Layer: Current oral healthcare is fragmented in terms of the demographic, healthcare, and behavioural spheres. Clinical dentistry remains largely episodic and procedure-based within a closed system that is not linked to the public health infrastructure, and surveillance trends are regularly gathered on a demographic basis that has minimal connection to healthcare. In the case of behavioural approaches, they are often short-run and generic to healthcare. The consequence of this subspecialty is a lack of room to address the more-associated causes of oral illness, a healthcare interruption, or late detection of the disease. Although there are similarities in the risk factors in relation to the biological associations, the health promotion program on oral health in non-communicable disease prevention programs is usually regarded as an independent one. The behaviours associated with oral health in this age of modern technology are still exhibiting the very drastically changing trends or the erroneous trends in relation to the model and the trends in sociocultural aspects, which even the existing healthcare networks cannot address effectively. Using such tools as natural language processing, trend detection, and checking the overall sentiment towards something, we can notice the warning signs early. This assists us in becoming aware of such things as the appearance of more fake news (such as the antifluoride stories), people becoming more interested in self-care that is dangerous, or people losing their confidence in dentists. Such hints come in so handy in cases where we do not have a lot of official or current dental data. AI also helps improve the situation with the help of location maps and risk information. Combining internet hints with data concerning the location of inhabitants and their identity, AI can locate at-risk communities, predict where the illness may be concentrated, and assist in the planning of particular actions to assist. In EpiDentomics, digital info used in this manner transforms simple observation of what happens to valuable information about the health of the people.

Dentomics and Clinical Integration: Dentomics is the scientific combination of clinical information of the oral cavity, molecular pathomarkers, behavioural indicators, and contextual information during the development of a holistic image of oral health in the context of systemic health. Dentomics is a congruent approach to an interdisciplinary approach to the conception of precision medicine, unlike traditional dentistry that addresses pathology at a tooth level. Examples of clinical data inputs include EHRs, periodontal measurements, caries measurements, salivary biomarkers, inflammatory measurements and patient-reported outcomes (Khoury et al., 2016). The data will be used to contextualize systemic health indicators like glycemic management, cardiovascular risk profiles and pregnancy status. As an example, mouth infections in pregnant patients can give indications of heightened risks of adverse outcomes, and periodontal inflammation could be an indicator of metabolism mismanagement in diabetics. Dentomics bridges the gap between dentistry and medicine, and two-way clinical integration is possible. Doctors understand that the health of the mouth can be altered to determine health. The dentists are in a better position to comprehend issues of the system that modify the progress of oral diseases. In the EpiDentomics model, Dentomics ensures that treatments, behavioural as well as digital, are biologically sound and clinically relevant.

One of the premises of the model of EpiDentomics analysis is a representation of the artificial intelligence of the Insight Engine. It produces predictive insights, risk stratification, and data to support decisions using information from both digital epidemiology and dentomics. It determines individuals and groups of people with different vulnerability to topical and systemic diseases through the implementation of the risk scoring process through machine learning algorithms. Prospective models are done on disease progression, non-adherence by choice, and response to treatment. Above all, these models continuously enhance their forecasts with the new developments. It implies that the primary task of this layer is the personalization and segmentation. Instead of sending a unified message, the AI engine decides, looking at behavioural readiness, risk profile and others, whom to send what message using what method of communication and when. An example would be when one who has early gum disease fails to attend appointments, he or she might be reminded. In case an individual consumes much sugar, they may be advised on the changes in diet. This AI device is not going to substitute experts; it is only going to assist them in making better decisions. It assists in ensuring that oral health programs are effective, more precise, and equitable by informing the authors of the resources and the steps to be implemented. Improvements in the Digital Health Communication Pathway are planned to be provided to patients in the area.

Figure 2. Framework of Epidentomics

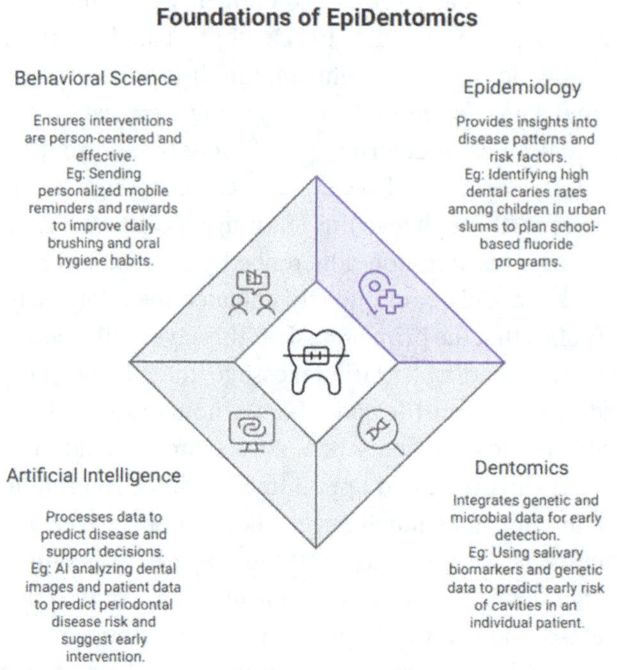

Source: *(Primary)*

DIGITAL HEALTH COMMUNICATION PATHWAY

It is intended to offer better enhancements of the Digital Health Communication Pathway to patients in the area. The information that becomes available after analysis is operationalized to be engaged through the Digital Health Communication Pathway. Some of the pathways that fall under this are chatbots, SMS alerts, mobile applications, teleconsultations, and learning environments. EpiDentomics tends to be more concerned with the micro-message, the communication that can be easily fitted in the busy schedule and is not based on the traditional approach of treating dental disease by means of education. Brushing, appointment reminders, suggestions regarding the reduction of sugar in the diet, and eliminating fears of seeing the dentist are only some of the examples of what these may encompass. The benefit of being able to continue with clinic visits is one of the strengths that this pathway provides. Cyber communications minimize reliance on physical gatherings at intervals as the clients are kept up to date on the treatment and also by offering qualified and real-time consultation. This strategy prospers the dental care outside settings where there is a scarcity of dental facilities.

Behavioural Nudging Engine

The Behavioural Nudging Engine facilitates effective, but subtle, change in oral healthcare practice by applying concepts that are a result of behavioural economics and psychology. Nudging alters the environment where the choices are changed to create an environment or area where the preferred choices are viable and alluring instead of forcing a person to make a particular choice. General techniques might include nudges concerning cues and prompts, defaults (i.e., automatic recall appointment reminders), gamification, and social proof messages. Dental-specific nudges may include visual cue reminder notices in regard to the practice of brushing and flossing and messages giving comparisons in regard to the dedication of the dental community to preventive measures. Although this layer is most important in the low- and middle-income country environment, where norms, literacy, and access to technology, among others, are very much dependent, cultural sensitivity is central to this layer. To ensure that no force or stigma is developed, the design of the nudge must be of high ethical standards and linguistic needs. Nudging Applicability Epistemology of EpiDentomics in practice.

Behavioural Response: "Behavioural response" refers to the fact that people do begin to act and maintain good dental habits. It encompasses such issues as brushing your teeth, reducing the amount of sugar in your diet, quitting smoking, visiting the dentist, and ensuring that the problems are addressed promptly. EpiDentomics is virtually obsessed with monitoring behavioural of individuals. They also focus on what is measurable, like when individuals report that they have sticking to their behaviours, whether they are adhering to a plan, the frequency of using the app, and whether they attend their appointments. These statistics provide good evidence that the approaches are effective and contribute to the enhancement of the system continuously.

Oral systemic health outcomes: Once they do permanent modifications to habits, it contributes to health in most ways; fewer cavities, healthy gums, and the capacity to control blood sugar better. They are also less painful, more functional, and happier. Such positive outcomes also result in the reduction of medical expenditure, equitable care access, and the superiority of dental and general care coordination. The EpiDentomics approach demonstrates how our behaviour can be altered to prevent illness and enhance well-being. It creates a clear connection between our actions, what happens in our bodies, and the effect of that on our system.

Feedback Loop: There is an EpiDentomics as a learning health system due to its feedback loop. The AI Insight Engine continuously receives information on what people are doing and how they are doing in the clinic, which allows the system to improve itself over time. This feedback will allow the system to recover fast in case of new threats, people getting weary of modifying their actions, or false information being transmitted. The model improves over time, is more accurate, learns the cultural differences, and is more effective in promoting good oral as well as total health.

The uses of the EpiDentomics conceptual framework extend beyond the theoretical description, as it is backed up by the empirical data that points to the relevance of the digital communication strategies to boost health. This section discusses some of the critical trends that have been discovered during research on communication strategy-based interventions through the power of influencers and application of health initiatives on the internet in India. To show how the level is applicable in real life, all the illustrations are connected with the level.

Evidence-based Digital Oral Health Interventions:

In the last 10 years, digital oral health programs have not only abandoned simple and unaltered teaching aids but also more interactive platforms that emphasize behaviour. It has been demonstrated that such features as mobile applications, text notifications, and web-based programs may significantly help improve the way individuals brush their teeth, control plaque, and make dental appointments, in contrast to traditional instructional strategies alone (Fedele et al., 2020; Scheerman et al., 2018). Indeed, certain studies have discovered that mobile tooth brushing applications with reminders, feedback, and tracking of progress may make kids and teens brush more frequently and with less plaque. There is no need to merely provide information, but these programs enable the creation of good habits through providing reminders at the appropriate time. Likewise, it has been demonstrated that text message reminder systems can make people, in particular, underserved groups of people, visit the dentist more frequently and receive preventive care.

Mapping to EpiDentomics Layers

Digital Epidemiology Layer: The usage data and self-reports reveal the existence of the poor brushing frequency, missed appointments, poor brushing frequency, etc.

AI Insight Engine: The users are divided according to levels of adherence and risk profiles.

Digital Health Communication Pathway: Individualized feedback messages and all reminders are provided through apps or SMS.

Behavioural Nudging Engine: Prompts, goal tracking, and positive feedback strengthen the formation of habits.

Behavioural Response & Outcomes: Better oral hygiene practices lead to plgingivalgingivial reduction.

These findings offer the background evidence that digitally mediated, behaviour-based interventions are highly consistent with the logic of the EpiDentomics model. We take self-reports and data to detect normal behaviour, such as the failure to brush teeth or attend appointments. After that, AI organizes users into categories according to the risk and adherence to the program. Thereafter, we send reminders and suggestions in the form of apps or texts that are customized to them. We encourage, track goals, and give tips to assist people in developing better habits. The result? Improved oral health will result in less plaque and swollen gums. These findings will provide a clear picture of the fact that concentrating on behaviour with the help of digital means will be effective with the EpiDentomics model.

Figure 3. Epidentomics Approach

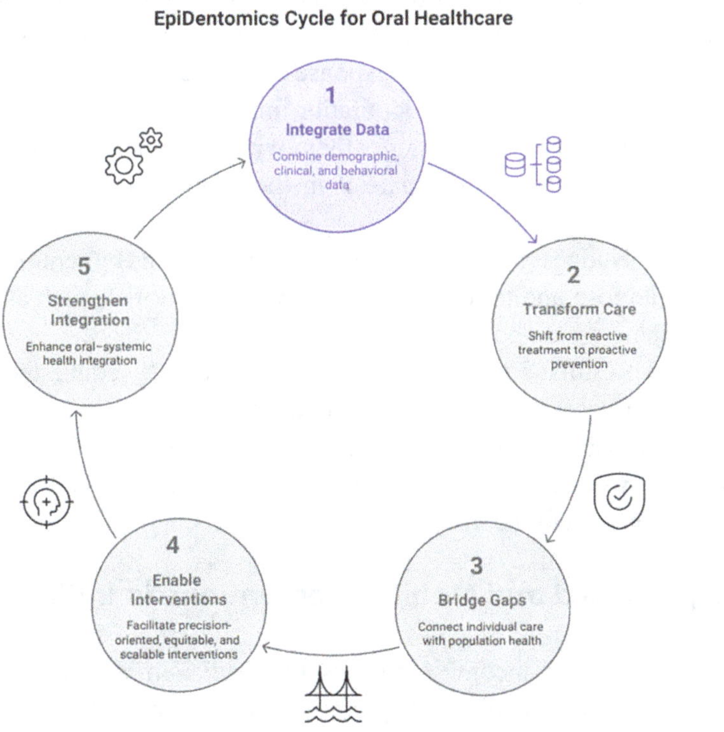

Source: *(Primary)*

Public Health Multimedia Programs

Social media has become an excellent source of passing health information, particularly when discussing the matters that leave your body and mouth in trouble. To illustrate, Facebook, Instagram, and YouTube anti-smoking advertisements have actually altered the manner in which individuals perceive smoking, the level of their knowledge about it, and whether they desire to quit smoking (Majmundar et al., 2020). Common teaching techniques are not as effective as displaying stories, getting people to relate their experiences, and messages that appeal to the emotions. The same happens with the programs that attempt to make people reduce their sugar consumption (typically in order to avoid obesity and diabetes), which indirectly benefit the teeth. Such factors as sugar taxes and smoking the campaign to reveal the fact of how much sugar is in food have taken their effect. It is discussed more, and people are behaving differently, thus resulting in less consumption of sugary drinks in certain places (Falbe et al., 2022).

Digital Epidemiology: We follow the trending topics with the use of social media or detect fake news. We examine the response of people to posts on sugar or tobacco.

AI Insights: We segment the population into segments, such as teenagers or high-risk segments, to be able to target them with the appropriate messages.

Digital Communication: We share it in the form of short videos, posts, and hashtags.

Behavioural Nudges: So we very quietly steer decisions by reminding people of what they could lose and telling them about what is normal, such as the majority of people of their age do not smoke.

The Health Results: Reduced sugar and tobacco will reduce the risk of such things as gum disease, cavities, and certain cancers.

These advertisements endorse the concept of Shared Risk Factor Approach of EpiDentomics by illustrating the possibility of using one digital intervention to treat multiple diseases simultaneously.

WhatsApp-Based and Mobile Interventions in India

In low- and middle-income countries like India, in which smartphones are used widely, WhatsApp and mobile phone-based interventions are acceptable and widely used as well. A collection of community-based tests has reported how useful WhatsApp-based health communications messages could become in terms of eliminating tobacco use and controlling diabetes and maternity treatment (Arora et al., 2024).

Health Communication Campaigns

One of the emerging trends in the sphere of healthcare communication, especially among the younger generation, is healthcare advertising with the help of the influencers. Health communication done by credible influencers such as the gym or health-related blogger or health professionals is more effective as compared to the health communication done by the healthcare institution itself. Influencers have been utilized in the promotion of orthodontic adherence, smoking, and oral care as well as cosmetic dental practice in the situation (oral health). Shorter videos may be simple to involve the audiences in demonstrating how to brush their teeth, the falsehoods regarding fluorides, or the personal experience of dropping the habit of using smokeless tobacco.

How Epidemics Connect:

The Digital Epidemiology: Likes, shares, and comments present how individuals feel and what they think.

AI Insights: Content is presented to users that have similar interests or risky behaviours through platform algorithms.

The influencers pass information in a simple yet effective manner that attracts the attention of people.

Behavioural Nudges: As an observer, one may be strongly affected by the idea that this is how people like me behave.

Behavioural Change: This may be able to get people to desire to challenge poor behaviours and begin good ones.

Planning the content of an influencer ethically and supporting it with data will correspond with the intention of EpiDentomics to target the real-world behaviour and specific circumstances.

Public Health Surveillance and Planning

One of the critical uses of the EpiDentomics approach is improvement in the oral health surveillance and strategic planning. Traditional surveillance systems involve regular data gathering and reporting based on clinical locations, which in most occasions are expensive and time-consuming, besides being limited in their regions. By further developing digital epidemiology, EpiDentomics offers an extension and a further enhancement to conventional surveillance systems by allowing practically real-time dental health surveillance on risks and behaviours. With merely a glance at what people are discussing on social media, what they are searching on the internet and the level of their engagement in their localities, the public health folks can identify when there is something amiss. By way of example, they may realize that more people are complaining of toothaches, that there was an influx of misinformation, or that fewer people were getting check-ups. Through this information, politicians will be able to allocate the resources more effectively, targeting those who require help the most, and strategize in advance. AI-based maps provide an opportunity to locate underserved regions and disease concentration areas, which simplifies exceptionally local planning. EpiDentomics decides on public health in a better, fairer, and quicker way. It transforms the post-factum checking of oral health into the pre-factum planning.

Integrated Medical-Dental Care

EpiDentomics provides us with a good path to close the excavation between medical and dental care, hence allowing the integration of medical and dental care. Combining dental and medical data makes oral health an important component of the overall condition of a person, as well as their healthcare. Because clinics can share dentists, NIC health records, and use AI to assist in decision-making, this creates an opportunity to have two-way referrals and more coordinated care. As an illustration, when one has a severe gum infection, he or she may be referred to test the presence of metabolic or cardiac factors. And diabetes patients who do not have their glucose levels under control may be referred to a gum test. Online technologies are additional to anchoring the work of doctors and dentists, making it seem simpler to adhere to the treatment plan during the intervals between the appointments. This plan helps oral health to be taken more seriously in the case of a long-term illness, reduces the number of repeated services, and ensures that your care is consistent. EpiDentomics is an initiative that advocates the full healthcare system, which is patient-centered by integrating dental health into larger healthcare systems.

Rural, Remote, and Underserved Populations

EpiDentomics is effective in rural or isolated areas that do not have sufficient dentists or resources or that are simply too distant to dental offices. These communities can be truly connected to healthcare by means of digital tools. With the texts or messaging apps, the individuals can be informed on how to avoid the issue of dental problems, be reminded about the appointments with the dentist, and be informed about potential hazards, all without having to meet a dentist on a regular basis. In addition, these online prompts can make individuals start caring more about their teeth and gums, which can prevent the acceleration of tooth decay and reduce the number of visits to the emergency room. Electronic information can also be used to determine what type of dental services a community requires the most. The most important thing about the model is that it aims at adapting to various cultures and circumstances. In this manner, the messages are read in the appropriate language and that which is mindful of local practices. EpiDentomics can bridge this gap by spreading oral health awareness beyond the clinic setting and ensuring that preventive care is more equitable to all.

Non-Communicable Disease (NCD) Program Integration

Dental problems and big health issues such as diabetes can be linked in the same risks and biology, and therefore, EpiDentomics can be useful in programs that aim at preventing and curing non-communicable diseases (NCDs), particularly among moms and those with diabetes. Such aspects as gum health can be used in dealing with diabetes, and it will reveal early whether a person has unregulated sugar in the blood. Integrated care can facilitate getting people to visit a dentist on time, and reminders can ensure that people care about their teeth and visit a dentist. Message dispatching on dental health will reduce the risk of gum issues in the course of pregnancy and poor outcomes in mom programs. EpiDentomics can enhance the existing NCD plans when we integrate oral health into the plans. This increases the significance of dental health to the overall health, and it assists us in dealing with the common risk factors. The EpiDentomics model is flexible, scalable, and applicable to various areas of application. Citizens can use the paradigm to promote oral health in a data-driven, behaviour-based, and equity-driven manner, regardless of whether it is applied in surveillance, integrated care, education, or chronic disease management. One of the strongest points is its capacity to convert rather complex theoretical concepts into practical and context-sensitive interventions that can be used to enhance the current public health priorities.

Analysis and Implementation

To adequately apply the findings of oral health to the oral health in the population and consequently change the manner in which the findings influence the population through their related reactions, it is essential that one employ configuration procedures, having taken into account ethics, contextual ethics, and systematics. Ethical nudges are non-compelling but helpful treatments that allow people to make more effective decisions without impairing their autonomy and their informed consent. Some examples of nudges in the specialty of oral health can include simplification of intricate treatment options frameworks, default appointment alerts to preventive check-ups, and visual prompts to desirable habits, including quitting smoking or brushing your teeth twice in one day. Nudges should be morally right, and this means that they should be transparent and beneficial. The right to choose should be offered to people, and people should not be obliged to change their behaviour, but rather, based on solid behaviour data, intervention should be made. The specific type of nudging, ethical nudging, can play the role of not only bridging the gap between knowing and doing when it aligns with the goals of public health without further widening inequalities or diminishing trust in healthcare systems.

Countering Misinformation

The fact that evidence-based preventive programs on oral health are highly sabotaged by the swift dissemination of falsehoods about health information, especially in the digital and social space (Sekhar & Prabakar, 2023). Misconceptions regarding the complementary treatments, overestimation of dangers of the dentures, or insufficient confidence in the health care of the professionals may damage the health-seeking behaviours. The right approaches to reduce such problems involve connecting with trusted messengers, proper information dispersion in due time, and keeping track of the trends in health information dispersion. A simple, uniform, and ready form of communication would be the debunking of digital platforms and presented health information, and this is what dental and health organizations should take on. The most notable aspect to observe here is that instead of engaging in a conflict, engagement and education need to be the center of attention in order to develop the required health literacy in countering health misinformation.

RESULTS AND IMPLICATIONS

The individuals who are to design, implement, and effect the oral health care should also be taken into consideration in the translation of the conceptual ideas into the practical impact. The real-life applications of the ideas presented in this work have not only a scientific viewpoint but can also be viewed according to the human perspective. This point of view recognizes the fact of the influence of the ideas on the human condition.

The main task of the policymakers is to establish the favourable environment in which innovation can do justice to equity, morality, and credibility. The regulators must be updated to adapt to emerging digital oral health products, including tele dentistry, AI-based risk assessment, and mobile health apps, and do it with the dual role of safeguarding patient rights and data protection. Definite standards on interoperability, ethical use of information, and responsibility will be necessary so as not to be fragmented or abused.

Among the opportunities is the implementation of oral health in the regional and national digital health strategies. Dental health might be incorporated into the digital health systems of the future, which can facilitate information sharing, care continuum, and surveillance at the population level. Historically, oral health has not been part and parcel of bigger health systems. Oral health indicators should be prioritized in digital health dashboards by policymakers to develop prevention and early detection services, which are equal in importance to curative ones. The policymaking should integrate community voices simultaneously, as there is a great gap between the level of digital inclusion, knowledge, and access among various communities.

The implications are more personal to the physician considering that he/she has direct experience with the impact on patient interaction. The task of the professional becomes to broaden his or her area of work beyond the technical sphere of work to provide advice and speak in the context of the change of a new standard of preventive and digitally enabled oral healthcare. A patient-engagement approach can be used to optimize outcomes by involving the patient as a partner instead of an object.

To maintain continuity of care, technology like teleconsultation, electronic record systems, and reminder services may be well applied, particularly in chronic cases and cases that are distant to services. Technology must complement the therapeutic bond, rather than replace the bond. It is necessary to strike such a balance between being efficient and being empathetic so as to prevent the negative effects of interfaces on the human interface required of all therapeutic success. To this end, the aspect of professional growth in digital and patient communication skills will have to be pursued.

Oral health systems remind the citizen of his/her continued significance to them through the daily intercourse of the citizen and the daily choices made; citizens do exert a greater influence upon a citizen's health status as compared to infrequent clinical visits. Empowering those individuals who have the right to define and actively engage in maintaining their oral health throughout their lives by equipping them with the appropriate knowledge, skills, and resources to maintain their oral health in a productive way.

The digital systems can develop the potential to alter the manner in which the citizen develops an active interaction with her/his oral health using personalized reminders, educational content, and self-monitoring equipment to facilitate preventive behaviours. Empowerment should be all-inclusive. Consequently, the self-care behaviour is influenced by social determinants, e.g., the level of education, income level, and cultural viewpoint, and should be considered in the development of the Oral Health Empowerment Solution. Social elements of peer support, community involvement, and culturally relevant messaging have the capacity of boosting motivation and confidence in the capacity to assume responsibility for taking care of his or her oral health through self-care. A citizen will be more willing to seek health services and will always practice healthy behaviour when he or she feels empowered.

In the end, these beneficial outcomes disclose that every person has a role to play in ensuring that oral health is improved. Clinicians offer caring, administrators are functional, policymakers are visionary and protectionary, and the citizens offer self-agency to their lives. The anthropocentric approach acknowledges that relationships, trust, and a sense of commitment to a common purpose of health equity is what, more than technological innovations or regulations, makes a system operable.

Data Privacy Concerns

The core of digital oral health systems is personal health information, which can be gathered in a multi-platform and continuous way. The increased application of technology in dental information, habits, and photos, as well as lifestyle aspects, is a threat and an opportunity. There is always a possibility that people do not know about the ways their information is gathered, stored, and once more spread about. Violation of confidentiality has serious repercussions. Ethical data management should also take into account transparency, permission, and proportionality, not to mention technical methods. Only data that is required to help in treatment and in the interest of the public health is supposed to be facilitated, and the individuals must provide full and complete information regarding the data being obtained and the purpose of the same.

Relevance of DPDPA 2023 and GDPR

The practice of ethical use of digital health technologies has become critically protected through legal frameworks, which establish protection such as the General Data Protection Regulation (GDPR) of the European Union and the Digital Personal Data Protection Act 2023 (DPDPA) of India. Considering the review, the GDPR and DPDPA are based on the same fundamental themes: legal processing, data minimization, limiting purpose and the rights of individuals to their personal data. Both are not only regulatory but also powerful ethical requirements of any system of oral health to operate within or between jurisdictions. In India the DPDPA 2023 is necessary because it imposes a duty on data fiduciaries to safeguard the personal data of individuals and gives individuals the right to access, rectify, and amend their personal data. The international implication of the GDPR puts an increased focus on the necessity to consider the implications of privacy-by-design and accountability. When they combine these structures, they pressurize health systems to integrate ethical structures in their systems, rather than consider compliance as a secondary consideration.

Digital Inequality

Digital transformation might amplify the level of the digital divide between potential and non-potential users of technology. Other factors leading to the digital divide are technological factors such as low digital literacy levels, inconsistency in technology use, affordability of technology at low cost, and the language, culture/beliefs, and values. Consequently, oral health disparities would deny certain groups/societies access to and utilization of digital services to make appointments, tele dentistry services, and preventative messaging.

Ethical application of technology must stipulate that there would be deliberate design planning to guarantee fair dispensation. It is possible to fill this gap by using community-based facilitation, regionally relevant content, and the combination of in-person and online services with the help of hybrid care models.

Ethical Limits of Nudging

Behavioural nudges have been adopted as a result of the need to advance preventive measures in reference to oral healthcare. Nonetheless, the ethical standards should be followed. Even well-intentioned and persuasive, ambiguous, or manipulative behavioural nudges can place healthcare environments at risk of transitioning between offering advice and coercion despite the presence of gentle forms of persuasion in healthcare environments.

Ethically acceptable nudging has such characteristics as clarity, moderation, and the respect of choice. Nudges must not violate health advantages, but may not exploit health benefits of an organization, and the option to refuse. Oral health nudges need to strengthen self-efficacy as opposed to addressing the vices of cognition. On the one hand, there is the need to achieve a balance between innovation and responsibility. Pragmatically, all systems of innovation and sustainability are required to have social and legal issues. The level of trust in the Ethical OS system should be equal to the level of trust in technology, as both offer added value to the stakeholders by ensuring human welfare is protected and social values, as well as individual rights, are considered using privacy protection, legal compliance, equity, and ethical reflection.

Future Scope

The advent of new frontiers in improving the oral health systems has been rendered possible by the speedy convergence of technologies, behavioural disciplines, and population health. Current models appear to be good, but further research and innovation in this field will be vital in ensuring that they are successful. The future developments give the potential that we will be in a position to make a radical change in the promotion, prevention, and treatment of oral health in the upcoming years. Despite the growing use of behavioural nudges that promote preventive oral health behaviour practices, their effectiveness is strongly related to cultural norms, social values, and environmental forces. What is considered to be the motive of one population in causing behavioural change might very well not work or even be detrimental to another population. Due to this reason, intercultural validation is necessary to achieve ethical and effective delivery. The application of mixed-methods and comparative approaches is necessary in future research to be able to check the functioning of nudges in various cultural contexts. Such studies are able to aid in the establishment of inclusive and culturally sensitive oral health programs by identifying the universal principles behind the same behaviour modification as well as permitting respect for the local norms. It has also been demonstrated that long-term digital and behavioural oral health interventions have the potential (and are often positive) effect, though the long-term effects are not yet understood. Longitudinal research is required to gain a better insight into the sustainability of interventions in the long term, the unforeseen consequences that can arise, and their practical long-term efficacy. Long-term follow-up studies to determine long-term viability of behaviour change, system-level effects, and cost-benefit analysis should be clearly placed in the agenda of future research.

CONCLUSION

This chapter have promoted a vision that integrates empowered bicultural technologies, growth, and ethical governing to revolutionize the oral health systems in the future in this chapter with the concept of EpiDentomics, an integrative framework, which combines epidemiology, digital technologies, behavioural sciences, and ethical governance. The chapter has plotted the reconstitution of oral health as a fundamental element of population health embedded within larger digital health ecologies and sensitive to social, cultural, and behavioural vectors by shifting the paradigm to its more traditional, treatment-based conceptualization. Its connection of the methodologies of implementing strategies, implications, and ethics, as well as a future agenda, is one of the main strengths of the chapter. As pointed out in the chapter, there is a relationship between digital technologies, nudges, and health technologies, and the systems perspective is needed over the emphasis of standalone solutions. According to the holistic approach described in this chapter, there is no innovation on its own that can result in successful outcomes in the field of oral health but rather policy alignment, an empowered workforce, an engaged community, and morally responsible data and technology practices.

The discussion of EpiDentomics in this chapter can be deemed operational and useful analytically. Regarding its operation, it plays a part in designing the action in the form of customized and preventive action. Analytically it assists in the interpretation of intricate relationships between individual conduct and the reaction of a health system as far as risk and treatment interventions are concerned. Also, EpiDentomics is a prospective model of health care founded on digital epidemiology and behavioural data and information. It is also required that there be a shift towards predictive and preventative dentistry. This change in oral health systems remains emphasized in the future by the necessity of early detection and engagement and self-management support in life. This transformation does not only enhance performance but also makes oral health policies in alignment with non-communicable disease strategies and universal health care and health equity agendas.

REFERENCES

Abidin, C. (2018). *Internet celebrity: Understanding fame online*. Emerald., DOI: 10.1108/9781787560765

Arora, V., Mishra, S. S., Sahoo, J., Gupta, M., Joshi, A., Bajaj, K., Joshi, V., & Joshi, N. K. (2024). Effectiveness of M-Health in Improving Physical Activity: An Indian Perspective. *National Journal of Community Medicine*, *1*(15), 1. DOI: 10.55489/njcm.150120243345

Baima, G., Arce, M., Romandini, M., & Van Dyke, T. (2025). Inflammatory and immunological basis of periodontal diseases. *Journal of Periodontal Research*, jre.70040. Advance online publication. DOI: 10.1111/jre.70040 PMID: 41065279

Falbe, J., Grummon, A. H., & Krieger, J. W. (2022). Sugar-sweetened beverage taxes and population health outcomes. *JAMA Pediatrics*, *176*(2), 129–131. DOI: 10.1001/jamapediatrics.2021.5051 PMID: 34902011

Fathima, F., & Sakthi, D. S. (2023, March). Personality Traits and Its Effect On Oral Health of Outpatients Visiting a Private Dental Institution in Chennai. In *2023 International Conference on Business Analytics for Technology and Security (ICBATS)* (pp. 1-4). IEEE. https://doi.org/DOI: 10.1109/ICBATS57792.2023.10111302

Fedele, D. A.. (2020). Mobile apps for oral health promotion. *Community Dentistry and Oral Epidemiology*, *48*(5), 432–440. DOI: 10.2196/11432

Keesara, S., Jonas, A., & Schulman, K. (2020). Covid-19 and health care's digital revolution. *The New England Journal of Medicine*, *382*(23), e82. DOI: 10.1056/NEJMp2005835 PMID: 32240581

Khoury, M. J., Iademarco, M. F., & Riley, W. T. (2016). Precision public health. *American Journal of Preventive Medicine*, *50*(3), 398–400. DOI: 10.1016/j.amepre.2015.08.031 PMID: 26547538

Majmundar, A., Le, N., Moran, M. B., Unger, J. B., & Reuter, K. (2020). Public response to a social media tobacco prevention campaign: Content analysis. *JMIR Public Health and Surveillance*, *6*(4), e20649. DOI: 10.2196/20649 PMID: 33284120

Michie, S., Van Stralen, M. M., & West, R. (2011). The behaviour change wheel. *Implementation Science : IS*, *6*(1), 42. DOI: 10.1186/1748-5908-6-42 PMID: 21513547

Oyekunle, D. O. T., Okwudili Matthew, U., Preston, D., & Boohene, D. (2024). Trust beyond technology algorithms: A theoretical exploration of consumer trust and behaviour in technological consumption and AI projects. *Journal of Computer and Communications*, *12*(06), 10–4236. DOI: 10.4236/jcc.2024.126006

Salathe, M., Bengtsson, L., Bodnar, T. J., Brewer, D. D., Brownstein, J. S., Buckee, C., Campbell, E. M., Cattuto, C., Khandelwal, S., Mabry, P. L., & Vespignani, A. (2012). Digital epidemiology. https://doi.org/DOI: 10.1371/journal.pcbi.1002616

Sanz, M., Marco Del Castillo, A., Jepsen, S., Gonzalez-Juanatey, J. R., D'Aiuto, F., Bouchard, P., Chapple, I., Dietrich, T., Gotsman, I., Graziani, F., Herrera, D., Loos, B., Madianos, P., Michel, J.-B., Perel, P., Pieske, B., Shapira, L., Shechter, M., Tonetti, M., & Wimmer, G. (2020). Periodontitis and cardiovascular diseases. *Journal of Clinical Periodontology*, *47*(3), 268–288. DOI: 10.1111/jcpe.13189 PMID: 32011025

Scheerman, J. F. M., Meijel, B. V., Empelen, P. V., Verrips, G. H. W., Loveren, C. V., Twisk, J. W. R., Pakpour, J. H., Braak, V. N., & Kramer, G. J. C. (2018). Digital interventions for oral health behaviour. *Caries Research*, *52*(6), 507–517. DOI: 10.1111/idh.12415 PMID: 31291683

Sekhar, P., & Prabakar, J. (2023). Knowledge and Practice of Preventive Measures for Oral Health Care among 14-16 Year Old School Children in Chennai - An Observational Study. *2nd International Conference on Business Analytics for Technology and Security, ICBATS 2023*. DOI: 10.1109/ICBATS57792.2023.10111394

Sheiham, A., & Watt, R. G. (2000). The common risk factor approach. *Community Dentistry and Oral Epidemiology*, *28*(6), 399–406. DOI: 10.1034/j.1600-0528.2000.028006399.x PMID: 11106011

Taylor, G. W., & Borgnakke, W. S. (2008). Periodontal disease: Associations with diabetes, glycemic control and complications. *Oral Diseases*, *14*(3), 191–203. DOI: 10.1111/j.1601-0825.2008.01442.x PMID: 18336370

Thaler, R. H., & Sunstein, C. R. (2008). *Nudge*. Yale University Press., DOI: 10.1016/j.soscij.2008.09.003

Tu, C., Wang, G., Hu, Z., Wang, S., Yan, Q., & Liu, X. (2023). Burden of oral disorders, 1990–2019: Estimates from the global burden of disease study 2019. *Archives of Medical Science : AMS*, *19*(4), 930–940. DOI: 10.5114/aoms/165962 PMID: 37560733

KEY TERMS AND DEFINITIONS

Behavioural Nudging: This enmeshes using elusive, non-coercive intercessions to impact healthy behaviour without controlling choices.

Dentomics: It is the scientific combination of clinical information of the oral cavity, molecular pathomarkers, behavioural indicators, and contextual information during the development of a holistic image of oral health in the context of systemic health.

Digital Epidemiology: This involves the usage of digital data sources to track disease patterns, risk factors, and health behaviours in real time and enhances traditional epidemiology by permitting faster results.

EpiDentomics: It is an integrative conceptual framework that conglomerates epidemiology, dentomics (oral biological data), artificial intelligence, and behavioural science to recuperate oral health prevention and maintenance.

Health Communication: The strategic use of communication approaches and media to update, impact, and motivate individuals and communities to implement healthy behaviours.

Health Technology: This refers to the usage of digital tools, medical devices, software, data systems, and platforms to advance healthcare delivery

Infodemiology: It is the study of health information patterns on the internet, incorporating how health information spreads, is disbursed, or misinterpreted online. It benefits public health authorities to recognize misinformation and understand public concerns to design effectual communication strategies during health emergencies.

Non-Communicable Diseases (NCDs): They are chronic diseases spreading from person to person, such as diabetes, cardiovascular diseases, cancer, and chronic respiratory diseases.

Oral Health: The inclusive health of the teeth, gums, tongue, and oral tissues, and their capability to function without discomfort, infection, or disease. This is closely connected to general health.

Preventive Health Programs: They are systematized efforts aimed at averting disease before it happens, rather than handling illness after onset. These agendas focus on vaccination, screening, lifestyle modification, early detection, and health education to condense long-term healthcare expenditures and disease encumbrance.

Public Health Multimedia Programs: The use of audio, video, graphics, animations, and digital platforms to transfer health messages to larger audiences. These programs increase engagement and understanding by exhibiting health information in simple formats, for preventive health and behaviour change.

Chapter 9
Psychodental Interactions:
A Comprehensive Review of Oral Hygiene and Its Impact on Mental Health

Awais Farid
http://orcid.org/0009-0002-7549-4079
James Cook University, Australia

Zahra Fatima
http://orcid.org/0009-0008-8252-0822
Hong Kong University of Science and Technology, Hong Kong

Zeeshan Fareed
http://orcid.org/0009-0000-9272-2067
Hong Kong University of Science and Technology, Hong Kong

Muhammad Farhan Sheharyar Hassan
http://orcid.org/0009-0008-9401-8602
Nishtar Medical University, Pakistan

Aisha Manzoor
Lahore College for Women University, Pakistan

Sakhaudiin Ahmed Mohamud
Wellshare International, USA

ABSTRACT

This chapter examines the bidirectional relationship between oral hygiene and mental health through a comprehensive review of current evidence on psychodental interactions. It synthesizes epidemiological findings, biological mechanisms, behavioural pathways, psychosocial consequences, and shared social determinants linking oral health and psychological wellbeing. This chapter further discusses the influence of mental illness on oral hygiene behaviours, identifies vulnerable populations, and explores emerging innovations, including digital health and integrated models of care. An Integrated Psychodental Framework is proposed to illustrate the multidi-

DOI: 10.4018/979-8-3373-8402-3.ch009

rectional pathways connecting oral hygiene, biological mediators, mental health outcomes, and broader social determinants. This chapter highlights the importance of interdisciplinary collaboration and holistic healthcare approaches to improve oral health, mental wellbeing, and future research in psychodentistry.

1. INTRODUCTION

Oral hygiene is commonly understood as a basic component of personal care, disease prevention, and physical wellbeing. Traditionally, its importance has been discussed in relation to dental caries, periodontal disease, tooth loss, oral pain, and broader systemic conditions such as diabetes and cardiovascular disease (Ray, 2023). However, growing interdisciplinary evidence suggests that oral hygiene may also be closely connected with mental health, emotional wellbeing, social functioning, and quality of life (Malicka et al., 2022). This emerging area of enquiry highlights the need to move beyond a narrow dental model and consider oral health as part of a broader biopsychosocial system.

Mental health disorders, including depression, anxiety, stress-related conditions, substance use disorders, eating disorders, and severe mental illness, represent a major global public health burden (Zhao et al., 2024). These conditions influence daily routines, motivation, self-care capacity, diet, sleep, social participation, and engagement with health services. Oral hygiene behaviours, such as toothbrushing, flossing, dental attendance, dietary choices, and avoidance of tobacco or harmful substances, are deeply shaped by these same behavioural and psychosocial factors (Prabhu et al., 2026). As a result, oral hygiene and mental health should not be viewed as separate domains, but as interconnected aspects of human health.

The relationship between oral hygiene and mental health appears to be bidirectional. On one hand, poor mental health can contribute to deterioration in oral hygiene. Individuals experiencing depression may have reduced motivation, fatigue, impaired concentration, and diminished interest in self-care, all of which can affect regular toothbrushing and dental attendance. Anxiety, dental fear, trauma histories, and social avoidance may delay dental treatment and increase the risk of untreated oral disease (Avramova, 2022). People living with severe mental illness may also experience additional challenges, including medication-related dry mouth, altered diet, substance use, poverty, stigma, and fragmented access to healthcare (Bida et al., 2025). These factors can combine to increase the risk of caries, periodontal disease, oral infections, pain, and tooth loss.

On the other hand, poor oral hygiene and oral disease may contribute to psychological distress and poorer mental health outcomes. Oral pain, halitosis, visible dental decay, missing teeth, and poor oral appearance can affect confidence, body image, communication, employment opportunities, intimate relationships, and social participation. For many people, oral health is closely linked to dignity, identity, and self-esteem. When oral disease becomes visible or painful, it may reinforce shame, isolation, embarrassment, and reduced quality of life (Yactayo-Alburquerque et al., 2021). In this way, oral hygiene is not only a clinical behaviour but also a socially and psychologically meaningful practice.

Several biological pathways may help explain the connection between oral hygiene and mental health. Poor oral hygiene can contribute to dysbiosis of the oral microbiome, periodontal inflammation, and systemic inflammatory responses (Di Stefano et al., 2022). Chronic inflammation has been implicated in the pathophysiology of depression, cognitive decline, and other neuropsychiatric outcomes. Periodontal pathogens and inflammatory mediators may influence systemic immune activation, vascular function, oxidative stress, and potentially neuroinflammatory processes (Hajishengallis & Chavakis, 2021). Although causal pathways remain under investigation, these mechanisms provide a plausible biological foundation for psychodental interactions.

Stress-related pathways are also important. Psychological stress can alter immune function, salivary flow, cortisol levels, oral microbial balance, and health behaviours. Behaviours and physiological changes can worsen oral health while simultaneously contributing to psychological distress. This creates a reinforcing cycle in which stress affects oral hygiene, oral disease affects wellbeing, and both are shaped by wider social determinants.

Social determinants further complicate the relationship between oral hygiene and mental health. Poverty, housing insecurity, low health literacy, limited access to dental care, rurality, disability, cultural barriers, and experiences of discrimination can increase vulnerability to both poor oral health and poor mental health (Peres et al., 2019). Dental services are often separated from mental health services, and oral health is frequently neglected in mental health assessment and care planning (Peres et al., 2019; Johansson et al., 2025). Similarly, dental practitioners may not always feel equipped to identify psychological distress, trauma, or mental health-related barriers to oral hygiene. This separation contributes to missed opportunities for prevention, early intervention, and integrated care.

The concept of "psychodental interactions" provides a useful framework for understanding these overlapping biological, behavioural, psychological, and social pathways. Psychodental interactions refer to the ways in which oral health, oral hygiene behaviours, mental health, emotional wellbeing, and psychosocial functioning influence one another. This concept recognises that oral hygiene is not merely an individual habit, but a behaviour embedded within motivation, cognition, culture, social support, service access, and structural conditions. It also recognises that oral disease can have consequences beyond the mouth, affecting identity, participation, and mental wellbeing.

Despite increasing recognition of the oral–mental health connection, important gaps remain in the literature. Much of the existing evidence is cross-sectional, making it difficult to determine causality or directionality (Khammissa & Andriankaja, 2025). There is also variation in how oral hygiene, oral health status, and mental health outcomes are measured across studies. Vulnerable populations, including adolescents, older adults, people with disabilities, culturally diverse communities, refugees, Indigenous populations, and people living with severe mental illness, require greater research attention. Furthermore, few models fully integrate biological mechanisms with behavioural and social determinants.

This chapter aims to provide a comprehensive review of oral hygiene and its impact on mental health through a psychodental lens. It will examine epidemiological evidence, biological mechanisms, behavioural pathways, psychosocial consequences, shared determinants, and implications for clinical practice and public health. The chapter will also consider how emerging technologies, integrated care models, and interdisciplinary research may support more holistic approaches to prevention and treatment. By bringing together dental, psychological, biomedical, and public health perspectives, this chapter seeks to advance understanding of the mind–mouth connection and highlight the importance of oral hygiene as part of mental health promotion.

Ultimately, oral hygiene should be understood not only as a dental practice but also as a meaningful determinant and reflection of mental wellbeing. Recognising psychodental interactions may help clinicians, researchers, and policymakers design more integrated, person-centred, and equitable approaches to health. Such approaches are particularly important for populations experiencing complex needs, where oral disease and mental health difficulties often coexist and reinforce one another (Khairunnisa et al., 2024).

2. CONCEPTUALISING PSYCHODENTAL INTERACTIONS

2.1 Defining Psychodental Interactions

The relationship between oral health and mental health has historically been examined within separate disciplinary boundaries, with dentistry primarily focusing on oral diseases and psychiatry concentrating on psychological and behavioural disorders. However, increasing evidence suggests that these domains are intricately linked and cannot be fully understood in isolation (Afroz et al., 2025). The emerging concept of psychodental interactions seeks to bridge this gap by acknowledging the dynamic and reciprocal influences between oral hygiene behaviours, oral diseases, psychological wellbeing, and social functioning.

For the purpose of this chapter, psychodental interactions are defined as the multidirectional biological, behavioural, psychological, and social processes through which oral hygiene practices and oral health status influence mental health outcomes and vice versa. This conceptualisation extends beyond a simple association between oral disease and mental illness, recognising that oral hygiene is a behaviour shaped by motivation, cognition, emotional states, social environments, cultural norms, and access to healthcare services.

The concept aligns closely with person-centred healthcare models that recognise the interconnectedness of physical, psychological, and social dimensions of health. It also reflects broader trends towards interdisciplinary approaches that encourage collaboration between dental professionals, psychologists, psychiatrists, primary care practitioners, and public health specialists (Chan et al., 2026). Despite growing interest in this area, psychodentistry remains a relatively underdeveloped field, and there is currently no universally accepted framework for understanding the complex pathways linking oral hygiene and mental wellbeing.

2.2 The Biopsychosocial Perspective

The biopsychosocial model provides an appropriate theoretical framework for conceptualising psychodental interactions. Originally proposed to overcome limitations associated with the traditional biomedical model, the biopsychosocial perspective emphasises that health outcomes are influenced by interactions among biological processes, psychological characteristics, and social determinants (Bolton & Gillett, 2019).

Within a psychodental context, biological factors include oral microbial composition, periodontal inflammation, systemic immune responses, neuroendocrine pathways, salivary function, genetic susceptibility, and medication-related physiological changes. These biological mechanisms may contribute to both oral diseases and psychiatric conditions, suggesting common pathophysiological pathways (Martínez et al., 2022).

Psychological factors encompass cognition, emotions, motivation, stress responses, self-esteem, body image perceptions, coping strategies, and health-related behaviours. Individuals experiencing symptoms of depression or anxiety may have reduced motivation to maintain oral hygiene routines, while poor oral health may contribute to negative self-perceptions, embarrassment, and social withdrawal (Ganesan et al., 2024). Psychological distress can therefore function both as a cause and consequence of deteriorating oral health.

Social determinants represent another critical dimension of psychodental interactions. Socioeconomic disadvantage, educational attainment, employment status, social support networks, housing stability, cultural beliefs, and access to healthcare services can significantly influence oral hygiene practices and mental wellbeing (Foláyan et al., 2025). Populations experiencing marginalisation often face multiple barriers that increase susceptibility to both poor oral health and psychological distress.

The biopsychosocial model therefore provides a holistic framework capable of explaining why oral hygiene behaviours cannot be understood solely as individual choices. Instead, these behaviours should be considered within broader social contexts that influence opportunities, resources, and health outcomes.

2.3 Behavioural Pathways Linking Oral Hygiene and Mental Health

Health behaviours constitute one of the most immediate pathways connecting oral hygiene and mental health. Oral hygiene practices such as tooth brushing, flossing, tongue cleaning, mouth rinsing, regular dental attendance, and dietary control require sustained behavioural engagement and self-regulation (Rogers et al., 2022). Mental health disorders frequently impair these capacities.

Depressive symptoms, including anhedonia, fatigue, hopelessness, reduced concentration, and psychomotor slowing, may reduce an individual's willingness or ability to engage in routine oral hygiene activities (Barranca-Enríquez & Romo-González, 2022). Anxiety disorders may contribute to avoidance of dental appointments due to fear of treatment, pain anticipation, or previous traumatic experiences associated with dental care. Similarly, chronic stress may promote maladaptive coping behaviours, including smoking, excessive sugar intake, alcohol consumption, and poor dietary habits, all of which increase oral disease risk.

Behavioural theories may offer additional insights into psychodental interactions. Models such as the Health Belief Model, Theory of Planned Behaviour, Self-Determination Theory, and Social Cognitive Theory suggest that oral hygiene behaviours are influenced by perceived susceptibility, self-efficacy, social norms, and intrinsic motivation (McDowell, 2023). Understanding these determinants may facilitate the design of behavioural interventions aimed at improving both oral health outcomes and psychological wellbeing.

2.4 Emerging Recognition of the Mind–Mouth Connection

Interest in the relationship between oral health and systemic health has expanded considerably over the past two decades. The oral-systemic health paradigm acknowledges associations between periodontal disease and conditions such as cardiovascular disease, diabetes mellitus, adverse pregnancy outcomes, and respiratory illnesses (Kapila, 2021). More recently, researchers have begun exploring potential connections between oral diseases and neuropsychiatric outcomes.

Several hypotheses have been proposed to explain the mind–mouth connection. These include inflammatory theories, microbial dysbiosis models, neuroendocrine mechanisms, psychosocial pathways, and behavioural explanations (Marwaha et al., 2025). Chronic oral inflammation may influence systemic cytokine production and contribute to neuroinflammatory processes implicated in depression and cognitive decline. Alterations in oral microbial communities, particularly those prevalent in hospital settings and long-term care facilities(LTCF) among older adults, may also affect immune regulation and metabolic pathways that influence oral and general health. (Farid et al., 2025a; Farid et al., 2026; Farid et al., 2025b).

Although evidence supporting these mechanisms is still evolving, the available literature suggests that oral hygiene represents a potentially modifiable factor capable of influencing mental wellbeing. Improved understanding of psychodental interactions may therefore create opportunities for integrated prevention strategies, interdisciplinary clinical care, and more comprehensive approaches to health promotion.

Overall, psychodental interactions should be considered an emerging interdisciplinary field that seeks to understand how oral hygiene behaviours, oral diseases, psychological wellbeing, and social determinants collectively shape health outcomes. Establishing a clearer conceptual foundation for this field may help guide future research, facilitate collaboration among health professionals, and support the development of holistic interventions aimed at improving both oral and mental health.

Table 1. Conceptual Components of Psychodental Interactions

Domain	Oral Health Components	Mental Health Components	Examples of Interactions
Biological	Periodontal disease, oral microbiome, salivary function	Neuroinflammation, HPA-axis activation, immune dysregulation	Periodontal inflammation contributing to depressive symptoms
Psychological	Oral hygiene behaviours, dental attendance	Motivation, self-esteem, anxiety, stress	Depression reducing toothbrushing frequency
Behavioural	Diet, smoking, alcohol use, oral self-care	Coping mechanisms, health behaviours	Stress-induced smoking worsening periodontal disease
Social	Access to dental care, socioeconomic status, social support	Social isolation, stigma, quality of life	Poverty limiting access to oral and mental healthcare
Healthcare Systems	Dental services, preventive programs	Mental health services, counselling	Integrated psychodental screening and referral pathways

3. ORAL HYGIENE AND MENTAL HEALTH: EPIDEMIOLOGICAL EVIDENCE

Epidemiological studies conducted over the past two decades have increasingly identified significant associations between oral hygiene practices, oral disease burden, and adverse mental health outcomes (Kisely et al., 2016). Although causality remains difficult to establish due to the predominance of cross-sectional and observational studies, the consistency of findings across different populations and settings suggests a meaningful relationship between oral health behaviours and psychological wellbeing. This section reviews evidence linking oral hygiene with depression, anxiety, stress, cognitive impairment, social isolation, sleep disturbances, and overall quality of life.

3.1 Oral Hygiene and Depression

Depression is among the most frequently studied mental health conditions in relation to oral health. Characterised by persistent low mood, diminished interest or pleasure, fatigue, impaired concentration, altered sleep patterns, and reduced motivation, depression can substantially interfere with self-care behaviours, including oral hygiene maintenance. Several population-based studies have reported that individuals with depressive symptoms are more likely to exhibit poor oral hygiene practices, infrequent tooth brushing, irregular dental attendance, and increased prevalence of untreated dental caries and periodontal disease (Cademartori et al., 2018).

Conversely, poor oral health may also contribute to depressive symptoms. Individuals with visible dental decay, halitosis, tooth loss, and oral pain may experience embarrassment, low self-esteem, social withdrawal, and feelings of hopelessness (Kisely, 2016). Such experiences may reduce participation in social activities, negatively affect interpersonal relationships, and contribute to psychological distress. Longitudinal studies have suggested that tooth loss and deteriorating oral health may predict the development of depressive symptoms among older adults, although the directionality of these associations requires further investigation.

Several studies have demonstrated a dose-response relationship, whereby worsening periodontal status is associated with increasing severity of depressive symptoms (Kisely, 2023). However, many investigations rely on self-reported oral health indicators and screening tools for depression, which may introduce reporting biases and limit comparability across studies. Future prospective studies incorporating clinical oral examinations and validated psychiatric assessments may provide stronger evidence regarding causal pathways.

3.2 Anxiety Disorders and Oral Hygiene

Anxiety disorders constitute another important domain within psychodental research. Generalised anxiety disorder, social anxiety disorder, panic disorder, and specific phobias can influence oral hygiene behaviours through multiple mechanisms (Kisely et al., 2016). Dental anxiety has been widely recognised as a major barrier to seeking preventive and therapeutic dental care.

Individuals with high levels of dental fear may postpone or completely avoid dental visits, often until symptoms become severe and require emergency treatment. This avoidance pattern contributes to progressive oral disease, pain, and functional impairment, which may further reinforce anxiety and avoidance behaviours. The concept of the "vicious cycle of dental anxiety" has been proposed to explain how fear leads to avoidance, worsening oral conditions, increased embarrassment, and heightened anxiety during subsequent encounters with dental services (Alkan et al., 2015).

Social anxiety may also influence oral hygiene indirectly. Concerns regarding appearance, fear of negative evaluation, and difficulties engaging in healthcare interactions may reduce help-seeking behaviours and adherence to oral hygiene recommendations. Studies have shown that individuals with anxiety disorders often report poorer oral health-related quality of life compared with those without psychological distress (Ng & Leung, 2008).

Moreover, anxiety-related physiological changes, including increased sympathetic nervous system activity, alterations in salivary composition, and parafunctional habits such as bruxism, may contribute to oral health deterioration. Bruxism has been particularly associated with stress, anxiety, and emotional dysregulation, potentially leading to temporomandibular disorders, tooth wear, and chronic facial pain (Pavlou et al., 2024).

3.3 Psychological Stress and Oral Health

Psychological stress has emerged as an important determinant of oral hygiene and oral disease. Stressful life events, occupational demands, financial difficulties, caregiving responsibilities, and chronic psychosocial adversity can influence oral hygiene behaviours through behavioural, hormonal, and immunological pathways. Individuals experiencing chronic stress may be more likely to engage in unhealthy coping strategies such as smoking, alcohol consumption, excessive sugar intake, and irregular sleep patterns, all of which increase susceptibility to oral disease. Stress may also reduce adherence to preventive oral hygiene practices, including tooth brushing and routine dental check-ups (Cao et al., 2023).

Biologically, stress is associated with activation of the hypothalamic-pituitary-adrenal (HPA) axis and increased secretion of cortisol, which may influence immune function, salivary flow rates, and inflammatory responses (Nunez et al., 2025). Elevated cortisol concentrations have been associated with increased risk of periodontal inflammation and impaired wound healing. Although these associations do not necessarily imply causation, they provide plausible explanations for the observed relationships between stress and oral health outcomes. University students, healthcare workers, and caregivers have frequently been studied as populations vulnerable to stress-related oral health problems (Antoniadou et al., 2024).

3.4 Cognitive Decline and Dementia

Emerging evidence suggests that oral hygiene and oral health status may be associated with cognitive functioning and neurodegenerative disorders (Borsa et al., 2021). Older adults with poor oral hygiene, advanced periodontal disease, and significant tooth loss have been reported to experience higher rates of cognitive impairment and dementia compared with individuals maintaining good oral health (Borsa et al., 2021).

Several hypotheses have been proposed to explain these associations. Chronic periodontal inflammation may contribute to systemic inflammatory burden and neuroinflammation, potentially accelerating neurodegenerative processes. Oral pathogens and their metabolic products may also gain access to the bloodstream and central nervous system, influencing brain function through direct and indirect pathways (Eicher & Mohajeri, 2022).

In addition, tooth loss may affect nutritional status and mastication efficiency, leading to reduced dietary quality and diminished sensory stimulation, both of which have been implicated in cognitive decline. Nonetheless, evidence remains inconclusive, and reverse causality must also be considered. Individuals with cognitive impairment may struggle to maintain adequate oral hygiene due to memory deficits, impaired executive functioning, and dependence on caregivers.

3.5 Oral Hygiene, Social Isolation, and Quality of Life

Oral hygiene has important implications for social participation and quality of life. Oral conditions such as halitosis, tooth discoloration, missing teeth, periodontal disease, and visible dental decay may adversely affect communication, confidence, and social interactions. These factors can contribute to feelings of embarrassment, social withdrawal, loneliness, and reduced life satisfaction.

Oral health-related quality of life has become an increasingly important outcome measure in psychodental research. Instruments such as the Oral Health Impact Profile (OHIP), General Oral Health Assessment Index (GOHAI), and various patient-reported outcome measures have demonstrated associations between poor oral health and impaired psychosocial wellbeing (Borg-Bartolo et al., 2025). Studies consistently indicate that individuals with untreated oral diseases report lower levels of self-esteem, reduced social functioning, and poorer perceptions of general health (Salvador & Toassi, 2021).

3.6 Limitations of Existing Epidemiological Evidence

Despite substantial progress in psychodental research, several limitations remain. Many studies employ cross-sectional designs that preclude determination of temporal relationships (Dao et al., 2025). Considerable heterogeneity exists regarding oral health assessments, mental health screening tools, study populations, and analytical methods, making comparisons difficult. Residual confounding related to socioeconomic status, smoking, comorbid conditions, and healthcare access may also influence observed associations.

Future research should prioritise prospective cohort studies, standardised outcome measures, and interdisciplinary methodologies that integrate dental, psychological, biological, and public health perspectives. Such approaches may strengthen understanding of psychodental interactions and inform evidence-based interventions aimed at promoting both oral hygiene and mental wellbeing.

Table 2. Major Epidemiological Themes Linking Oral Hygiene and Mental Health Outcomes

Mental Health Outcome	Oral Health Indicators Examined	Reported Association	Common Limitations
Depression	Toothbrushing frequency, periodontal disease, tooth loss	Poor oral hygiene associated with increased depressive symptoms	Predominantly cross-sectional studies
Anxiety	Dental attendance, dental fear, oral health-related quality of life	Anxiety linked to dental avoidance and poorer oral health	Self-reported anxiety measures
Stress	Bruxism, gingival inflammation, oral ulcers	Chronic stress associated with adverse oral behaviours and inflammatory changes	Confounding lifestyle factors

continued on following page

Table 2. Continued

Mental Health Outcome	Oral Health Indicators Examined	Reported Association	Common Limitations
Cognitive Decline	Tooth loss, periodontal disease, oral hygiene status	Associations reported with dementia and cognitive impairment	Unclear causal direction
Social Isolation	Missing teeth, halitosis, oral appearance	Poor oral health associated with reduced social participation	Limited longitudinal evidence
Quality of Life	OHIP scores, oral symptoms	Oral disease negatively affects psychosocial wellbeing	Variation in assessment tools

4. BIOLOGICAL MECHANISMS UNDERPINNING PSYCHODENTAL INTERACTIONS

Understanding the relationship between oral hygiene and mental health requires consideration of the biological pathways that may mediate these interactions. While behavioural and psychosocial mechanisms undoubtedly contribute to psychodental associations, emerging evidence suggests that oral diseases and poor oral hygiene may also influence neurological, endocrine, inflammatory, and immunological processes associated with mental wellbeing (Ganesan et al., 2024). Although causal relationships remain incompletely understood, several interconnected biological pathways have been proposed, including the oral microbiome-brain axis, systemic inflammation, hypothalamic-pituitary-adrenal (HPA) axis dysregulation, oxidative stress, and pain-related neurophysiological mechanisms.

4.1 The Oral Microbiome–Brain Axis

The human oral cavity hosts one of the most diverse microbial ecosystems in the body, comprising hundreds of bacterial, viral, fungal, and protozoal species that collectively contribute to oral and systemic health. Under physiological conditions, the oral microbiome exists in a relatively balanced state, supporting host immunity, maintaining mucosal integrity, and preventing colonisation by pathogenic organisms. However, poor oral hygiene practices can disrupt this microbial equilibrium, resulting in dysbiosis characterised by increased abundance of pathogenic bacteria associated with dental caries and periodontal disease.

Recent studies have proposed the existence of an oral microbiome-brain axis analogous to the better-established gut-brain axis (Bisht et al., 2024). According to this hypothesis, oral microorganisms may influence neurological function through several pathways, including direct microbial invasion, systemic dissemination of bacterial products, modulation of immune responses, and production of neuroactive metabolites.

Periodontal pathogens such as *Porphyromonas gingivalis*, *Treponema denticola*, and *Tannerella forsythia* have attracted particular attention because of their potential involvement in neurodegenerative disorders (Visentin et al., 2023). Bacterial lipopolysaccharides, gingipains, and other virulence factors produced by these organisms may contribute to chronic systemic inflammation and potentially cross compromised blood-brain barriers under certain pathological conditions (Visentin et al., 2023).

In addition to pathogenic mechanisms, oral microorganisms may indirectly influence mental health by affecting immune homeostasis, cytokine production, and metabolic pathways associated with neurotransmitter regulation. While current evidence remains largely observational, advances in metagenomics, transcriptomics, and microbiome profiling technologies may further elucidate the role of oral microbial communities in psychological wellbeing.

4.2 Neuroinflammation and Cytokine-Mediated Pathways

Inflammation has increasingly been recognised as a common feature linking oral diseases and psychiatric disorders. Periodontal disease is characterised by chronic inflammatory responses triggered by bacterial biofilms accumulating along gingival margins. Persistent periodontal inflammation results in local tissue destruction and release of pro-inflammatory mediators into systemic circulation.

Several cytokines implicated in periodontal disease have also been associated with depression, anxiety, cognitive impairment, and stress-related disorders. Elevated concentrations of interleukin-1 beta (IL-1β), interleukin-6 (IL-6), tumour necrosis factor-alpha (TNF-α), and C-reactive protein (CRP) have been reported among individuals experiencing depressive symptoms (Zavala-Medina et al., 2026). These inflammatory markers may influence neurotransmitter metabolism, neuroplasticity, and neuronal survival, potentially contributing to behavioural and emotional disturbances.

Neuroinflammation is increasingly considered a potential mechanism underlying psychiatric illnesses. Activated microglia and inflammatory cytokines may disrupt synaptic functioning, reduce neurogenesis, and alter signalling pathways involved in mood regulation. Consequently, chronic periodontal inflammation resulting from inadequate oral hygiene may represent a modifiable source of systemic inflammatory burden capable of influencing neuropsychiatric outcomes.

Nevertheless, it remains difficult to determine whether inflammation acts as a causal factor, mediator, or consequence within psychodental interactions. Longitudinal investigations and interventional studies assessing changes in mental health following periodontal treatment may provide valuable insights into these relationships.

4.3 Hypothalamic–Pituitary–Adrenal Axis Dysregulation

The HPA axis serves as a central component of the body's stress response system and has been implicated in both oral health and mental health disorders. Exposure to acute or chronic psychological stress stimulates secretion of corticotropin-releasing hormone, adrenocorticotropic hormone, and cortisol, resulting in widespread physiological effects.

Sustained elevations in cortisol concentrations may impair immune responses, alter inflammatory pathways, and reduce salivary secretion. Reduced salivary flow can diminish antimicrobial activity within the oral cavity, increase plaque accumulation, and promote conditions favourable for periodontal disease development. Cortisol-induced immune dysregulation may further exacerbate gingival inflammation and impair healing processes.

Conversely, chronic oral pain and severe periodontal disease may themselves function as physiological stressors capable of activating HPA axis responses (Nunez et al., 2025). Recurrent pain, functional limitations, and concerns regarding oral appearance may contribute to psychological stress, thereby reinforcing bidirectional pathways between oral health and emotional wellbeing.

The HPA axis therefore represents an important biological interface through which psychological stress may influence oral hygiene behaviours and oral disease progression, while oral health conditions may reciprocally affect stress-related neuroendocrine functioning.

4.4 Oxidative Stress and Cellular Damage

Oxidative stress refers to an imbalance between reactive oxygen species production and antioxidant defence mechanisms, resulting in cellular injury and tissue dysfunction. Increased oxidative stress has been implicated in numerous chronic diseases, including cardiovascular disorders, diabetes mellitus, neurodegenerative conditions, and depression (Borg-Bartolo et al., 2025).

Periodontal disease is associated with enhanced oxidative activity and elevated concentrations of reactive oxygen metabolites within gingival tissues (Bisht et al., 2024). Persistent oxidative stress may contribute to endothelial dysfunction, neuronal injury, and impaired cellular signalling pathways involved in emotional regulation and cognition.

Several researchers have suggested that oxidative stress may represent another common biological denominator linking oral diseases with psychiatric disorders (Visentin et al., 2023). However, evidence remains preliminary, and further studies are required to determine whether antioxidant interventions or improvements in oral hygiene can modify psychological outcomes.

4.5 Pain Perception and Neurobehavioural Responses

Pain constitutes an important yet frequently overlooked component of psychodental interactions. Dental caries, pulpitis, temporomandibular disorders, periodontal abscesses, and oral ulcerations may produce acute or chronic pain capable of affecting mood, sleep quality, cognitive functioning, and daily activities.

Chronic pain conditions have been strongly associated with depression and anxiety, with bidirectional relationships commonly observed (Visscher et al., 2018). Persistent oral pain may disrupt social participation, impair work productivity, and reduce overall quality of life. Simultaneously, psychological distress may amplify pain perception through mechanisms involving central sensitisation, altered neurotransmitter pathways, and maladaptive coping strategies.

Taken together, these biological mechanisms suggest that oral hygiene should not merely be considered a local preventive practice aimed at preserving dentition. Rather, oral hygiene may represent an important determinant of systemic health capable of influencing neurobiological processes associated with emotional wellbeing and mental health outcomes. Although additional research is needed to clarify causal pathways, existing evidence supports the notion that biological processes contribute substantially to psychodental interactions and warrant consideration within integrated models of healthcare.

Table 3. Proposed Biological Mechanisms Linking Oral Hygiene and Mental Health

Mechanism	Oral Health Process	Potential Mental Health Impact	Proposed Pathway
Oral Microbiome Dysbiosis	Periodontal pathogens, plaque accumulation	Depression, cognitive decline	Immune modulation, microbial metabolites
Neuroinflammation	Periodontal inflammation	Mood disorders, neurodegeneration	Elevated IL-1β, IL-6, TNF-α
HPA Axis Dysregulation	Chronic stress, reduced salivary flow	Anxiety, depression	Cortisol-mediated immune changes
Oxidative Stress	Tissue destruction, chronic inflammation	Cognitive dysfunction	Reactive oxygen species and neuronal injury
Chronic Oral Pain	Caries, TMD, periodontal abscess	Anxiety, sleep disturbance, depression	Central sensitisation and behavioural impairment

5. MENTAL HEALTH DISORDERS AS DETERMINANTS OF POOR ORAL HYGIENE

The relationship between oral hygiene and mental health is increasingly recognised as bidirectional. While poor oral hygiene may contribute to adverse psychological outcomes, mental health disorders themselves can substantially impair oral self-care behaviours, increase susceptibility to oral diseases, and hinder access to preventive and therapeutic dental services (Alkan et al., 2015). Understanding how psychiatric conditions influence oral hygiene is critical for developing integrated interventions that address both mental and oral health needs.

Mental illnesses can affect oral hygiene through multiple pathways, including reduced motivation, impaired executive functioning, medication side effects, unhealthy coping behaviours, social isolation, financial hardship, and fragmented healthcare utilisation. The cumulative effect of these factors often results in increased prevalence of dental caries, periodontal disease, tooth loss, oral infections, xerostomia, halitosis, and reduced oral health-related quality of life (Kisely, 2016).

5.1 Mental Health Disorders and Their Impact on Oral Hygiene

Mental health disorders can substantially influence oral hygiene behaviours through a combination of psychological, behavioural, social, and biological mechanisms. Conditions such as depression, anxiety disorders, schizophrenia, bipolar disorder, and substance use disorders frequently reduce an individual's motivation, cognitive functioning, emotional regulation, and capacity to maintain routine self-care practices. Consequently, regular toothbrushing, flossing, healthy dietary habits, and preventive dental attendance may be neglected, increasing the risk of plaque accumulation, dental caries, periodontal disease, halitosis, oral pain, and eventual tooth loss.

The relationship is further complicated by behavioural avoidance and social disadvantage. Individuals experiencing anxiety may postpone dental visits because of fear of treatment, while those living with severe mental illness often encounter additional barriers related to impaired cognition, social isolation, financial hardship, unstable housing, and reduced access to healthcare services. Substance misuse may further accelerate oral deterioration through direct biological effects, poor nutrition, smoking, and neglect of personal hygiene. Collectively, these factors contribute to disproportionately poor oral health among people living with mental illness and reinforce the bidirectional relationship between oral hygiene and psychological wellbeing.

In addition to the effects of mental illness itself, psychotropic medications may adversely influence oral health. Antidepressants, antipsychotics, anxiolytics, mood stabilisers, and medications used in addiction treatment commonly produce xerostomia, reducing the protective functions of saliva and increasing susceptibility to dental caries, periodontal disease, oral infections, and halitosis. Other adverse effects, including bruxism, taste disturbances, gingival enlargement, dysphagia, and sedation, may further compromise oral hygiene behaviours and quality of life. These interacting biological and behavioural factors emphasise the importance of considering oral health as an integral component of mental healthcare.

5.2 Implications for Clinical Practice

Recognition of the close relationship between mental illness and oral hygiene has important implications for clinical practice. Mental health professionals should routinely encourage oral self-care behaviours, identify barriers to accessing dental services, and facilitate timely referrals when oral health concerns are identified. Likewise, dental practitioners should be aware of the behavioural manifestations of mental illness, medication-related oral complications, and the psychosocial challenges that may influence treatment adherence. Collaborative care involving dentists, psychiatrists, psychologists, primary care physicians, nurses, and allied health professionals has the potential to improve both oral and mental health outcomes through earlier intervention, preventive education, and coordinated person-centred care.

Table 4. Mental Health Disorders and Their Potential Impact on Oral Hygiene

Mental Health Condition	Mechanisms Affecting Oral Hygiene	Common Oral Manifestations
Depression	Reduced motivation, fatigue, social withdrawal	Plaque accumulation, caries, periodontal disease
Anxiety Disorders	Dental avoidance, bruxism, stress behaviours	Tooth wear, TMD, xerostomia
Schizophrenia	Cognitive impairment, apathy, poor healthcare engagement	Severe periodontal disease, tooth loss
Bipolar Disorder	Disrupted routines, impulsivity, substance use	Gingivitis, untreated caries
Substance Use Disorders	Neglect of self-care, direct toxic effects	Extensive caries, oral infections, xerostomia
Psychotropic Medication Use	Reduced salivary flow, sedation, taste changes	Dry mouth, candidiasis, halitosis

6. SHARED DETERMINANTS AND RISK FACTORS

Psychodental interactions are influenced by a broad range of social, behavioural, and environmental determinants that simultaneously affect oral hygiene behaviours and mental wellbeing. Rather than acting independently, these determinants often interact throughout the life course, contributing to health inequalities and reinforcing the bidirectional relationship between oral and mental health.

6.1 Socioeconomic Status and Poverty

Socioeconomic disadvantage remains one of the strongest shared determinants of poor oral hygiene and mental illness. Financial hardship, food insecurity, unstable housing, and limited access to preventive healthcare may reduce opportunities for maintaining oral hygiene while increasing psychological stress and vulnerability to mental disorders. Consequently, poverty often perpetuates a cycle of poor oral health, reduced quality of life, and worsening mental wellbeing.

6.2 Health Literacy

Health literacy influences an individual's ability to understand health information, adopt preventive behaviours, and navigate healthcare systems. Limited oral and mental health literacy may contribute to poor oral hygiene practices, delayed healthcare utilisation, reduced treatment adherence, and persistent stigma surrounding mental illness. Improving accessible and culturally appropriate health education remains an important public health priority.

6.3 Lifestyle and Behavioural Factors

Several modifiable lifestyle behaviours contribute to both oral disease and psychological distress. Smoking, alcohol misuse, unhealthy diets, poor sleep, and physical inactivity increase susceptibility to periodontal disease while also influencing stress responses, emotional wellbeing, and chronic disease risk. These shared behavioural determinants provide opportunities for integrated prevention strategies targeting both oral and mental health.

6.4 Trauma and Chronic Stress

Exposure to trauma, adverse childhood experiences, and chronic psychosocial stress may influence lifelong health behaviours and emotional regulation. Individuals affected by persistent stress often experience greater difficulty maintaining oral hygiene, increased engagement in unhealthy coping behaviours, and reduced healthcare utilisation. Trauma-informed healthcare approaches may therefore improve both patient engagement and long-term psychodental outcomes.

6.5 Cultural and Healthcare Factors

Cultural beliefs, stigma, language barriers, and geographic location can substantially influence oral hygiene practices and access to healthcare. Migrants, Indigenous populations, and individuals living in rural or remote communities frequently encounter barriers to both dental and mental health services. Addressing these inequities requires culturally responsive care, community engagement, and innovative service delivery models that improve access to integrated healthcare.

6.6 Public Health Perspective

The evidence presented throughout this chapter suggests that psychodental interactions are shaped not only by individual behaviours but also by broader social determinants of health. Consequently, interventions focused solely on behaviour change are unlikely to achieve sustained improvements. Effective psychodental strategies should combine preventive oral healthcare, mental health promotion, health literacy initiatives, trauma-informed practice, and equitable healthcare policies to address the upstream determinants of both oral disease and psychological wellbeing.

Table 5. Shared Determinants Influencing Oral Hygiene and Mental Health

Determinant	Impact on Oral Hygiene	Impact on Mental Health	Potential Interventions
Poverty	Reduced access to dental services, delayed treatment	Increased stress, depression, anxiety	Subsidised services, social protection policies
Health Literacy	Poor oral hygiene knowledge and practices	Reduced help-seeking, stigma	Community education, plain language materials
Smoking and Alcohol	Periodontal disease, oral cancer risk	Substance dependence, mood disorders	Behavioural interventions, cessation programs
Trauma and ACEs	Dental avoidance, neglected oral care	PTSD, anxiety, depression	Trauma-informed healthcare
Cultural Barriers	Delayed care utilisation	Reduced engagement with mental health services	Culturally responsive programs
Rurality	Limited dental workforce availability	Reduced access to specialised mental healthcare	Telehealth and outreach services

7. PSYCHOSOCIAL CONSEQUENCES OF POOR ORAL HYGIENE

Poor oral hygiene influences far more than oral health, affecting psychological wellbeing, social participation, self-confidence, and overall quality of life. Conditions such as dental pain, halitosis, periodontal disease, tooth loss, and visible dental decay may negatively affect interpersonal relationships, emotional wellbeing, and daily functioning, creating a reinforcing cycle between poor oral health and psychological distress.

7.1 Self-Esteem and Body Image

Oral appearance plays an important role in self-esteem and body image, particularly among adolescents and young adults. Visible oral diseases, missing teeth, halitosis, and dental discoloration may reduce confidence, increase embarrassment, and contribute to social anxiety or negative self-perception. Contemporary beauty standards and increased exposure to idealised smiles through digital media may further amplify these psychological effects.

7.2 Social Participation and Relationships

Oral health problems may affect communication, eating, smiling, and social interactions. Individuals experiencing oral pain, halitosis, or visible dental disease may avoid conversations, social gatherings, or intimate relationships due to embarrassment or fear of negative judgement. Such social withdrawal may increase loneliness, reduce social connectedness, and contribute to poorer mental wellbeing.

7.3 Employment and Daily Functioning

Poor oral health may also influence educational achievement, employability, and workplace performance. Oral pain, functional limitations, and concerns regarding appearance can affect communication, productivity, attendance, and professional confidence. Consequently, untreated oral diseases may contribute to both economic disadvantage and reduced quality of life.

7.4 Oral Health-Related Quality of Life

Oral health-related quality of life (OHRQoL) provides a patient-centred measure of how oral conditions affect physical, emotional, and social wellbeing. Research consistently demonstrates that poor oral hygiene is associated with reduced OHRQoL, reflecting difficulties with eating, sleeping, communication, self-confidence, and social participation. Standardised instruments such as the Oral Health Impact Profile (OHIP) and General Oral Health Assessment Index (GOHAI) are widely used to evaluate these outcomes and complement traditional clinical assessments.

7.5 Clinical Implications

The psychosocial consequences of poor oral hygiene reinforce the need for person-centred and integrated models of care. Dental practitioners should recognise the psychological and social impacts of oral diseases, while mental health professionals should consider oral hygiene as an important component of overall wellbeing. Routine assessment of oral health-related quality of life, self-care behaviours, and psychosocial concerns may facilitate earlier intervention, improve patient engagement, and strengthen collaboration between dental and mental healthcare services.

Table 6. Psychosocial Consequences Associated with Poor Oral Hygiene

Domain	Potential Consequences	Mental Health Implications
Self-Esteem	Reduced confidence, negative self-image	Depression, social anxiety
Body Image	Dissatisfaction with smile and appearance	Emotional distress, low self-worth
Social Participation	Avoidance of gatherings, isolation	Loneliness, reduced wellbeing
Relationships	Communication difficulties, embarrassment	Relationship strain, withdrawal
Employment	Perceived discrimination, absenteeism	Financial stress, anxiety
Quality of Life	Pain, functional limitations, sleep disturbance	Reduced life satisfaction

8. VULNERABLE POPULATIONS AND PSYCHODENTAL CONSIDERATIONS

Although psychodental interactions can affect individuals across the lifespan, certain populations appear particularly vulnerable due to biological susceptibility, psychosocial stressors, limited healthcare access, and complex support needs. Understanding the unique challenges experienced by these groups is important for designing equitable prevention strategies and integrated interventions.

8.1 Children and Adolescents

Childhood and adolescence represent important developmental periods during which oral hygiene habits, self-care behaviours, and psychological wellbeing are established. Oral diseases experienced during these stages may influence school attendance, sleep quality, social participation, and self-esteem. Adolescents are particularly sensitive to issues related to physical appearance, peer acceptance, and body image. Conditions such as visible dental decay, malocclusion, halitosis, and tooth discoloration may contribute to embarrassment, bullying, social anxiety, and reduced confidence. Mental health difficulties emerging during adolescence, including depression, anxiety, and eating disorders, may further interfere with oral hygiene maintenance and preventive dental attendance.

8.2 Older Adults

Older adults often experience cumulative oral disease burden, tooth loss, xerostomia, chronic illnesses, and functional limitations that may compromise oral hygiene practices. Simultaneously, ageing is associated with increased risks of loneliness, depression, bereavement, and cognitive decline. Cognitive impairment may reduce an individual's ability to maintain oral hygiene routines, increasing reliance on caregivers and healthcare providers. Poor oral health among older adults may also contribute to nutritional deficiencies, speech difficulties, reduced social engagement, and diminished quality of life (Lipsky et al., 2024). Oral health promotion within community and residential aged care settings may therefore provide opportunities to improve both oral and psychological wellbeing.

8.3 People Living with Disabilities and Severe Mental Illness

Individuals living with physical, intellectual, developmental, or psychosocial disabilities frequently experience oral health disparities. Mobility limitations, communication challenges, sensory sensitivities, behavioural difficulties, medication side effects, and dependence on caregivers may hinder effective oral hygiene practices and access to dental services. People living with severe mental illnesses, including schizophrenia and bipolar disorder, often encounter additional barriers related to social disadvantage, stigma, fragmented healthcare systems, and reduced motivation for self-care. Integrating oral health assessments and education into disability and mental health services may help reduce these inequalities.

8.4 Culturally Diverse, Indigenous, and Remote Communities

Migrants, refugees, Indigenous populations, and individuals residing in rural and remote areas may experience disproportionate burdens of poor oral health and mental illness due to historical disadvantage, socioeconomic inequities, language barriers, and limited access to healthcare services. Experiences of migration, displacement, trauma, and cultural stigma may further influence oral hygiene behaviours and healthcare utilisation patterns. Community-led initiatives, culturally safe healthcare practices, and innovative service delivery models such as telehealth may support improved psychodental outcomes among these populations.

9. INNOVATIONS AND FUTURE DIRECTIONS IN PSYCHODENTAL RESEARCH

Psychodentistry remains an emerging interdisciplinary field with significant opportunities for innovation. Advances in digital health technologies, microbiome science, artificial intelligence (AI), and precision medicine may enhance understanding of psychodental interactions and support more personalised approaches to prevention and care (Zhu et al., 2025).

Digital technologies such as tele-dentistry platforms, mobile applications, smart toothbrushes, and wearable devices may improve oral hygiene monitoring, patient engagement, and access to preventive services, particularly among underserved populations. AI-assisted tools may facilitate early identification of oral diseases, behavioural risk factors, and individuals at increased risk of psychological distress, thereby supporting targeted interventions.

Rapid developments in microbiome research also offer promising opportunities. Improved understanding of oral microbial communities and their relationship with inflammation, neurobiology, and mental health may contribute to novel preventive approaches, including microbiome modulation therapies and personalised oral healthcare strategies (Kosan et al., 2022).

Future psychodental research should move beyond predominantly cross-sectional studies and prioritise longitudinal investigations, intervention trials, implementation research, and mixed-methods approaches that explore lived experiences and contextual influences. Standardisation of outcome measures and evaluation of integrated care models involving dental practitioners, psychologists, psychiatrists, nurses, and public health professionals may further strengthen the evidence base.

Ultimately, the continued evolution of psychodentistry will depend upon interdisciplinary collaboration, methodological innovation, and a commitment to addressing oral and mental health inequalities through holistic and person-centred approaches.

10. TOWARDS AN INTEGRATED PSYCHODENTAL FRAMEWORK: CLINICAL, PUBLIC HEALTH, AND POLICY IMPLICATIONS

The evidence presented throughout this chapter supports the notion that oral hygiene and mental health are interconnected through a complex network of biological, behavioural, psychological, and social pathways. Existing studies have predominantly examined individual components of these relationships; however, few attempts have been made to conceptualise psychodental interactions within a unified model. To address this gap, an Integrated Psychodental Framework (IPF) is proposed to facilitate understanding of the multidirectional mechanisms linking oral hygiene behaviours and mental wellbeing.

The proposed framework recognises oral hygiene as both a determinant and consequence of mental health outcomes. At the individual level, oral hygiene practices are influenced by psychological factors such as motivation, self-efficacy, emotional regulation, cognitive functioning, stress responses, and health beliefs. These behavioural determinants directly affect oral health status, including plaque accumulation, periodontal inflammation, dental caries, oral pain, halitosis, and tooth loss.

Biological mediators constitute a second component of the framework. Poor oral hygiene may contribute to dysbiosis of the oral microbiome, chronic inflammatory responses, oxidative stress, immune dysregulation, and activation of neuroendocrine pathways, including the hypothalamic-pituitary-adrenal axis. These processes may influence neurotransmitter systems, neuroplasticity, and neuroinflammatory pathways implicated in depression, anxiety disorders, cognitive decline, and stress-related conditions.

Mental health outcomes represent the third component of the framework. Psychological distress, depressive symptoms, anxiety, impaired self-esteem, social withdrawal, loneliness, and reduced quality of life may arise directly or indirectly from oral diseases and their psychosocial consequences. At the same time, pre-existing mental health disorders may impair self-care behaviours, reduce engagement with dental services, and increase vulnerability to poor oral hygiene. This reciprocal relationship reinforces a cyclical process in which oral and psychological conditions perpetuate one another over time.

Importantly, psychodental interactions do not occur independently of broader social environments. Social determinants such as socioeconomic disadvantage, educational attainment, trauma exposure, cultural beliefs, healthcare accessibility, housing insecurity, and social support systems influence opportunities for maintaining oral hygiene and accessing mental healthcare. These determinants may either mitigate or exacerbate psychodental risks and therefore represent important targets for prevention strategies and policy interventions.

The Integrated Psychodental Framework also highlights opportunities for clinical integration. Dental practitioners may be among the first healthcare professionals to identify symptoms of psychological distress, social isolation, or deteriorating self-care behaviours during routine examinations. Incorporating brief mental wellbeing screening tools into dental practice may facilitate early referral pathways and improve continuity of care. Similarly, psychiatrists, psychologists, primary care physicians, nurses, and allied health professionals may benefit from routinely assessing oral hygiene practices, oral discomfort, and barriers to accessing dental services, particularly among vulnerable populations.

From a public health perspective, psychodental interactions warrant greater attention within health promotion initiatives and national oral health strategies. Community-based interventions that combine oral health education, mental health literacy, behavioural counselling, and social support may offer more comprehensive approaches to disease prevention. School-based programs, aged care initiatives, disability support services, and culturally responsive community outreach activities may provide effective settings for integrated psychodental interventions.

Policy implications should also be considered. Fragmentation between dental and mental healthcare systems may contribute to missed opportunities for prevention, delayed treatment, and widening health inequalities (Watt et al., 2019). Policymakers should therefore consider mechanisms to improve interdisciplinary collaboration, strengthen workforce training, expand access to preventive services, and support implementation of integrated models of care. Investment in telehealth technologies, digital behavioural interventions, and community navigation services may further enhance accessibility, particularly in rural and underserved regions.

The Integrated Psychodental Framework proposed in this chapter should be considered a conceptual model intended to guide future research, clinical innovation, and health policy development. Empirical validation through longitudinal studies, intervention trials, and implementation research will be necessary to evaluate its applicability across diverse populations and healthcare settings. Nevertheless, the framework provides a foundation for understanding psychodental interactions as a dynamic and multifaceted phenomenon that extends beyond traditional disciplinary boundaries and supports a more holistic understanding of human health and wellbeing.

Figure 1. Integrated Psychodental Framework illustrating the multidirectional relationships between social determinants, psychological factors, oral hygiene behaviours, biological mediators, and mental health outcomes. The framework emphasises the bidirectional feedback mechanisms linking oral health and psychological wellbeing.

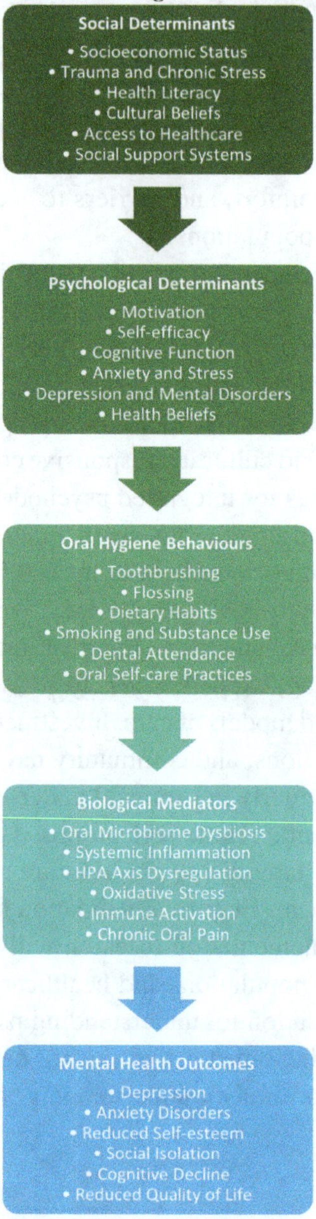

11. CONCLUSION

Oral hygiene has traditionally been viewed as a preventive practice aimed primarily at maintaining oral health and reducing the burden of dental diseases. However, the evidence reviewed throughout this chapter suggests that oral hygiene should also be recognised as an important determinant, correlate, and consequence of mental health and psychological wellbeing. Emerging findings indicate that oral health and mental health are interconnected through complex biological, behavioural, psychological, and social mechanisms, supporting the concept of psychodental interactions.

This review demonstrates that poor oral hygiene and oral diseases are associated with a range of adverse mental health outcomes, including depression, anxiety, chronic stress, social isolation, reduced self-esteem, impaired quality of life, and potentially cognitive decline. Conversely, mental health disorders may substantially compromise oral hygiene behaviours through reduced motivation, impaired cognition, medication-related side effects, unhealthy coping behaviours, and barriers to accessing healthcare services. These bidirectional relationships highlight the importance of moving beyond traditional disciplinary boundaries and adopting more holistic approaches to health promotion and disease prevention.

Several biological mechanisms may contribute to psychodental interactions, including oral microbiome dysbiosis, chronic systemic inflammation, neuroinflammatory pathways, oxidative stress, hypothalamic-pituitary-adrenal axis dysregulation, and pain-related neurophysiological responses. At the same time, social determinants such as poverty, trauma exposure, low health literacy, cultural barriers, stigma, and inequitable access to healthcare services significantly shape oral hygiene behaviours and mental wellbeing. Vulnerable populations, including children, older adults, people living with disabilities, individuals with severe mental illness, and culturally diverse communities, may experience disproportionate burdens of psychodental challenges and require targeted interventions.

Despite growing recognition of the relationship between oral hygiene and mental health, the evidence base remains limited by methodological heterogeneity, reliance on cross-sectional study designs, and inconsistent measurement approaches. Future investigations should prioritise longitudinal studies, intervention trials, implementation research, and mixed-methods methodologies capable of examining causal pathways and contextual influences. Advances in artificial intelligence, microbiome science, precision medicine, and digital health technologies may further enhance understanding of psychodental interactions and facilitate the development of personalised and integrated models of care.

The Integrated Psychodental Framework proposed in this chapter provides a conceptual basis for understanding the multidirectional pathways linking oral hygiene behaviours, biological mediators, mental health outcomes, and social determinants of health. Although further empirical validation is required, this framework may support future research, clinical innovation, and policy development aimed at improving both oral and psychological wellbeing.

Ultimately, oral hygiene should no longer be regarded solely as a dental concern but rather as an essential component of holistic health and wellbeing. Strengthening collaboration among dental professionals, mental health practitioners, primary healthcare providers, researchers, policymakers, and communities may contribute to more equitable, person-centred, and integrated healthcare systems capable of addressing the interconnected challenges of oral and mental health in the twenty-first century.

REFERENCES

Alkan, A., Cakmak, O., Yilmaz, S., Cebi, T., & Gurgan, C. (2015). Relationship between psychological factors and oral health status and behaviours. *Oral Health & Preventive Dentistry*, *13*(4), 331–339. PMID: 25197739

Antoniadou, M., Manta, G., Kanellopoulou, A., Kalogerakou, T., Satta, A., & Mangoulia, P. (2024, December). Managing stress and somatization symptoms among students in demanding academic healthcare environments. [). MDPI.]. *Health Care*, *12*(24), 2522. PMID: 39765949

Avramova, N. T. (2022). Dental fear, anxiety, and phobia; causes, diagnostic criteria and the medical and social impact. *Journal of Mind and Medical Sciences*, *9*(2), 23. DOI: 10.22543/2392-7674.1348

Barranca-Enríquez, A., & Romo-Gonzâlez, T. (2022). Your health is in your mouth: A comprehensive view to promote general wellness. *Frontiers in Oral Health*, *3*, 971223. DOI: 10.3389/froh.2022.971223 PMID: 36186536

Bida, S. M., Cre u, O. C., Bida, C., Tudorici, T., & Chirita, R. (2025). ORAL HEALTH CHALLENGES IN PATIENTS WITH PSYCHIATRIC DISORDERS: RISKS, BARRIERS, AND CLINICAL IMPLICATIONS. *Romanian Journal of Medical and Dental Education*, *14*(2).

Bisht, V., Das, B., Hussain, A., Kumar, V., & Navani, N. K. (2024). Understanding of probiotic origin antimicrobial peptides: a sustainable approach ensuring food safety. *npj Science of Food*, *8*(1), 67.

Bolton, D., & Gillett, G. (2019). *The biopsychosocial model of health and disease: New philosophical and scientific developments*. Springer. DOI: 10.1007/978-3-030-11899-0

Borg-Bartolo, R., Roccuzzo, A., Tennert, C., Prasinou, M., Jäggi, M., Molinero-Mourelle, P., Bornstein, M. M., & Campus, G. (2025). Oral health-related quality of life of community-dwellers in the canton of Bern, Switzerland. *Acta Odontologica Scandinavica*, *84*, 42707. DOI: 10.2340/aos.v84.42707

Borsa, L., Dubois, M., Sacco, G., & Lupi, L. (2021). Analysis the link between periodontal diseases and Alzheimer's disease: A systematic review. *International Journal of Environmental Research and Public Health*, *18*(17), 9312. DOI: 10.3390/ijerph18179312 PMID: 34501899

Cademartori, M. G., Gastal, M. T., Nascimento, G. G., Demarco, F. F., & Correa, M. B. (2018). Is depression associated with oral health outcomes in adults and elders? A systematic review and meta-analysis. *Clinical Oral Investigations*, *22*(8), 2685–2702. DOI: 10.1007/s00784-018-2611-y PMID: 30191327

Cao, R., Lai, J., Fu, X., Qiu, P., Chen, J., & Liu, W. (2023). Association between psychological stress, anxiety and oral health status among college students during the Omicron wave: A cross-sectional study. *BMC Oral Health*, *23*(1), 470. DOI: 10.1186/s12903-023-03151-3 PMID: 37424009

Chan, A. K. Y., Hui, J. C. Y., Hu, L. L., & Chu, C. H. (2026). The Mouth–Mind Connection: Interplay of Oral and Mental Health in Older Adults. *Geriatrics (Basel, Switzerland)*, *11*(1), 8. DOI: 10.3390/geriatrics11010008 PMID: 41562791

Dao, A. T., Do, L. G., Stormon, N., Dhanapriyanka, M., & Ha, D. H. (2025). Causal analyses in longitudinal observational studies in oral health: A scoping review. *Community Dentistry and Oral Epidemiology*, *53*(1), 7–16. DOI: 10.1111/cdoe.13002 PMID: 39248439

Di Stefano, M., Polizzi, A., Santonocito, S., Romano, A., Lombardi, T., & Isola, G. (2022). Impact of oral microbiome in periodontal health and periodontitis: A critical review on prevention and treatment. *International Journal of Molecular Sciences*, *23*(9), 5142. DOI: 10.3390/ijms23095142 PMID: 35563531

Eicher, T. P., & Mohajeri, M. H. (2022). Overlapping mechanisms of action of brain-active bacteria and bacterial metabolites in the pathogenesis of common brain diseases. *Nutrients*, *14*(13), 2661. DOI: 10.3390/nu14132661 PMID: 35807841

Farid, A., Fatima, Z., Fareed, Z., Athar, Z., Manzoor, A., & Sheharyar, M. F. H. (2026). Emerging Infectious Control Technologies: A Global Perspective Surveillance and Response to Hospital Acquired Infections. In *Innovation and Transformation of Public Health* (pp. 459-496). IGI Global Scientific Publishing.

Farid, A., Han, W., Kwan, J. K., & Yeung, K. L. (2025). Enhancing bedding hygiene in long-term care facilities: Investigating the impact of multilevel antimicrobial polymers (MAP-1) on bacterial and MDRO reduction. *Antimicrobial Resistance and Infection Control*, *14*(1), 36. DOI: 10.1186/s13756-025-01555-0 PMID: 40270052

Farid, A., Han, W., Lai, C. K. C., Kwan, J. K. C., & Yeung, K. L. (2025). Clinical evaluation of MAP-1 antimicrobial coating on patient privacy curtains: Insights from a randomized trial in a Hong Kong hospital. *The Journal of Hospital Infection*, *162*, 223–231. DOI: 10.1016/j.jhin.2025.05.012 PMID: 40456490

Folấyan, M. O., Bernard, O. T., Titus, O. S., Alade, O., Aliyu, T. K., Bhayat, A., Ndembi, N., Fasiku, G., & El Tantawi, M. (2025). Cultural practices, oral health service utilisation and oral health policy and guidelines development in Africa: Insights from the yorùbá ethnic group. *Frontiers in Oral Health, 6*, 1539827. DOI: 10.3389/froh.2025.1539827 PMID: 40045959

Ganesan, A., Kumar, G., Gauthaman, J., Lakshmi, K. C., & Kumbalaparambil, Y. A. (2024). Exploring the relationship between psychoneuroimmunology and oral diseases: A comprehensive review and analysis. *Journal of Lifestyle Medicine, 14*(1), 13–19. DOI: 10.15280/jlm.2024.14.1.13 PMID: 38665319

Hajishengallis, G., & Chavakis, T. (2021). Local and systemic mechanisms linking periodontal disease and inflammatory comorbidities. *Nature Reviews. Immunology, 21*(7), 426–440. DOI: 10.1038/s41577-020-00488-6 PMID: 33510490

Johansson, C., Beckman, L., Rystedt, I., Kramer, A. C. A., & Lindmark, U. (2025). Oral health and oral health needs among patients with serious mental illness: Reflections and experiences of psychiatric staff in Sweden. *BMC Psychology, 13*(1), 446. DOI: 10.1186/s40359-025-02780-3 PMID: 40296173

Kapila, Y. L. (2021). Oral health's inextricable connection to systemic health: Special populations bring to bear multimodal relationships and factors connecting periodontal disease to systemic diseases and conditions. *Periodontology 2000, 87*(1), 11–16. DOI: 10.1111/prd.12398 PMID: 34463994

Khairunnisa, Z., Siluvai, S., Kanakavelan, K., Agnes, L., Indumathi, K. P., & Krishnaprakash, G. (2024). Mental and oral health: a dual frontier in healthcare integration and prevention. *Cureus, 16*(12). Afroz, T., Beyene, J., Zaheer, K., Alameddine, M., Nabi, M. H., Hawlader, M. D. H., & Hossain, A. (2025). Oral health care challenges in individuals with severe mental illness: a qualitative meta-synthesis. *Frontiers in Oral Health, 6*, 1655450.

Khammissa, R. A. G., & Andriankaja, O. M. (2025). Deepening the relationship between diabetes, oral health and periodontal disease. *Frontiers in Oral Health, 6*, 1752592. DOI: 10.3389/froh.2025.1752592 PMID: 41584962

Kisely, S. (2016). No mental health without oral health. *Canadian Journal of Psychiatry. Revue Canadienne de Psychiatrie, 61*(5), 277–282. DOI: 10.1177/0706743716632523 PMID: 27254802

Kisely, S. (2023). Periodontal health and psychiatric disorders. *Current Oral Health Reports, 10*(3), 111–116. DOI: 10.1007/s40496-023-00339-y

Kisely, S., Sawyer, E., Siskind, D., & Lalloo, R. (2016). The oral health of people with anxiety and depressive disorders–a systematic review and meta-analysis. *Journal of Affective Disorders, 200*, 119–132. DOI: 10.1016/j.jad.2016.04.040 PMID: 27130961

Kosan, E., Krois, J., Wingenfeld, K., Deuter, C. E., Gaudin, R., & Schwendicke, F. (2022). Patients' perspectives on artificial intelligence in dentistry: A controlled study. *Journal of Clinical Medicine, 11*(8), 2143. DOI: 10.3390/jcm11082143 PMID: 35456236

Lipsky, M. S., Singh, T., Zakeri, G., & Hung, M. (2024). Oral health and older adults: A narrative review. *Dentistry Journal, 12*(2), 30. DOI: 10.3390/dj12020030 PMID: 38392234

Malicka, B., Skośkiewicz-Malinowska, K., & Kaczmarek, U. (2022). The impact of socioeconomic status, general health and oral health on health-related quality of life, oral health-related quality of life and mental health among Polish older adults. *BMC Geriatrics, 22*(1), 2. DOI: 10.1186/s12877-021-02716-7 PMID: 34979959

Martínez, M., Postolache, T. T., García-Bueno, B., Leza, J. C., Figuero, E., Lowry, C. A., & Malan-Müller, S. (2022). The role of the oral microbiota related to periodontal diseases in anxiety, mood and trauma-and stress-related disorders. *Frontiers in Psychiatry, 12*, 814177. DOI: 10.3389/fpsyt.2021.814177 PMID: 35153869

Marwaha, K., Cain, R., Asmis, K., Czaplinski, K., Holland, N., Mayer, D. C. G., & Chacon, J. (2025). Exploring the complex relationship between psychosocial stress and the gut microbiome: Implications for inflammation and immune modulation. *Journal of Applied Physiology (Bethesda, Md.), 138*(2), 518–535. DOI: 10.1152/japplphysiol.00652.2024 PMID: 39813028

McDowell, I. (2023). Theoretical models of health behavior. *Understanding health determinants: Explanatory theories for social epidemiology*, 253-306.

Ng, S. K., & Leung, W. K. (2008). A community study on the relationship of dental anxiety with oral health status and oral health-related quality of life. *Community Dentistry and Oral Epidemiology, 36*(4), 347–356. DOI: 10.1111/j.1600-0528.2007.00412.x PMID: 19145721

Nunez, S. G., Rabelo, S. P., Subotic, N., Caruso, J. W., & Knezevic, N. N. (2025). Chronic stress and autoimmunity: The role of HPA axis and cortisol dysregulation. *International Journal of Molecular Sciences, 26*(20), 9994. DOI: 10.3390/ijms26209994 PMID: 41155288

Pavlou, I. A., Spandidos, D. A., Zoumpourlis, V., & Papakosta, V. K. (2024). Neurobiology of bruxism: The impact of stress. *Biomedical Reports*, *20*(4), 1–10. DOI: 10.3892/br.2024.1747 PMID: 38414628

Peres, M. A., Macpherson, L. M., Weyant, R. J., Daly, B., Venturelli, R., Mathur, M. R., Listl, S., Celeste, R. K., Guarnizo-Herreño, C. C., Kearns, C., Benzian, H., Allison, P., & Watt, R. G. (2019). Oral diseases: A global public health challenge. *Lancet*, *394*(10194), 249–260. DOI: 10.1016/S0140-6736(19)31146-8 PMID: 31327369

Prabhu, S. R., Warnakulasuriya, S., & Bhardwaj, S. (Eds.). (2026). *Lifestyle in Oral Health and Disease: A Comprehensive Guide for Oral Healthcare Providers*. Springer Nature.

Ray, R. R. (2023). Periodontitis: An oral disease with severe consequences. *Applied Biochemistry and Biotechnology*, *195*(1), 17–32. DOI: 10.1007/s12010-022-04127-9 PMID: 36098930

Rogers, A. A., Willumsen, T., Strømme, H., & Johnsen, J. A. K. (2022). Top-down self-regulation processes as determinants of oral hygiene self-care behaviour: A systematic scoping review. *Clinical and Experimental Dental Research*, *8*(4), 807–826. DOI: 10.1002/cre2.548 PMID: 35396799

Salvador, S. M., & Toassi, R. F. C. (2021). Oral health self-perception: Physical, social and cultural expressions of a body in interaction with the world. *Physis (Rio de Janeiro, Brazil)*, *31*(1), e310122. DOI: 10.1590/s0103-73312021310122

Visentin, D., Gobin, I., & Maglica, Ž. (2023). Periodontal pathogens and their links to neuroinflammation and neurodegeneration. *Microorganisms*, *11*(7), 1832. DOI: 10.3390/microorganisms11071832 PMID: 37513004

Visscher, C. M., Baad-Hansen, L., Durham, J., Goulet, J. P., Michelotti, A., Barraza, C. R., & Raphael, K. G. (2018). Benefits of implementing pain-related disability and psychological assessment in dental practice for patients with temporomandibular pain and other oral health conditions. *The Journal of the American Dental Association*, *149*(6), 422–431. DOI: 10.1016/j.adaj.2017.12.031 PMID: 29653670

Watt, R. G., Daly, B., Allison, P., Macpherson, L. M., Venturelli, R., Listl, S., Weyant, R. J., Mathur, M. R., Guarnizo-Herreño, C. C., Celeste, R. K., Peres, M. A., Kearns, C., & Benzian, H. (2019). Ending the neglect of global oral health: Time for radical action. *Lancet*, *394*(10194), 261–272. DOI: 10.1016/S0140-6736(19)31133-X PMID: 31327370

Yactayo-Alburquerque, M. T., Alen-Méndez, M. L., Azañedo, D., Comandé, D., & Hernández-Vásquez, A. (2021). Impact of oral diseases on oral health-related quality of life: A systematic review of studies conducted in Latin America and the Caribbean. *PLoS One*, *16*(6), e0252578. DOI: 10.1371/journal.pone.0252578 PMID: 34077473

Zavala-Medina, L. C., Salas-Leiva, J. S., Villegas-Mercado, C. E., Arreguín-Cano, J. A., Soto-Barreras, U., Santana-Delgado, S. A., Larrinua-Pacheco, A. D., García-Vega, M. F., & Bermúdez, M. (2026). Oral Dysbiosis and Neuroinflammation: Implications for Alzheimer's, Parkinson's and Mood Disorders. *Microorganisms*, *14*(1), 143. DOI: 10.3390/microorganisms14010143 PMID: 41597661

Zhao, X., Liu, L., Zhao, P., Jiang, W., & Nahata, M. (2024). The Global Burden and Trends of Mental Disorders and Substance Use Disorders Among Adolescents and Young Adults: Findings from the Global Burden of Disease Study 1990–2021. *Available at SSRN* 4957498. DOI: 10.2139/ssrn.4957498

Zhu, N., Bian, J., Dong, Z., & Zhu, N. (2025). An empirical study on the psychological impact of medical AI on patients undergoing dental surgery. *Scientific Reports*, *16*(1), 401. DOI: 10.1038/s41598-025-29754-0 PMID: 41339456

Chapter 10

Integrative Omics Approaches to Oral-Systemic Health Epidemiology

R. Alfiya Roofi
Department of Microbiology, Sacred Heart College, Tirupattur, India

B. Lokeshwari
http://orcid.org/0009-0005-6612-5134
Department of Microbiology, Sacred Heart College, Tirupattur, India

P. Saranraj
http://orcid.org/0000-0002-5052-6532
Department of Microbiology, Sacred Heart College, Tirupattur, India

A. Mubarak Ali
http://orcid.org/0009-0009-6367-7864
Department of Microbiology, Sacred Heart College, Tirupattur, India

S. Mayilazhagan
http://orcid.org/0009-0007-4750-6905
Department of Microbiology, Sacred Heart College, Tirupattur, India

ABSTRACT

Oral mucositis (OM) is a pain and suffering condition associated with cancer treatment, negatively affecting the patient's quality of life and treatment outcomes. The oral cavity houses the second largest community of microbes in the human body, and the perturbation of this microbiome has been shown to be associated with many

DOI: 10.4018/979-8-3373-8402-3.ch010

systemic diseases, including cardiovascular, diabetes, and inflammatory diseases. Studies of transcriptome and proteome of Candida albicans infection have identified immune responses in hosts and strategies used by fungi to escape, offering targets for potential therapies. Although there have been remarkable developments in the field, there are still challenges such as cost, lack of standardization, and need for validation studies.

1. INTRODUCTION

Oral microbiota represents the second most significant microbial community within the human body, following the gut microbiota. Over 772 bacterial species have been identified in the oral cavity (Hobson et al., 2021). The oral cavity comprises several distinct ecological niches, including the tongue, oral mucosa, buccal surfaces, tooth surfaces, gingiva, and sub- and supragingival sites. Saliva represents a key component within these niches. Diverse microbial strains with various activities and different susceptibilities to diseases are present in each of the above-mentioned niches. The oral microbiota generates various primary and secondary metabolites that participate in the initial stages of food digestion. Bacteria from the mouth along with their metabolites, such as microbial metabolites and endotoxins, may get into the blood circulation system causing systemic inflammation (Eichner & Dietz, 2003). Poor oral hygiene contributes to various systemic conditions, and conversely, systemic diseases can exacerbate oral health problems. This bidirectional relationship is particularly evident in connections between oral diseases and conditions such as rheumatoid arthritis, diabetes, cardiovascular disease, and pneumonia. Moreover, the mouth is a model structure for other regions of the body, and the complicated biological ecosystem of the mouth could give insight on the mechanisms behind diseases. Patients with HNSCC suffer from a very painful and debilitating condition known as Oral Mucositis (OM) due to the treatment they receive (Reynolds et al., 2006).

Oral Mucositis (OM) is one of the common conditions that result from the treatment of cancers, particularly among HNSCC patients receiving chemotherapy or radiotherapy. Cancer treatments can lead to inflammation and damage of the mucosal membranes in the mouth and pharynx. The oral microbiome is considered the second largest collection of microbes within the human body. Additionally, as part of the body's immune system response, these microorganisms release host-derived anti-inflammatory cytokines that contribute to inflammation and affect various human tissues and organs (Miura et al., 2022). Accumulating evidence from epidemiological studies and clinical research supports the association between oral bacteria, their products, and the development of cardiovascular diseases. As part of the immune response, oral microorganisms release host-derived cytokines that contribute to inflammation and affect various tissues and organs. Accumulating evidence from epidemiological studies and clinical research supports the association between oral bacteria, their products, and the development of cardiovascular diseases.

2. PERSONALIZED THERAPIES FOR RISK MANAGEMENT IN OMICS

Oral Mucositis (OM) exemplifies a complex human trait requiring both host genetic predisposition and an initiating event—such as drugs, radiation, or therapy—making it an ideal model for studying gene-environment interactions. As a complex trait, OM is likely influenced by multiple genes (Galié et al., 2021). Moreover, assessing the interactions of these genes with other clinical, behavioural, and epidemiologic traits provides a good approach to identify novel biomarkers and tools to improve OM risk prediction. Moreover, assessing the interactions of these genes with other clinical, behavioural, and epidemiologic traits provides a good approach to identify novel biomarkers and tools to improve OM risk prediction.

2.1 Genomics

Host genetic susceptibility to OM has been investigated using candidate gene studies, pathway-based analyses, and Genome-Wide Association Approaches (GWAS). To determine the potential role in the specific disease, candidate gene studies focus on significant genes that had been previously selected on basis of knowledge or hypothesis (Alemán et al., 2018). On the other hand, pathway-based studies analyze a set of genes that may be involved in common biological processes or functions, and hence a combined effect on a certain trait. Genome-Wide Association Studies (GWAS) perform comprehensive whole-genome scans without prior hypotheses regarding specific genes or pathways (Uffelmann et al., 2021). Genes and SNPs or single nucleotide polymorphisms that are associated with OM in HNSCC patients have been documented through several genomic approaches.

2.2 Genome-Wide Approach

The whole genome association studies without any hypothesis are good for finding out the genetic factors involved in complex diseases. However, this approach requires large sample sizes and incurs high costs for reliable replication, limiting its widespread application. Schack et al. reported the Stimulator of IF Response gene Acting Interactor 1 (STING1) to have a strong association with OM in their three-cohort study (1183 Danes, finding phase; 597 Danes, replicate phase; and

235 Asians, confirmation phase). STING1 (also known as TMEM173) is associated with infection, inflammation, immunity, autophagy, and apoptosis. In an earlier genome-wide analysis by Yang et al., SNP rs117157809 located in the protein coding gene, TNKS (tankyrase), has been found to increase OM by over three-folds among patients having nasopharyngeal cancer. TNKS is involved in radiation damage. Depletion of TNKS has been found to cause sensitivity to ionizing radiation-induced mutation, chromosomal aberration, telomere fusion, and cell death (Figure 1) This figure illustrates how omics technologies (genomics, transcriptomics, proteomics, and metabolomics) are integrated to understand an individual's biological profile and identify disease-related genetic variations. Genome-wide analysis examines the complete genetic information to assess disease risk and detect potential health problems at an early stage. Based on these findings, personalized therapies are designed to provide targeted treatments and effective risk management tailored to each patient's genetic profile. This approach improves early diagnosis, prevention, treatment outcomes, and overall healthcare by delivering precision medicine.

Figure 1. Personalized Therapies for Risk Management in Omics

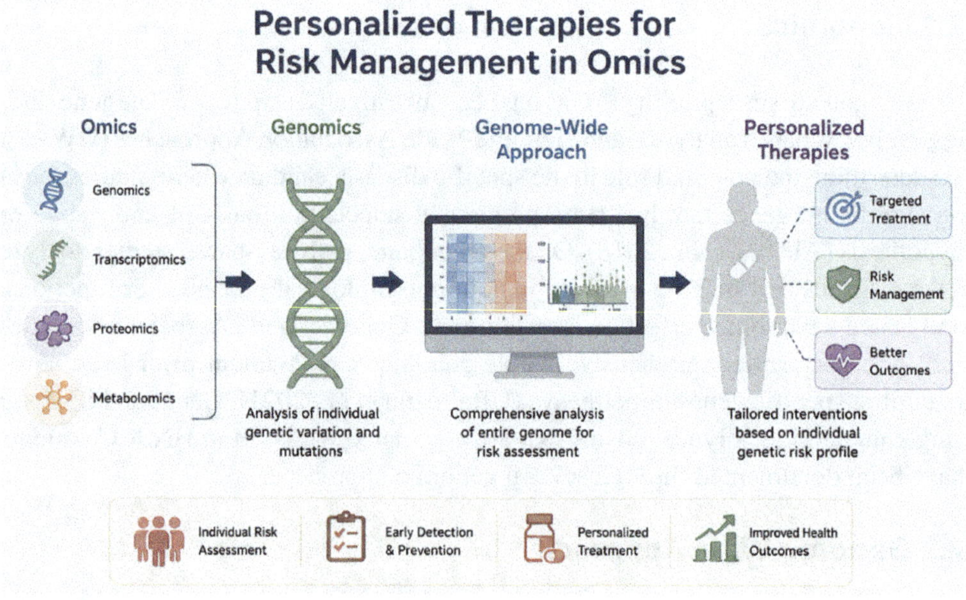

3. METAGENOMICS AND MULTI-OMICS INTEGRATION

Metagenomic sequencing has revealed gut microbial communities that vary across different physiological and pathological states. Furthermore, multi-omic studies—including microbial transcriptomics (RNA), metaproteomics (proteins), and metabolomics (metabolites)—have advanced our understanding of microbiome ecology, unculturable microorganisms, and the complex interactions among the host, gut microbes, and environmental factors that influence health. For instance, A clinical study demonstrated that daily administration of 12 g of prebiotic fiber for 4 weeks significantly enhanced beneficial bacterial metabolite production and increased Bifidobacteria populations in healthy subjects (Kang et al., 2022). Several genes responsible for prebiotic consumption, acetate production, and oxidation of choline to betaine. In addition, the amounts of plasma protein components involved in blood vessel activity, fibrosis response, immune cell communication, and hormonal regulation associated with obesity were associated with the abundances of genes of carbohydrate-active enzymes in the specific microbiome of subjects whose regular diet was supplemented with foods containing fibres from peas and oranges over ten weeks. In contrast, a very low-calorie diet (800 kcal per day) in obese postmenopausal women affected some microbiome components in correlation with changes in the composition of specific bile acids, plasma metabolites, and the expression pathways of genes in adipose tissue (Djekic et al., 2020).

A change to a Mediterranean diet for two months in contrast to nut consumption alone, metabolic changes were related to microbiota genus (Lachnospira, NK4A136 and wild-type Ruminococcus) together with focal metabolite classes (cholate and cadaverine). A 4-week vegetarian diet in heart disease with ischemia positively impacted cardiovascular and metabolic risk factors and shifted gut microbial composition (predominantly determined by several strains of Ruminococcus) and metabolites of plasma (for example, l-carnitine, acylcarnitine and typical phospholipids) (Zhou et al., 2023). Furthermore, differential gut microbial proteins were found in the stools from persons on diets with different amount of fiber and glycaemic index for 28 days, among them being involved in synthesis and breakdown of fatty acids. Importantly, a switch from a beef to a chicken-based diet within two weeks predominantly altered the number of Bacteroides genus, and therefore likely caused immunoglobulins in faeces, especially in high- and middle-BMI Chinese volunteers.

Cross-sectional analysis revealed that intake of plant-based nutrients or artificial sweeteners correlated with metabolic differences—primarily involving bile acids—based on gut microbiome enterotypes (Krüger et al., 2015). Gut microbiota composition also affected correlations between soy isoflavones intake and plasma and fecal metabolites, including 2-hydroxybutyrate, glycine, and liquiritigenin, that had significance in the development of hypertension and diabetes. Female twins were found to have remarkable correlation of yogurt consumption with reduced visceral fat deposition as well as changes in the focal metabolome (higher 3-hydroxyoctanoic acid) and gut microbiome (temporary increase of A. thermophilus and B. lactis species) (Zaas et al., 2010). Interestingly, chicken eaters had more diverse gut microbiota and increased concentrations of Prevotella types 2 and 9, which were positively correlated with focal concentration of indole and skatole. Moreover, modifications in the gut flora resulting from the meal quality at the same time affected the concentrations of metabolites responsible for cardiovascular or intestinal diseases. Moreover, differences in the gastrointestinal metabolome, including microbial co-metabolites produced by the gut microbiota, correlated with the diet of vegans and omnivores (Jafari & Azuaje, 2006).

It has usually been shown that vegans have higher amounts of potentially beneficial host microbiome metabolites (short- and medium-chain fatty acids and their derivatives) than omnivores. Also, microbial genes and proteins responsible for cell motility, nutrient breakdown and transport, and amino acid and mineral synthesis were demonstrated to be more prevalent in the vegan or vegetarian diet. In vegetarians, an increased amount of microbial pathway associated with utilization of branched chain amino acids was observed together with decreased circulation of BCAAs. Therefore, in comparison with other populations, Indian patients possessed different gut microbiota and serum metabolome compositions, which were associated with diet, based on multi-omics data (Donia et al., 2014). At the same time, increased levels of the targeted short-chain fatty acids and favourable microbiome-associated metabolome profile were correlated with high adherence to the Mediterranean diet (mainly plant-based). It was also demonstrated that gut microbes could utilize metabolic pathways affecting epigenome to influence the impact of the diet on human health. Thus, the expression level of epigenetically relevant enzymes, including DNA methyltransferase, protein acetyltransferase, deacetylases, and demethylases can be influenced by microbes in the diet through metabolites such as phenolic acids, isothiocyanates, and short-chain fatty acids (Segata et al., 2012). In this connection, one recent study explored the impact of common diets on the composition of gut microbiota and the epigenetic state of a person. Nevertheless, further clinical research is required for the investigation of the food-microbiota-epigenetics axis and the application of nutritional precision approaches, since most of the information is gathered through animal studies and laboratory experiments. Moreover, it was found that malnutrition of the gut microbiota can negatively influence miRNA expression, which can result in the development of various illnesses (Cheung et al., 2022).

The microbial structure (abundance of Proteobacteria species and Gammaproteobacteria) and miRNA expression (hsa-let-7g-5p, hsa-miR-170, and hsa-miR-186-3p) were likely responsible for the connection between poor diet quality and increased risk of developing mild cognitive impairment in middle-aged and older Chinese individuals. Interestingly, human obesity is known to be related to the interplay between circulating miRNAs (miR-130b-3p, miR-185-5p, and miR-21-5p) and the number of bacterial species (such as Bacteroides Geerthi). Also, vegetarians, vegans, and omnivores in healthy people can be easily differentiated by combining analysis of 25 miRNAs, 25 taxa, and 7 dietary components (Murugesan et al., 2020). Moreover, plant-derived miRNAs (xenomas) in diets were found to change the composition of the gut microbiota and the permeability of gut epithelium (Table 1) This table summarizes the integration of metagenomics with other omics technologies to provide a comprehensive understanding of microbial communities. Each omics approach contributes unique information, such as genetic material, gene regulation, RNA expression, proteins, and metabolites, enabling a complete analysis of microbial functions. Integrating these datasets improves the identification of active microorganisms, enzymes, biomarkers, and ecosystem functions. Overall, multi-omics integration supports precision microbiome research and advances applications in biotechnology, healthcare, and environmental monitoring.

Table 1. Metagenomics and Multi-Omics Integration

Omics Approach	Role in Metagenomics Integration	Applications
Metagenomics	Analyzes genetic material from microbial communities	Microbial ecology, environmental monitoring
Epigenomics	Studies DNA modifications and gene regulation	Understanding microbial adaptation and gene expression control
Transcriptomics	Examines RNA transcripts produced by microbes	Identifying metabolically active microorganisms
Proteomics	Analyzes proteins expressed by microbial communities	Enzyme discovery, pathway characterization
Metabolomics	Investigates small-molecule metabolites	Biomarker discovery, ecosystem function analysis
Integrated multi-omics	Combines data from multiple omics platforms	Precision microbiome studies, biotechnology, health and environmental applications

4. CLINICAL IMPLICATIONS

It has become clear that the oral-gut axis is a bi-directional pathway where the bacterial balance is critical for disease prevention. Oral bacteria such as Porphyromonas gingivalis and Fusobacterium nucleatum may migrate to the gut, disturb the delicate balance in the intestines, and increase the levels of inflammation in the system, which contributes to autoimmune and metabolic disorders. Dysbiosis crosstalk could be harnessed to devise novel diagnostics and therapy approaches (Schmidt et al., 2019). Studying saliva and faecal microbiota provides an invasive method to identify the presence of predictive biomarkers associated with some diseases, such as Inflammatory Bowel Disease (IBD) and colorectal cancer. There are different therapies targeted at the restoration of microbial balance that include antibiotics and probiotics, FMT for extreme cases of bacterial imbalance, and some pharmaceuticals, including metformin and allopurinol, proven to affect gut microbiome (Dong et al., 2021). Notably, for patients suffering from biochemical and autoimmune diseases, prevention of oral health is a key aspect of therapy that can help disrupt this vicious cycle and decrease the levels of systemic inflammation. It is necessary to understand the exact dynamics involved in this phenomenon to create precise diagnostic tools and treatments which will tackle the disease at its core (Pietiainen et al., 2018).

5. OMICS PERSPECTIVE ON CANDIDA-HOST INFECTION

The host-pathogen interaction has become "the epitome of biomedical research" due to advances in both innate and regulatory immunology. Furthermore, host-pathogen interaction in a standard Candida infection can be studied in an objective and quantitative manner due to the advancement in the science of systems biology and omics technology. Understanding host-pathogen interaction in Candida albicans virulence and innate immunity interactions and understanding the roles that each of these processes play in the development of Candida albicans would be essential to gain full understanding of host-pathogen interaction. This might lead to the development of new therapies targeting host immune response to infection (Abusleme et al., 2013).

6. CHALLENGES APART FROM OMICS AND SYSTEMS BIOLOGY APPROACHES

The study of the host-pathogen system is still faced with challenges because of the emergence of systems biology and omics technologies. The challenges that should be considered in the proteomic analysis of the direct interaction between immune response cells of a parasitic host and fungi have been mentioned by Krüger et al. (Buhlin et al., 2009). They are associated with the extreme complexity of proteins (including the extended dynamic range), choosing appropriate donors of blood for the research, choosing the right Multiplicity Of Infection (MOI) without reducing the quality of the result of relative analysis, demands from isolation techniques for immunological effector cells, demands from culturing conditions for immunological effector cells, and homogeneity of the cytoplasm suspension for inoculation. In the future, transcriptomic profiling may prove useful for fungal diagnostics.

It has been argued by some researchers that the induced transcriptional profile can be utilized to differentiate bacterial and Candida infections (Moran et al., 1996). However, there are certain challenges that should be considered. For verification purposes, the transcriptome profiles should be replicated in other research involving large patient cohorts with candidemia. Moreover, the high costs and time that is needed for conducting transcriptomics analysis form an additional challenge. Since the transcriptomics data is complex, each of such experiments requires standardization and validation (Fitzgerald & Kagan, 2020). In the case of research of fungi, the development of the appropriate protocol becomes a necessity. Such approach may cause certain techniques to be ineffective owing to the specific anatomy of fungi and especially the fungal cell wall. In some cases, the presence of the fungal cell wall may prevent from effective lysis of fungal cells, resulting in incomplete lysis (Edfeldt et al., 2002). Moreover, the wall of the fungi may interfere with the process of metabolic labelling necessary for such techniques as Stable Isotope Labelling by Amino Acids in Cell Culture (SILAC), as mentioned by Colibri et al. (2005). Nevertheless, new techniques are being applied in the field of systems biology and omics. The effectiveness and the precision of these techniques have not been validated even though recently reported.

7. ORAL MICROBIOME AND GUT MICROBIOME

Similarity between the gut and the oral microbiota has been observed. It is believed that about 45% of the microorganisms in these two ecosystems are common. The five predominant phyla in the oral microbiota include Proteobacteria, Firmicutes, Bacteroidetes, Actinobacteria, and Fusobacteria among others (Kaptoge et al., 2014). Similarly, there are certain types of bacteria that are dominant in the gut microbiota such as Actinobacteria, Bacteroidetes, and Firmicutes. The prevalent bacteria in the oral cavity vary among individuals from different geographical locations. For example, Neisseria is the common genus in the Chinese population while Veillonella is the common genus in the Canadian population and Prevotella in the Qatari population. Studies have shown that there exists oral microbiota capable of causing gut dysbiosis either through systemic mechanisms or direct transfer of oral microbiota to the gut. According to a bioinformatic study on the microbes in both oral and gut of five different countries' populations, about 10% of the oral microbiota successfully transfers to the gut (Pushalkar et al., 2020). One such well-known oral pathogen, Fusobacterium nucleatum, which is sporadic, has also been detected in the gut, according to our previous studies involving gut microbiota. The formation of arterial plaques has been favourably associated with Fusobacterium nucleatum in the gut. Mostly all studies related to this topic are done in animal models in which bacteria are provided orally to mice and then the change in gut microbiota is observed therefore. For example, when Fusobacterium nucleatum was administered orally to healthy mice, there was an observed change in the focused microbiota including increase in apoptosis markers in colon tissue and increased abundance of Fusobacterium nucleatum.

Antibiotics such as metronidazole have been administered to reduce or even eliminate this effect (Joshi et al., 2014). There is an observation that patients with other health conditions tend to be susceptible to the transmission of opportunistic infections. Some infections, such as Fusobacterium nucleatum subtypes, can also cause this translocation thereby worsening the level of severity of the disease. The alterations in the levels of gut microbe and Firmicutes, who are the primary biomarkers for patients with coronary heart diseases and strokes, are also examples that show the relationship that exists between the mouth and microbes about Cardio Vascular Diseases (CVDs). Thus, our hypothesis is that the intestinal microbiota could have a tremendous therapeutic effect on the gut microbiome and even aid in causing CVDs. For example, the use of Oral Microbiota Transplantation (OMT) technique has shown promising results in reducing negative effects in gut and mouth bacteria, which might positively affect CVD treatment (Tang et al., 2017).

8. POTENTIAL MECHANISMS BY WHICH THE ORAL MICROBIOTA AFFECT CVDS

8.1 Inflammation and Immune Responses

The oral microbiota plays a considerable role in systemic and local inflammation that affects cardiometabolic health and facilitates the progression of CVDs. Dysbiosis of the oral microbiota and elevated periodontal pathogens trigger immune responses, including neutrophil and macrophage activation. Besides, immune response activates cells like gamma delta and dendritic cells that produce mediators leading to inflammation. The dysbiosis of oral microbiota and the extent of inflammatory process are closely interconnected, thus, forming a vicious circle (Fan & Pedersen, 2021). The blood contains pro-inflammatory cytokines because of oral inflammation and high concentrations of certain oral bacteria; the release of mediators of inflammation leads to the creation of atheromatous plaque. It is characterized by an abundance of acute phase-related proteins, pro-inflammatory cytokines and chemokines like fibrinogen and Inter Leukin (IL)-6. Moreover, alterations in the gut microbiota due to mouth-gut microbial transfer and the presence of oral bacteria in blood can increase the systemic inflammation and lead to heart disease (Chen et al., 2023).

8.2 Lipopolysaccharide

The gram-negative bacteria's outer membrane consists of Lipo-Polysaccharide (LPS) or endotoxin. Earlier studies indicated that the LPS is the significant mediator of inflammation and might contribute to the pathogenesis of atherosclerosis. Endotoxemia and the dysfunction of endothelial cells may happen due to the role of the LPS as an immunomodulator or immune stimulator that migrates from the oral cavity to the blood (Hünniger et al., 2014). After migration, LPS targets Lipopolysaccharide Binding Protein (LBP), CD14, and Toll-Like Receptor 4 (TLR4). Because of their binding, the inflammatory process is started, which triggers the release of pro-inflammatory cytokines. It has already been shown that the TLR4 stimulates the pathogenesis of atherosclerosis in mouse models and has been detected in the plaques formed because of atherosclerosis. Moreover, the increasing serum levels of LPS or LBP have been related to increased cardiovascular disease risk. The keystone pathogen *P. gingivalis* secretes lipopolysaccharide (LPS), which modulates adhesion molecules (ICAM-1 and E-selectin) and impairs polymorphonuclear leukocyte function. Therefore, the immunological reaction is suppressed, and leukocyte recruitment is hindered (Dühring et al., 2015).

8.3 Cytokines

Pro-inflammatory cytokines serve as key mediators linking oral microbiota to atherosclerotic inflammation. The higher levels of pro-inflammatory cytokines such as TNF, IL-1, and IL-6 have been reported to be correlated with an increased risk of developing cardiovascular disease in epidemiological studies. Several well-known oral infections have been found to correlate with pro-inflammatory cytokines. For example, oral Porphyromonas has been favourably correlated with pro-inflammatory cytokines in saliva such as IL-1β, IL-2, IL-8, and IL-13 in human studies using 16S sequencing data while Fusobacterium has been correlated with IL-1β. In addition, several pro-inflammatory cytokines such as IL-1β, IL-2, IL-4, IL-6, IL-7, IL-9, IL-12, and IL-17 have been positively correlated with oral *Streptococcus* bacteria. Autoinducer 2, which is released by *P. gingivalis* (a known oral pathogen), induces the secretion of IL-8 from oral epithelial cells (Durmuş et al., 2015).

It is known that this cytokine plays a role in endothelial dysfunction, which is characterized by elevated levels of cell adhesion molecules, pro-coagulant activity, and mononuclear cell adhesion, along with IL-6 and MCP1. Also, *P. gingivalis* and *F. nucleatum* can induce the secretion of TNF-α, IL-6, and IL-8 in macrophages, neutrophils, and monocytes (Remmele et al., 2015). An animal study has demonstrated that *P. gingivalis* infection induces the accumulation of macrophages and inflammatory mediators including CD40, IFN, IL-1β, and IL-6 in the atherosclerotic lesions of mice. It appears that these responses occur less in the case of mice with immunodeficiency (Dix et al., 2015). The higher concentrations of bacteria on their surface contribute to both the systemic and local inflammatory processes, as well as cytokine and mediator production (Figure 2) This figure explains the potential mechanisms by which oral microbiota contribute to Cardiovascular Diseases (CVDs). During periodontal disease or oral dysbiosis, bacteria such as Porphyromonas gingivalis can enter the bloodstream and release Lipo-Polysaccharide (LPS), which activates immune cells through TLR4 and the NF-κB signalling pathway. This stimulation leads to the release of pro-inflammatory cytokines, including TNF-α, IL-1β, IL-6, IL-17, and CRP, causing chronic systemic inflammation. The resulting inflammation damages blood vessels, promotes atherosclerotic plaque formation and instability, and ultimately increases the risk of cardiovascular events such as heart attack (myocardial infarction) and stroke.

Figure 2. Potential Mechanisms of Oral Microbiota Affect CVDs

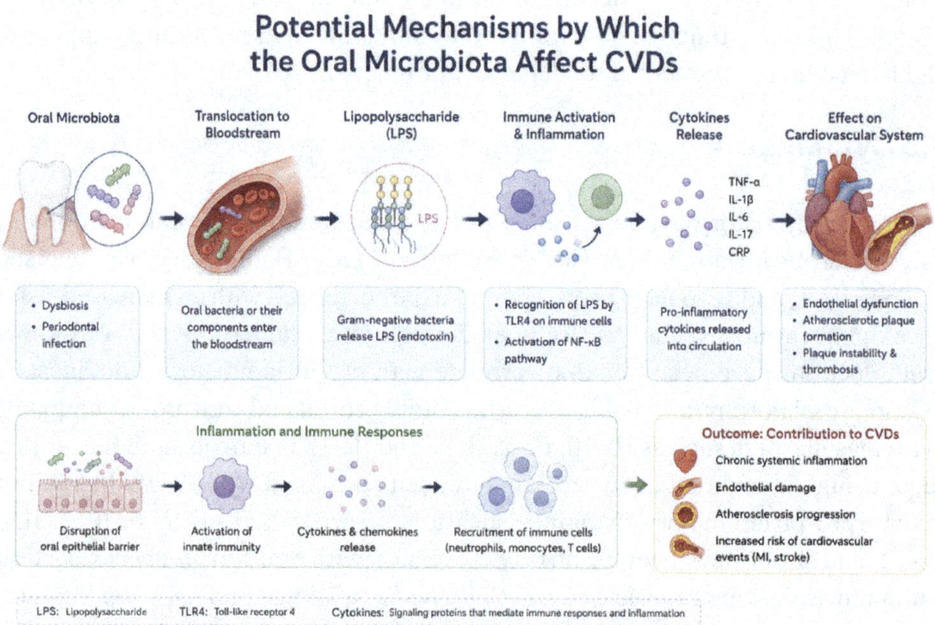

9. ORAL MICROBIOTA IN ATHEROMATOUS TISSUE

The pathophysiology of atherosclerosis has recently been associated with the oral microbiota, particularly through recurrent infections. Besides local gingival pathology, oral infections can trigger systemic processes due to bacteraemia and inflammation. Among the recent topics, one can highlight the identification of the components of oral microbiota in vascular lesions (Lehnert et al., 2015). Apart from systemic inflammation, the presence of the infections in the vascular lesions provides additional evidence of the association between oral and cardiovascular health. Apart from bacteria components circulating in the blood, periodontal infections secrete virulence factors, which is another factor, contributing to the vascular injury and imbalance of the host response. Pathogens such as *P. gingivalis*, *Treponema denticola*, and *Fusobacterium nucleatum* produce toxins and enzymes that degrade extracellular matrix proteins and epithelial intercellular junctions, facilitating bacterial entry into the bloodstream (Kim et al., 2005). Upon entering the circulation, they change immune cell signalling and cause an imbalance between the host and bacteria, resulting in chronic dysbiosis. This imbalance maintains low-grade inflammation, activates endothelium, and is involved in the vascular remodelling processes associated with early atherosclerosis (Table 2) The table explains the presence of oral microbiota in atherosclerotic (arterial plaque) tissue and their role in cardiovascular disease. It highlights those periodontal pathogens such as *Porphyromonas gingivalis, Aggregatibacter Actinomycetemcomitans, Fusobacterium nucleatum*, and *Treponema denticola* can enter the bloodstream through damaged gums and reach arterial walls. These bacteria trigger inflammation, damage endothelial cells, and promote lipid accumulation, leading to plaque formation and instability. Advanced techniques such as PCR, 16S rRNA sequencing, metagenomics, and FISH are used to detect these microbes, while microbiome profiling supports biomarker discovery and the development of preventive and therapeutic strategies for atherosclerosis.

Table 2. Oral Microbiota in Atheromatous Tissue

Aspect	Description	Significance in Atherosclerosis
Definition	Presence of oral microorganisms within atheromatous (arterial plaque) tissue.	Suggests a link between oral health and cardiovascular disease.
Major Oral Bacteria Detected	*Porphyromonas gingivalis, Aggregatibacter actinomycetemcomitans, Fusobacterium nucleatum, Treponema denticola.*	May contribute to plaque formation and vascular inflammation.
Route of Entry	Bacteria enter the bloodstream through periodontal lesions and damaged oral tissues.	Facilitates microbial dissemination to arterial walls.

continued on following page

Table 2. Continued

Aspect	Description	Significance in Atherosclerosis
Detection Methods	PCR, 16S rRNA sequencing, metagenomic analysis, fluorescence in situ hybridization (FISH).	Enables identification of microbial species in plaques.
Inflammatory Effects	Stimulates cytokine production and immune-cell activation.	Promotes chronic vascular inflammation.
Endothelial Dysfunction	Microbial toxins and inflammatory mediators damage endothelial cells.	Initiates and accelerates atherosclerotic processes.
Plaque Development	Oral bacteria may enhance lipid accumulation and foam-cell formation.	Contributes to plaque growth and instability.
Clinical Implications	Periodontal disease may increase cardiovascular risk.	Highlights the importance of oral hygiene in heart health.
Research Applications	Microbiome profiling and biomarker discovery.	Supports development of preventive and therapeutic strategies.

10. COMPUTATIONAL SYSTEMS BIOLOGY

The establishment of omics standards has increased the demand for computational tools to analyze omics datas. Omics data may include transcript, proteomic, and metabolomics data on fungal immunity to construct host-pathogen interaction networks and predict infection outcomes using them. There has been no relationship among the datasets of host-pathogen interactions, which have been gathered using direct experimentation quantification. Computational systems biology provides an approach for linking up these datasets for various factors to explore the significant features of host-pathogen interactions. The novel area in the research of fungal immunity is computational systems biology (Hünniger et al., 2014).

Neutrophils played a major role in the immune response, while monocytes contributed to a lesser extent. Dynamics of a Candida-host interaction in the whole blood could therefore be quantitatively and precisely predicted through a computational *Candida albicans* infection model developed by the researchers. To identify the main factors of antifungal immunity and make quantitative predictions about the a priori uncertain transition rates, time-resolved data were produced and simulated by means of the state-based approach combined with the Monte Carlo Annealing Simulation (MCAS) technique. The authors concluded that the neutrophils play a crucial role in the process of killing and immune response elicited by *Candida albicans* in human blood through intracellular killing and phagocytosis and that filamentation, activation, or exhaustion of the innate immune cells do not affect the capability of Candida albicans to escape the immune response. An infection in the bloodstream can be spread due to *Candida albicans* cell resistance to phagocytosis. In addition, the authors suggested that quantitative analysis of host-pathogen interaction in a complex environment like human blood could be facilitated through the experiment-model-experiment cycle described in this study (Müller et al., 2007). In contrast, Dühring et al. outlined various strategies for host defence, which comprised methods of fungal evasion, immunological response mechanisms, and general stress mechanisms. In addition, they talked about the use of computational and systems/ biology tools for studying these complex relationships using agent-based modeling and game theory approaches. Durmuş et al. reviewed the existing literature regarding computational analysis of Pathogen-Host Interaction (PHI) networks, which included computational prediction of PHIs, text-mining of PHI data, mathematical modeling, bioinformatics analysis of PHIs, and inference of PHI networks from omics data. Eno1, Phospho-Lipase B (PLB1), the above-mentioned Hsp70, and pyruvate kinase (CDC19) are some of the Candida virulence factors that interact with host factors like CD4, Alb and Amyloid β (A4) Precursor Protein (APP), Toll-Type Receptor 2 (Tlr2), and normal epidermal growth factor receptor (Eger), respectively, as noted by Remmele et al. in their network analysis of Candida albicans PHIs.

In the future, analysis of high-throughput of host-pathogen transcriptome or proteome data is going to be enhanced due to the integrated network. On the contrary, Lange et al. designed a random forest classifier algorithm to find out if a patient has an infection of either fungus, microbe or simulated infection using the transcriptomic data derived from the interaction of bacteria pathogenic organisms such as Staphylococcus aureus and Escherichia coli, and pathogenic fungi *Candida albicans* and *Aspergillus fumigatus* in the human whole-blood model (Lim et al., 2011). Such an approach provides new insights into host systemic responses and may lead to the development of innovative antimicrobial therapy in the future. Typical *C. albicans* infection in human blood sample model, Lehnert et al. have designed a bottom-up modelling approach that evolved from a state-driven model to an agent-driven model. Moreover, the authors predict that in the future diagnosis of infectious diseases would be facilitated greatly by using a systemic medicine approach that exploits the predictive powers of virtual infection models (MacCallum et al., 2009).

The use of both computational modeling and experiments by Peltz and his colleagues helped explore the applicability of computational modeling to predict the mortality of the host organism in the process of *C. albicans* infection. Next generation computational genomic mapping software that includes a variety of advanced components was developed within this study. It became clear through computational modeling that the classical complement pathway components including C1q, C1r, and C1s would influence the survival rate of mice in the mouse model of C. albicans infection, where the interaction of C1 and C. albicans along with the survival of chromosome substitution strains was strongly influenced from C1rs and C1rs alleles. The researchers noted that the survival in case of C. albicans infection that relies on the interplay between C5 and C1r/s alleles was predicted with success through the combination of an experimental mouse genetic model and a new generation of the computational genetic mapping technique. In addition, it was suggested that this combinatory approach to genetic modeling based on conditionality will help us better understand the genetic factors contributing to the development of autoimmune, infectious, and neurodegenerative disorders. In summary, because of the absence of relevant data, mathematical modeling of PHI pathways remains at its infancy stage. However, modeling of huge amounts of data obtained during transcriptome, proteome, and metabolomic studies may help us comprehend the process of infection, develop novel drugs to fight infections, and find biomarkers for disease diagnosis.

11. TRANSCRIPTOMICS

Host-Candida albicans interactions have been explored through various transcriptomic studies. Normal human monocytes co-cultured with *Candida albicans* resulted in the over-expression of certain genes involved in the generation of anti-inflammatory cytokines IL-1 and tumour necrosis factor, according to the microarray study. Further, it was observed that 56 genes involved in chemotaxis, cell death, and cytoplasmic signalling pathway were up regulated in primary human endothelial cells when they were cultured against Candida albicans in vitro (Vialas et al., 2009). It should be mentioned that our study on the comparison of transcriptome profiles of HUVEC infected with low and high concentrations of *Candida albicans* revealed significant differences in the expressions of genes associated with apoptosis and cell death. The concept of virulence being associated with yeast in its original form and merely serving to reproduce was contradicted by our results.

Immune-response genes were largely expressed throughout the process of infection ranging from invasion through injury. Nevertheless, MacCallum (2009) revealed that the immune response for the kidney in response to infection by virulent and attenuated *C. albicans* strains largely involves acute phase response, coagulation cascades and complement during the global response to *Candida albicans* infection. In addition, MacCallum (2009) established that whereas infection by a reduced strain of *Candida albicans* bacteria was associated with non-immune responses including metabolic pathways, infection by a virulent strain of Candida albicans bacteria leads to immune response in the kidney mainly innate immunity. Expression of chemokines early in the course of infection predicted the immunopathology of the kidney after systemic *C. albicans* infection as per MacCallum et al. (2009). Yet another study from Chin et al. (2014) found specific organ reactions of humans to infections, which were mainly due to the activation of innate immunity in response to *Candida albicans* infection and suggested the pathogenesis of infection with *Candida albicans* to be a multistage process. Studies conducted by Barker et al. (2008) have found that there is a specific response from the endothelial cells due to the infection with *C. albicans*, in addition to host immune genes being upregulated. Other non-immune responses like thrombosis, a stress response and apoptosis suppression have been noted. They might be induced because of the damage caused by Candida albicans to the cells of the endothelial layer.

This may have been due to the development of genes that facilitate angiogenesis and anti-apoptosis. In addition to this, studies done by Jose et al., (2013) indicate that Myeloid Tissue Leukemia 1 (Mcl1) which is a member of Bcl2 family is an anti-apoptosis factor. In phenotypic transition, Mcl1 plays a part in the promotion of cell survival through proliferation or differentiation. The anti-apoptosis factor includes the increased phosphorylation of Nucleo-Phosmin (NPM), which is a nucleolar protein, binds tumours specific inhibitors p19Arf and p53. NPM plays an important role in biogenesis, mitosis and DNA damage recovery. When all these factors are considered, most of the literature has suggested that the innate immune system which involves macrophages, neutrophils and monocytes is necessary for pathogen recognition, antimicrobial defence, activation of the adaptive immune system and eventually management of the disease course. On the contrary, investigations by Barker et al. (2008) suggested that for a deeper insight into the host immune responses to Candida infection, the contribution of angiogenesis in the development of Candida infection should be studied, along with the role of non-immune response pathways other than the classical immune response pathways. Nonetheless, since the survival of the macrophages against *Candida albicans* infection is promoted by the inhibition of apoptosis, inhibition of apoptosis could be one of the host immune strategies against the infection. Nonetheless, if the infected monocytes promote the proliferation and dissemination of *C. albicans*, which are still alive within them, inhibition of apoptosis could also be another virulence factor.

Further investigation is needed to determine whether the fungus or macrophages regulate this anti-apoptotic effect. By making use of RNA sequencing and siRNA technology, Liu et al. (2015) increased our understanding about the relation between the infection with *C. albicans* and host response. The research focused on the transcription profiles of *C. albicans* and normal host cells during the infection of oral epithelial cells and artery endothelial cells in vitro. Network analysis of the dataset helped identify a number of signalling proteins, which were not known to be associated with the host response to any infectious fungus. It was also noted that by controlling the uptake of *Candida albicans* by the host cells, PDGF BB and NEDD9 regulate the host-pathogen interaction.

12. PROTEOMICS

Although transcriptomic data provide gene-level information, they may not accurately reflect active effector molecules, as some transcripts may not be translated into functional proteins. However, the study on transcriptomics can bring about new knowledge on the interaction between the host and pathogen. Analysis of proteomics of interaction of *Candida albicans* with host immunity is vital to understand molecular interactions of host immunity defence mechanisms, understand how *Candida albicans* can escape host immunity and identify antigenic proteins during host-Candida interaction, which could be utilized in future as diagnostic and therapeutic treatment. Initially, Proto pathogen was focused on Candida albicans and its interaction with macrophages while Proteopathogen2 built on the concept and adopted the HUPO-PSI standards (Paul et al., 2010).

Changes in the expression of proteins in macrophages after stimulation with the wild-type strain of *C. albicans* SC5314 using the murine macrophage standardized cell line RAW264.7. The researchers found out that the expression of the Lydy, annexin type I, Hspa5, L-plasmin, and tropomyosin type 5 proteins were elevated, while the eif3s5, grp58, Hspa9a, Hip sixty years, and Hspa8a showed reduced expression. These variable results indicate that several cellular activities are involved, such as oxidation, protein synthesis, and folding, and cytoskeletal structure. However, in another separate experiment, for the effect of the interaction of heat-killed *Candida albicans* and macrophages RAW264.7 and found out that the result was anti-inflammatory response of the organism. In addition, hypothesized that the interaction of heat-killed *Candida albicans* cells can influence the normal proteomic response of a macrophage (Schirle et al., 2012). The interaction between *Candida albicans* in its normal form and RAW 264.7 macrophages by means of quantitative proteomics and classical phospho-proteomics. *Candida albicans* included inflammatory proteins as well as proteins involved in the process of oxidative stress formation. These proteins include the receptors, cytoskeletal cell proteins, mitochondrial ribosomal protein and normal transcriptional activators. In addition, these proteins involved in apoptosis and analyzed anti-apoptotic indicators.

Based on their findings, the authors proposed that the mechanism of apoptosis, apart from the inflammatory response, is necessary in host defence against *Candida albicans* (Clish et al., 2015). In the subsequent year, the changes that occur in protein synthesis in M1 or M2 types of macrophages stimulated by *Candida albicans*. It was found that M1 and M2 macrophages vary considerably in terms of metabolic and cytoskeletal reprogramming pathways. Fructose-1,6-biphosphatase 1, a key enzyme in gluconeogenesis, was also found to be present in higher amounts in M1 macrophages.

The authors have also found evidence of polarization switching from M1 to M2 when interacting with *Candida albicans*. Switching aids in the pathogenesis of Candida albicans by inhibiting the immune system response, leading either to fungal survival and colonization or the host's efforts to reduce the damage done by inflammation (Segers et al., 2019). The authors found 237 proteins from *Candida albicans* and 13 proteins from macrophages as potential interaction-specific compounds. The authors found that proteins from *Candida albicans* synthesized by macrophages are involved in glucose formation, membrane formation, stress response, and other unknown biological processes. Meanwhile, proteins from macrophages synthesized by *Candida albicans* are involved in a chaperone and death pathway. The authors hypothesized that *Candida albicans* could withstand the tough environment in macrophages by increasing stress proteins. Nonetheless, the process of formation of normal glucose via β-oxidation pathway and down regulation of regulator HSPA1A and apoptosis associated protein NOA1-synthesis in macrophages might have something to do with the escape of cytoplasmic candidiasis by macrophages. All in all, studies on the proteome in relation to host-pathogen interaction concerning Candidiasis are only at their infancy stage. Future studies are required to gain understanding of the pathogenic and virulence pathways of Candidiasis.

13. METABOLOMICS

Metabolomics involves the comprehensive characterization of metabolites and low-molecular-weight compounds in biological systems. It poses greater analytical challenges than genomics or proteomics due to the diverse physical and chemical properties of metabolites (Clish, 2015). The metabolome is analyzed with the help of different analytical platforms due to this challenge. Saliva is an attractive material for the diagnosis of systemic diseases and biomarkers of pathological states because the research used saliva, serum, and mobile organic molecules for different pathological states. Small molecular weight metabolites are usually characterized with the help of analytical platforms such as nuclear magnetic resonance spectroscopy, capillary electrophoresis-time-of-flight mass spectroscopy, gas chromatography with mass spectrometry, and liquid chromatography with mass spectrometry (Wang et al., 2017).

The application of Metabolomics provides great understanding about the biochemical changes that occur due to radiation or chemotherapy in the OM research. By using CE-TOF-MS technique, Matsuoka et al. (2021) studied the kinetics of saliva metabolic profile for nine male HNSCC patients who had undergone radiation therapy of 50 Gy. Levels Of Histidine, Aminobutyric Acid (GABA) or 2-Aminobutyric Acids (2AB) were found to be higher in high-grade OM compared to low-grade OM patients using partial least squares discriminant regression analysis. Although

2AB has been reported to increase in the state of high oxidative stress that may arise due to radiation, the GABA is known to be associated with the level of stress. They found higher levels of 9S-HEPE and 15-HETE in the patients undergoing MOM after radiation therapy. The metabolites are known to play a role in suppressing inflammation through different pathways (Geng et al., 2021).

The application of animal OM models in assessing the preclinical capability of pharmaceutical targets has equally been useful. Two different Chinese herbal medicines referred to as Huanghua Baihe Tablet (SBT), and Kou Yanqing Grains (KQG), have been used in two independent OM rat model investigations to establish the effects of the two treatments on OM symptoms alleviation and elucidating the underlying metabolic pathways. Geng et al. (2021) showed how SBT ameliorates OM inflammation symptoms through metabolic processes such as metabolism of cholic acid and linoleic acid (Chen et al., 2022). On the other hand, KQG gives promising results through alleviating OM symptoms through oxidative stress control, tryptophan metabolism, and neuro immunoendocrine system. Metabolomics profiling can help identify novel drug targets in OM through metabolic pathways associated with OM pathogenesis such as some amino acids and lipids. In addition, determining the existence of thousands of compounds that can be linked to OM clinical features to improve risk evaluation, and prediction is made possible by advances in metabolomics technology.

14. CONCLUSION

Integrative omics has transformed the investigation of oral–systemic health by linking genomic susceptibility, microbial ecology, host responses, metabolic alterations, and disease-associated signalling within a unified biological framework. The evidence presented in this chapter suggests that genomics, transcriptomics, proteomics, metabolomics, metagenomics, and computational systems biology can all help to explain the mechanisms behind oral mucositis, Candida-host interactions, oral-gut microbial communication, and cardiovascular outcomes of oral dysbiosis. Multi-omics integration can aid in the identification of risk variants, molecular biomarkers, inflammatory pathways, microbial virulence factors, and metabolite signatures that could aid in early diagnosis, patient stratification, treatment selection, and prediction of clinical outcomes. The oral microbiota could contribute to systemic disease via microbial translocation, activating immune system by lipopolysaccharide, the production of cytokines, endothelial dysfunction, and chronic low-grade inflammation. However, clinical translation remains limited due to high analytical costs, small cohort sizes, inconsistent study protocols, complex data integration challenges, and insufficient external validation. Standardized sampling, longitudinal multi-centre studies, harmonized bioinformatics pipelines, mechanistic validation and ethically regulated data sharing should be prioritised in future studies. The integration of AI and systems-level modelling could further enhance predictability and aid in precise prevention and personalized treatment for various patient populations globally. In summary, integrative omics offers a promising platform to gain insight into oral–systemic interactions and enhance multidisciplinary healthcare.

REFERENCES

Abusleme, L., Dupuy, A. K., Dutzan, N., Silva, N., Burleson, J. A., Strausbaugh, L. D., Gamonal, J., & Diaz, P. I. (2013). The subgingival microbiome in health and periodontitis and its relationship with community biomass and inflammation. *The ISME Journal*, *7*(5), 1016–1025. DOI: 10.1038/ismej.2012.174 PMID: 23303375

Alemán, J. O., Bokulich, N. A., Swann, J. R., Walker, J. M., De Rosa, J. C., Battaglia, T., Costabile, A., Pahlavans, A., Liang, Y., & Breslow, J. L. (2018). Fecal microbiota and bile acid interactions with systemic and adipose tissue metabolism in diet-induced weight loss of obese postmenopausal women. *Journal of Translational Medicine*, *16*(1), 244. DOI: 10.1186/s12967-018-1619-z PMID: 30176893

Buhlin, K., Hultin, M., Norderyd, O., Persson, L., Pockley, A. G., Rabe, P., Klinge, B., & Gustafsson, A. (2009). Risk factors for atherosclerosis in cases with severe periodontitis. *Journal of Clinical Periodontology*, *36*(7), 541–549. DOI: 10.1111/j.1600-051X.2009.01430.x PMID: 19538326

Chen, W., Li, C., Jin, D., Shi, Y., Zhang, M., Bo, M., Qian, D., Wang, M., & Li, G. (2022). Metabolomics combined with a network pharmacology-based strategy to reveal the underlying mechanism of Zhenhua submicron emulsion in treating oropharyngeal mucositis complications of radiation therapy for head and neck cancer. *Drug Design, Development and Therapy*, *16*, 3169–3182. DOI: 10.2147/DDDT.S376984 PMID: 36158237

Chen, W. A., Dou, Y., Fletcher, H. M., & Boskovic, D. S. (2023). Local and systemic effects of *Porphyromonas gingivalis* infection. *Microorganisms*, *11*(2), 470. DOI: 10.3390/microorganisms11020470 PMID: 36838435

Cheung, M. K., Chan, J. Y. K., Wong, M. C. S., Wong, P. Y., Lei, P., Cai, L., Lan, L., Ho, W. C. S., Yeung, A. C. M., Chan, P. K. S., & Chen, Z. (2022). Determinants and interactions of oral bacterial and fungal microbiota in healthy Chinese adults. *Microbiology Spectrum*, *10*(1), e0241021. DOI: 10.1128/spectrum.02410-21 PMID: 35107355

Clish, C. B. (2015). Metabolomics: An emerging but powerful tool for precision medicine. *Cold Spring Harbor Molecular Case Studies*, *1*(1), a000588. DOI: 10.1101/mcs.a000588 PMID: 27148576

Dix, A., Hünniger, K., Weber, M., Guthke, R., Kurzai, O., & Linde, J. (2015). Biomarker-based classification of bacterial and fungal whole-blood infections in a genome-wide expression study. *Frontiers in Microbiology*, *6*, 171. DOI: 10.3389/fmicb.2015.00171 PMID: 25814982

Djekic, D., Shi, L., Brolin, H., Carlsson, F., Särnqvist, C., Savolainen, O., Cao, Y., Bäckhed, F., Tremaroli, V., Landberg, R., & Frøbert, O. (2020). Effects of a vegetarian diet on cardiometabolic risk factors, gut microbiota, and plasma metabolome in subjects with ischemic heart disease: A randomized crossover study. *Journal of the American Heart Association*, *9*(18), e016518. DOI: 10.1161/JAHA.120.016518 PMID: 32893710

Dong, J., Li, Y., Xiao, H., Zhang, S., Wang, B., Wang, H., Li, Y., Fan, S., & Cui, M. (2021). Oral microbiota affects the efficacy and prognosis of radiotherapy for colorectal cancer in mouse models. *Cell Reports*, *37*(4), 109886. DOI: 10.1016/j.celrep.2021.109886 PMID: 34706245

Donia, M. S., Cimermancic, P., Schulze, C. J., Wieland Brown, L. C., Martin, J., Mitreva, M., Clardy, J., Linington, R. G., & Fischbach, M. A. (2014). A systematic analysis of biosynthetic gene clusters in the human microbiome reveals a common family of antibiotics. *Cell*, *158*(6), 1402–1414. DOI: 10.1016/j.cell.2014.08.032 PMID: 25215495

Dühring, S., Germerodt, S., Skerka, C., Zipfel, P. F., Dandekar, T., & Schuster, S. (2015). Host–pathogen interactions between the human innate immune system and *Candida albicans*: Understanding and modeling defense and evasion strategies. *Frontiers in Microbiology*, *6*, 625. DOI: 10.3389/fmicb.2015.00625 PMID: 26175718

Durmuş, S., Çakır, T., Özgür, A., & Guthke, R. (2015). A review on computational systems biology of pathogen–host interactions. *Frontiers in Microbiology*, *6*, 235. PMID: 25914674

Edfeldt, K., Swedenborg, J., Hansson, G. K., & Yan, Z. (2002). Expression of Toll-like receptors in human atherosclerotic lesions: A possible pathway for plaque activation. *Circulation*, *105*(10), 1158–1161. DOI: 10.1161/circ.105.10.1158 PMID: 11889007

Eichner, M., & Dietz, K. (2003). Transmission potential of smallpox: Estimates based on detailed data from an outbreak. *American Journal of Epidemiology*, *158*(2), 110–117. DOI: 10.1093/aje/kwg103 PMID: 12851223

Fan, Y., & Pedersen, O. (2021). Gut microbiota in human metabolic health and disease. *Nature Reviews. Microbiology*, *19*(1), 55–71. DOI: 10.1038/s41579-020-0433-9 PMID: 32887946

Fitzgerald, K. A., & Kagan, J. C. (2020). Toll-like receptors and the control of immunity. *Cell*, *180*(6), 1044–1066. DOI: 10.1016/j.cell.2020.02.041 PMID: 32164908

Galié, S., García-Gavilán, J., Camacho-Barcía, L., Atzeni, A., Muralidharan, J., Papandreou, C., Arcelin, P., Palau-Galindo, A., Garcia, D., Basora, J., Arias-Vasquez, A., & Bulló, M. (2021). Effects of the Mediterranean diet or nut consumption on gut microbiota composition and fecal metabolites and their relationship with cardiometabolic risk factors. *Molecular Nutrition & Food Research*, *65*(19), e2000982. DOI: 10.1002/mnfr.202000982 PMID: 34331403

Geng, Q. S., Liu, R. J., Shen, Z. B., Wei, Q., Zheng, Y. Y., Jia, L. Q., Wang, L. H., Li, L. F., Li, J., & Xue, W. H. (2021). Transcriptome sequencing and metabolome analysis reveal the mechanism of Huanghua Baihe Tablet in the treatment of oral mucositis. *Chinese Journal of Natural Medicines*, *19*(12), 930–943. DOI: 10.1016/S1875-5364(22)60150-X PMID: 34961591

Hobson, G., Adamson, J., Adler, H., Firth, R., Gould, S., Houlihan, C., Johnson, C., Porter, D., Rampling, T., Ratcliffe, L., Russell, K., Shankar, A. G., & Wingfield, T. (2021). Family cluster of three cases of monkeypox imported from Nigeria to the United Kingdom, May 2021. *Eurosurveillance*, *26*(32), 2100745. DOI: 10.2807/1560-7917.ES.2021.26.32.2100745 PMID: 34387184

Hünniger, K., Lehnert, T., Bieber, K., Martin, R., Figge, M. T., & Kurzai, O. (2014). A virtual infection model quantifies innate effector mechanisms and *Candida albicans* immune escape in human blood. *PLoS Computational Biology*, *10*(2), e1003479. DOI: 10.1371/journal.pcbi.1003479 PMID: 24586131

Jafari, P., & Azuaje, F. (2006). An assessment of recently published gene expression data analyses: Reporting experimental design and statistical factors. *BMC Medical Informatics and Decision Making*, *6*(1), 27. DOI: 10.1186/1472-6947-6-27 PMID: 16790051

Joshi, V., Matthews, C., Aspiras, M., de Jager, M., Ward, M., & Kumar, P. (2014). Smoking decreases structural and functional resilience in the subgingival ecosystem. *Journal of Clinical Periodontology*, *41*(11), 1037–1047. DOI: 10.1111/jcpe.12300 PMID: 25139209

Kang, J. W., Tang, X., Walton, C. J., Brown, M. J., Brewer, R. A., Maddela, R. L., Zheng, J. J., Agus, J. K., & Zivkovic, A. M. (2022). Multi-omic analyses reveal bifidogenic effects and metabolomic shifts in a healthy human cohort supplemented with a prebiotic dietary fiber blend. *Frontiers in Nutrition*, *9*, 908534. DOI: 10.3389/fnut.2022.908534 PMID: 35782954

Kaptoge, S., Seshasai, S. R. K., Gao, P., Freitag, D. F., Butterworth, A. S., Borglykke, A., Di Angelantonio, E., Gudnason, V., Rumley, A., Lowe, G. D. O., Jorgensen, T., & Danesh, J. (2014). Inflammatory cytokines and risk of coronary heart disease: New prospective study and updated meta-analysis. *European Heart Journal, 35*(9), 578–589. DOI: 10.1093/eurheartj/eht367 PMID: 24026779

Kim, H. S., Choi, E. H., Khan, J., Roilides, E., Francesconi, A., Kasai, M., Sein, T., Schaufele, R. L., Sakurai, K., Son, C. G., Greer, B. T., Chanock, S., Lyman, C. A., & Walsh, T. J. (2005). Expression of genes encoding innate host defense molecules in normal human monocytes in response to *Candida albicans. Infection and Immunity, 73*(6), 3714–3724. DOI: 10.1128/IAI.73.6.3714-3724.2005 PMID: 15908401

Krüger, T., Luo, T., Schmidt, H., Shopova, I., & Kniemeyer, O. (2015). Challenges and strategies for proteome analysis of the interaction of human pathogenic fungi with host immune cells. *Proteomes, 3*(4), 467–495. DOI: 10.3390/proteomes3040467 PMID: 28248281

Lehnert, T., Timme, S., Pollmächer, J., Hünniger, K., Kurzai, O., & Figge, M. T. (2015). Bottom-up modeling approach for the quantitative estimation of parameters in pathogen–host interactions. *Frontiers in Microbiology, 6*, 608. DOI: 10.3389/fmicb.2015.00608 PMID: 26150807

Lim, C. S., Rosli, R., Seow, H. F., & Chong, P. P. (2011). Transcriptome profiling of endothelial cells during infections with high and low densities of *Candida albicans* cells. *International Journal of Medical Microbiology : IJMM, 301*(6), 536–546. DOI: 10.1016/j.ijmm.2010.12.002 PMID: 21371935

MacCallum, D. M. (2009). Massive induction of innate immune response to *Candida albicans* in the kidney in a murine intravenous challenge model. *FEMS Yeast Research, 9*(7), 1111–1122. DOI: 10.1111/j.1567-1364.2009.00576.x PMID: 19845042

Miura, F., van Ewijk, C. E., Backer, J. A., Xiridou, M., Franz, E., de Coul, E. O., Banwart, D., van Cleef, B., van Rijckevorsel, G., & Swan, C. (2022). Estimated incubation period for monkeypox cases confirmed in the Netherlands, May 2022. *Eurosurveillance, 27*(24), 2200448. DOI: 10.2807/1560-7917.ES.2022.27.24.2200448 PMID: 35713026

Moran, A. P., Prendergast, M. M., & Appelmelk, B. J. (1996). Molecular mimicry of host structures by bacterial lipopolysaccharides and its contribution to disease. *FEMS Immunology and Medical Microbiology, 16*(2), 105–115. DOI: 10.1111/j.1574-695X.1996.tb00127.x PMID: 8988391

Müller, V., Viemann, D., Schmidt, M., Endres, N., Ludwig, S., Leverkus, M., Roth, J., & Goebeler, M. (2007). *Candida albicans* triggers activation of distinct signaling pathways to establish a proinflammatory gene expression program in primary human endothelial cells. *The Journal of Immunology : Official Journal of the American Association of Immunologists, 179*(12), 8435–8445. DOI: 10.4049/jimmunol.179.12.8435 PMID: 18056390

Murugesan, S., Al Ahmad, S. F., Singh, P., Saadaoui, M., Kumar, M., & Al Khodor, S. (2020). Profiling the salivary microbiome of the Qatari population. *Journal of Translational Medicine, 18*(1), 127. DOI: 10.1186/s12967-020-02291-2 PMID: 32169076

Paul, S. M., Mytelka, D. S., Dunwiddie, C. T., Persinger, C. C., Munos, B. H., Lindborg, S. R., & Schacht, A. L. (2010). How to improve R&D productivity: The pharmaceutical industry's grand challenge. *Nature Reviews. Drug Discovery, 9*(3), 203–214. DOI: 10.1038/nrd3078 PMID: 20168317

Pietiäinen, M., Liljestrand, J. M., Kopra, E., & Pussinen, P. J. (2018). Mediators between oral dysbiosis and cardiovascular diseases. *European Journal of Oral Sciences, 126*(S1, Suppl. 1), 26–36. DOI: 10.1111/eos.12423 PMID: 30178551

Pushalkar, S., Paul, B., Li, Q., Yang, J., Vasconcelos, R., Makwana, S., González, J. M., Shah, S., Xie, C., Janal, M. N., Queiroz, E., Bederoff, M., Leinwand, J., Solarewicz, J., Xu, F., Aboseria, E., Guo, Y., Aguallo, D., Gomez, C., & Saxena, D. (2020). Electronic cigarette aerosol modulates the oral microbiome and increases the risk of infection. *iScience, 23*(3), 100884. DOI: 10.1016/j.isci.2020.100884 PMID: 32105635

Remmele, C. W., Luther, C. H., Balkenhol, J., Dandekar, T., Müller, T., & Dittrich, M. T. (2015). Integrated inference and evaluation of host–fungi interaction networks. *Frontiers in Microbiology, 6*, 764. DOI: 10.3389/fmicb.2015.00764 PMID: 26300851

Reynolds, M. G., Yorita, K. L., Kuehnert, M. J., Davidson, W. B., Huhn, G. D., Holman, R. C., & Damon, I. K. (2006). Clinical manifestations of human monkeypox influenced by route of infection. *The Journal of Infectious Diseases, 194*(6), 773–780. DOI: 10.1086/505880 PMID: 16941343

Schack, L. M. H., Naderi, E., Fachal, L., Dorling, L., Luccarini, C., Dunning, A. M., Barnett, G., Barrera, M. E. A., Burnet, N. G., Calvo, L. M., Diergaarde, B., Dudding, T., Dunning, A., Duprez, F., Kerns, S. L., Kiang, M. C. L., Langendijk, H., Mehanna, H., Ness, A., & Alsner, J.The Head and Neck Group of the Radiogenomics Consortium. (2022). A genome-wide association study of radiotherapy-induced toxicity in head and neck cancer patients identifies a susceptibility locus associated with mucositis. *British Journal of Cancer*, *126*(7), 1082–1090. DOI: 10.1038/s41416-021-01670-w PMID: 35039627

Schirle, M., Bantscheff, M., & Kuster, B. (2012). Mass spectrometry-based proteomics in preclinical drug discovery. *Chemistry & Biology*, *19*(1), 72–84. DOI: 10.1016/j.chembiol.2012.01.002 PMID: 22284356

Schmidt, T. S. B., Hayward, M. R., Coelho, L. P., Li, S. S., Costea, P. I., Voigt, A. Y., Wirbel, J., Maistrenko, O. M., Alves, R. J., Bergsten, E., de Beaufort, C., Sobhani, I., Heintz-Buschart, A., Sunagawa, S., Zeller, G., Wilmes, P., & Bork, P. (2019). Extensive transmission of microbes along the gastrointestinal tract. *eLife*, *8*, e42693. DOI: 10.7554/eLife.42693 PMID: 30747106

Segata, N., Haake, S. K., Mannon, P., Lemon, K. P., Waldron, L., Gevers, D., Huttenhower, C., & Izard, J. (2012). Composition of the adult digestive tract bacterial microbiome based on seven mouth surfaces, tonsils, throat, and stool samples. *Genome Biology*, *13*(6), R42. DOI: 10.1186/gb-2012-13-6-r42 PMID: 22698087

Segers, K., Declerck, S., Mangelings, D., Van den Heyden, Y., & Van Eeckhaut, A. (2019). Analytical techniques for metabolomic studies: A review. *Bioanalysis*, *11*(24), 2297–2318. DOI: 10.4155/bio-2019-0014 PMID: 31845604

Tang, W. H. W., Kitai, T., & Hazen, S. L. (2017). Gut microbiota in cardiovascular health and disease. *Circulation Research*, *120*(7), 1183–1196. DOI: 10.1161/CIRCRESAHA.117.309715 PMID: 28360349

Uffelmann, E., Huang, Q. Q., Munung, N. S., de Vries, J., Okada, Y., Martin, A. R., Martin, H. C., Lappalainen, T., & Posthuma, D. (2021). Genome-wide association studies. *Nature Reviews. Methods Primers*, *1*(1), 59. DOI: 10.1038/s43586-021-00056-9

Vialas, V., Nogales-Cadenas, R., Nombela, C., Pascual-Montano, A., & Gil, C. (2009). Proteopathogen, a protein database for studying *Candida albicans*–host interaction. *Proteomics*, *9*(20), 4664–4668. DOI: 10.1002/pmic.200900023 PMID: 19743419

Wang, C., Liu, W., Yao, L., Zhang, X., Zhang, X., Ye, C., Jiang, H., He, J., Zhu, Y., & Ai, D. (2017). Hydroxyeicosapentaenoic acids and epoxyeicosatetraenoic acids attenuate the early occurrence of nonalcoholic fatty liver disease. *British Journal of Pharmacology*, *174*(14), 2358–2372. DOI: 10.1111/bph.13844 PMID: 28471490

Yang, D. W., Wang, T. M., Zhang, J. B., Li, X. Z., He, Y. Q., Xiao, R., Xue, W. Q., Zheng, X. H., Zhang, P. F., Zhang, S. D., Hu, Y.-Z., Shen, G.-P., Chen, M., Sun, Y., & Jia, W.-H. (2020). Genome-wide association study identifies genetic susceptibility loci and pathways of radiation-induced acute oral mucositis. *Journal of Translational Medicine*, *18*(1), 224. DOI: 10.1186/s12967-020-02390-0 PMID: 32503578

Yang, G., Feng, D., Li, F., Luo, B., Zhu, J., Yang, Q., Zheng, L., Dong, Q., Chen, M., Xu, Z., Li, L., Chen, P., & Sun, J. (2021). A randomized controlled phase II trial of maxillofacial and oral massage in attenuating severe radiotherapy-induced oral mucositis and lipid metabolite changes in nasopharyngeal carcinoma. *Radiotherapy and Oncology : Journal of the European Society for Therapeutic Radiology and Oncology*, *163*, 76–82. DOI: 10.1016/j.radonc.2021.07.024 PMID: 34343545

Zaas, A. K., Aziz, H., Lucas, J., Perfect, J. R., & Ginsburg, G. S. (2010). Blood gene expression signatures predict invasive candidiasis. *Science Translational Medicine*, *2*(21), 21ra17. DOI: 10.1126/scitranslmed.3000715 PMID: 20374997

Zhou, T., Xu, W., Wang, Q., Jiang, C., Li, H., Chao, Y., Sun, Y., & A, L. (2023). The effect of the "oral–gut" axis on periodontitis in inflammatory bowel disease: A review of microbe and immune mechanism associations. *Frontiers in Cellular and Infection Microbiology*, *13*, 1132420. DOI: 10.3389/fcimb.2023.1132420 PMID: 36923589

Chapter 11
Integrating Oral Health Biomarkers With Systemic Health Data Using AI

G. Imaiyavathi
Department of Microbiology, Sacred Heart College, Tirupattur, India

B. Lokeshwari
http://orcid.org/0009-0005-6612-5134
Department of Microbiology, Sacred Heart College, Tirupattur, India

P. Saranraj
http://orcid.org/0000-0002-5052-6532
Department of Microbiology, Sacred Heart College, Tirupattur, India

S. Kanshiya
Department of Microbiology, Sacred Heart College, Tirupattur, India

T. Elavarasi
http://orcid.org/0009-0003-0792-4484
Department of Microbiology, Sacred Heart College, Tirupattur, India

ABSTRACT

Artificial intelligence (AI) is rapidly transforming oral healthcare by enabling the integration of diverse oral biomarkers with systemic health information for more accurate, preventive, and personalized clinical decision-making. This chapter explores the potential applications of machine learning, deep learning, natural language processing and predictive analytics in analyzing multimodal data, such as dental radiographs, intraoral images, electronic health records, salivary protein profiles, oral microbiome, genomic data, outputs from wearable sensors, and patient-reported

DOI: 10.4018/979-8-3373-8402-3.ch011

data. Standardized collection of data, clear model development, prospective multi-center validation, data sharing systems, and ongoing professional supervision are needed to overcome these barriers. AI offers a promising pathway toward predictive, preventive, personalized, and participatory healthcare, while strengthening the role of oral health as an essential component of whole-body medicine.

1. INTRODUCTION

As AI becomes more integral to dentistry, its role is significant, especially when oral health issues are one of the most prevalent and expensive public-health challenges globally. Nutrition, communication, psychosocial health, productivity, and quality of life (QOL) are all impacted by dental caries, periodontal disease, tooth loss, oral mucosal lesions, and oropharyngeal cancer (Lv et al., 2024). Management of oral health is not just about solving clinical issues; it is all about the coordination of prevention, early detection, risk evaluation, treatment, education, monitoring and population surveillance. The ultimate objective here is to improve the health results and reduce any kind of disparity and waste in the resources of health care services. AI can assist in this context in such a way that it can analyze large volumes of complex and varied data, find out small signals of diseases, predict individual risks and ensure timely interventions. In practical terms, AI can support the analysis of x-rays and intraorals, help in developing a treatment plan, automate routine documentation processes and ensure patient-oriented communication (Wu et al., 2022). However, the adoption is very slow due to concerns about the quality of data, bias of algorithms, transparency, interoperability, privacy, ethical obligations, regulatory compliance and validation of AI in the real world. Thus, the adoption of AI in dental practice will depend upon clinical assessment, explainability, regulation of professionals and inclusiveness in using digital health technologies.

Nonetheless, the successful deployment of AI in public health goes beyond technical accuracy; it necessitates a specific emphasis on population-level impact and health inequity considerations. While high income countries might quickly embrace the use of digital diagnostics, LMICs have numerous challenges to overcome, such as insufficient digital infrastructure, poor internet connection, expensive commercial AI software, and lack of qualified individuals who can interpret the results of the AI (Murray et al., 2024). In other words, without careful planning and development of affordable open-source AI, these technologies might perpetuate the current oral health disparities among various populations. Therefore, from the policy perspective, governments and health agencies should create policies requiring external validation on different populations, encouraging the sharing of data, and creating reimbursement codes for preventive care assisted by AI technology. Consequently, taking the population health approach means that AI development is inseparable from implementation science and culturally appropriate interventions (Sun et al., 2025).

One of the primary scientific drivers behind combining AI with oral health care is the intimate connection between oral and systemic health. The oral cavity is an intricate microbial community and is often said to be a reflection of the body's physiology. Periodontal disease is a chronic inflammatory disease and can be associated with systemic diseases via the dispersion of microbes, immune system dysfunction and chronic release of inflammatory mediators. Common risk factors such as smoking, diabetes mellitus, obesity, and socioeconomic disadvantage can exacerbate periodontal inflammation and cause dysbiosis of the oral microbiome (Stephan et al., 2024). Extraoral disease associations include cardiovascular disease, adverse pregnancy outcomes, and several malignancies, and periodontal pathogens including *P. gingivalis, T. denticola* and *F. nucleatum* have been identified at extraoral locations. Chronic periodontal inflammation is also associated with higher levels of C-reactive protein, interleukins and tumour necrosis factor-alpha that could exacerbate insulin resistance, endothelial dysfunction, and coronary disease (Szabó et al., 2024). Epidemiologic studies have also been associated with myocardial infarction and stroke, highlighting the need for dental-medical integration assessment (Hung et al., 2019). With all the data from oral health, cardiovascular health, metabolic health, microbial health, and behavioural measurements, AI possesses the analytical power to integrate this information and enhance disease-risk stratification and more comprehensive models of preventive health care.

One such innovative use of AI in modern dentistry is the use of multimodal biomarkers. Oral health information could encompass subject-reported data, outputs from wearable devices, microbeomics, genomic and transcriptomic data, proteins, salivary metabolites, and three-dimensional and x-ray data. Metabolomic analysis has shown that changes in fatty-acid and amino-acid metabolic processes can mark a cardiometabolic dysfunction, and simultaneous measurements of salivary and plasma metabolic profiles indicate that saliva can be a convenient non-invasive index of systemic metabolic processes (Lan et al., 2024; Morze et al., 2022). Likewise, oral microbiome signatures could help identify systemic inflammatory diseases in early stages and help differentiate diseases (Menon et al., 2017). AI can assimilate these high-dimensional fields, identify nonlinear patterns, minimize interobserver variation, and produce digital biomarkers that more accurately reflect disease state and evolution than individual clinical parameters does. It can also assist in identification of biomarkers for Oral Squamous Cell Carcinoma (OSCC) and the association of imaging, molecular and histological features with immune response. However, there are some requirements for the introduction of new promising biomarkers into routine use, such as analytical validation, external clinical validation, and clinical utility assessment. Hence, the current chapter critically reviews the use of AI in oral health education, data collection and analysis, screening, diagnosis, treatment planning, monitoring of care, and biomarker integration, and highlights the scientific, ethical, regulatory, and translational necessities to foster precision oral-systemic healthcare.

2. AI-ENABLED PATIENT EDUCATION, VIRTUAL ASSISTANCE, AND PERSONALIZED ORAL HEALTH CARE

Education in oral health is a pivotal component of disease prevention and health promotion that strives to increase people's awareness about the reciprocal nature of oral disease outcomes and everyday habits. The goal of educational activities is to increase people's health literacy through teaching them how to perform proper tooth brushing and flossing, provide nutritional counseling, help quit smoking, and encourage regular dental checkups (Morze et al., 2022). Such programs not only serve to spread information about oral health issues but also to change attitudes, motivate people, raise self-efficacy, and change behavior. Education is especially important in terms of reaching out to vulnerable groups of people, such as children, elderly people, and poor populations who can benefit from culturally appropriate health information because it can help eliminate oral health inequalities among these groups. Through focusing on prevention, such education makes fewer complex and expensive restorative procedures unnecessary, thus improving people's lives, making them more involved in their treatment, and increasing the sustainability of public health systems (Murray et al., 2024).

2.1. Interactive Oral Health Education and Dissemination

Artificial Intelligence (AI) has led to a paradigm shift in the way oral health-related information is disseminated by replacing text-based and stagnant materials with interactive and visual presentations of information. Through advanced language processing and multimedia production techniques, AI is able to present clinically complex information in a more user-friendly and visually appealing form, thus making it easier for the general public to understand and retain (Sun et al., 2025). Another promising strategy includes AI-powered gamification, which utilizes behavioral psychology to encourage patient participation in preventive care services. In fact, research comparing standard mobile apps and gamification shows that although both approaches improve mothers' knowledge about oral hygiene and behaviors related to it, gamification leads to more significant decreases in the plaque index of children (Marashi et al., 2024).

Moreover, immersive technologies like Virtual Reality (VR) and Augmented Reality (AR) provide users with three-dimensional and multisensory learning spaces through which they can engage with virtual simulations of toothbrushes, flosses, and mouthwash. Experiential modes of learning encourage user participation in dental hygiene routines, fostering good practices for better oral health results in the future (Gottlieb et al., 2023). AI's ability to personalize content based on specific demographics such as children who require playful stories or senior citizens who need instructions in increases its efficacy as an educational tool in oral health.

2.2. AI-Powered Virtual Health Assistants and Chatbots

AI-powered chatbots and virtual assistants have emerged as scalable, round-the-clock digital tools designed to emulate human conversation and provide immediate, contextually relevant oral health guidance. These systems, deployable across mobile devices, social media platforms, and websites, are engineered to understand and interpret natural language inputs, enabling fluid and conversational user interactions (Uribe et al., 2024). They can address generic queries regarding oral hygiene practices, dietary recommendations, brushing and flossing techniques, and the interpretation of early warning signs, thereby democratizing access to preliminary dental advice.

In the more advanced versions, patients can be enabled to upload images from inside their mouth or describe their symptoms in great detail, which will be analyzed by the AI to provide preliminary health checks or triage suggestions. For instance, AI-powered self-monitoring applications like use of latest features of mobile phone selfies to identify early symptoms of gingivitis and other mucosal anomalies, providing personalized recommendations according to their visual analysis (Islam, 2025). The empirical tests of chatbots, such as Fun Dee chatbot, have shown impressive effectiveness in terms of lowering incidence of dental caries, reducing plaque, encouraging feeding habits, and overall oral health literacy, rendering them realistic and effective complements to traditional health care methods. However, it is crucial to stress that these digital aides should not replace the expertise of dental specialists in any way. They work best when used along with appropriate measures to secure patient's data and transparent information about technical limitations of the tool and procedures for escalating the process to in-person clinical assessment (Liu, 2025).

2.3. Personalized Recommendations and Self-Management

The capacity of AI to analyze multimodal user data—including demographic characteristics, medical and dental histories, treatment records, lifestyle patterns, and individual learning preferences—enables the generation of highly customized educational materials and behavioral interventions. By identifying user-specific learning modalities (e.g., visual versus textual), AI can prioritize the delivery of video tutorials, interactive simulations, or infographics over generic text, thereby enhancing comprehension and user engagement (Fanelli et al., 2025). Personalization extends beyond educational content to encompass actionable health recommendations, such as post-operative care instructions, tailored dietary modifications, medication adherence prompts, and customized oral hygiene regimens aligned with the user's specific risk profile.

Furthermore, AI-powered applications can offer timely corrective feedback about oral hygiene based on the analysis of input data from smart devices. This feedback motivates users to modify their brushing angle, brushing duration, or flossing procedures gradually. AI is also important in reducing dental phobia through empathic interaction and constant support (Marashi et al., 2024). The timely reminders about brushing, flossing, and regular dental check-ups, provided through mobile and smart devices, will ensure the development of good preventive habits, thus decreasing the probability of developing oral diseases. The users will be able to report on their oral health status periodically, and AI algorithms will analyze this information to produce health reports, identify problems, and propose evidence-based solutions. This feedback loop is beneficial for empowering patients and helping them become active participants of their oral healthcare rather than passive patients (Deng et al., 2024).

2.4. Integrated AI-Driven Workflow for Personalized Management

The intersection of education, virtual assistant, and personalized learning is most effectively illustrated through an AI-assisted workflow process as shown in Figure 1, which facilitates a smooth flow from data collection to continuous patient interaction. This process begins with the collection of different types of patient data, including intraoral imaging data, radiographic data, complete medical and dental history data, lifestyle and diet data, and data collected from wearables/IoT devices (Lei et al., 2025). The collected heterogeneous data is then integrated into a digital platform where they are organized, anonymized, and preprocessed for analysis.

Advanced machine learning and deep learning algorithms are then applied to this integrated dataset to identify clinically relevant patterns, such as carious lesions, plaque accumulation, periodontal bone loss, and early neoplastic changes. By uncovering nonlinear and intricate relationships that evade conventional clinical assessment, the AI system delivers a more thorough, standardized, and objective evaluation (Tuzo et al., 2019) . The analytical outputs inform a critical risk-stratification phase, categorizing patients according to their caries risk, periodontal risk, oral cancer susceptibility, and overall oral health status. This stratification transforms complex multimodal data into actionable, clinically meaningful categories that directly support decision-making.

Following risk stratification, the workflow translates AI-generated insights into personalized, patient-centric recommendations, including individualized oral hygiene instructions, nutritional and lifestyle modifications, tailored recall schedules, and specific preventive or therapeutic product suggestions. These recommendations are disseminated via mobile applications, patient portals, push notifications, and educational modules to facilitate active participation and adherence (Zhang et al., 2025). Importantly, as illustrated in Figure 1, the workflow is not a static, one-time event but a dynamic, adaptive loop of continuous monitoring and feedback. The system tracks patient progress, evaluates adherence to prescribed regimens, re-evaluates risk profiles in response to new data, and iteratively updates recommendations to reflect changes in symptoms, behavior, treatment response, or disease status.

This adaptive process transitions oral health management from episodic, visit-dependent care to a responsive, continuous, and patient-centered paradigm. Throughout this entire workflow, AI functions strictly as a supportive adjunct to clinical judgment, with treatment decisions and the management of complex conditions remaining under the purview of qualified dental professionals. Ultimately, this integrated architecture enhances early detection, reinforces preventive care, improves treatment adherence, and elevates both oral health outcomes and overall quality of life, underscoring the transformative potential of data-driven, AI-supported personalized dentistry (Gottlieb et al., 2023). Figure 1 illustrates a sequential AI-driven workflow for personalized oral health management, beginning with the acquisition of diverse patient data. It includes information from intraoral images, radiographs, medical and dental history, personal lifestyle and diet, and information from wearable technologies or IOT technologies.

Figure 1. AI-Driven Workflow for Personalized Oral Health Management

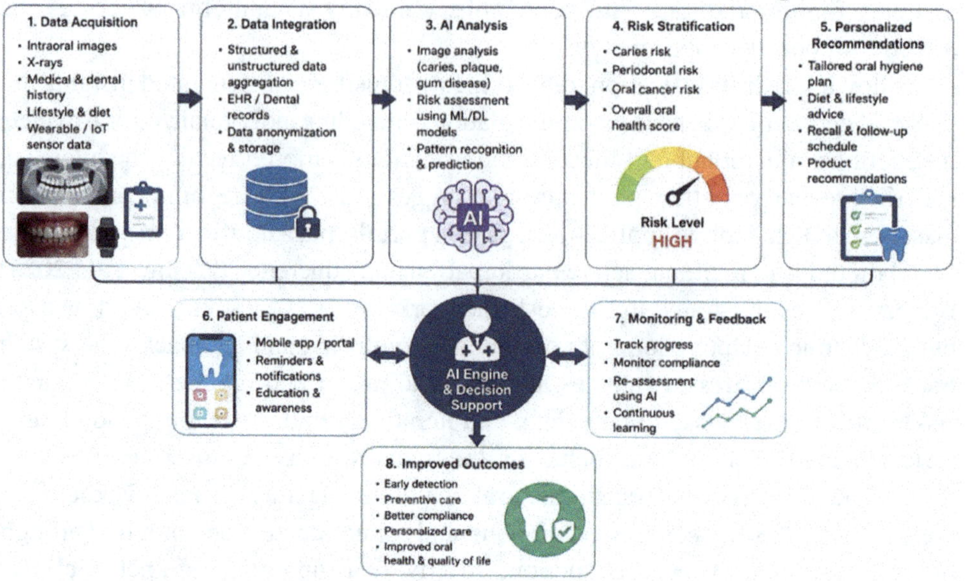

3. APPLICATIONS OF ARTIFICIAL INTELLIGENCE (AI) IN ORAL HEALTH

Artificial Intelligence (AI), digital health platforms, and smart devices have revolutionized the data types of oral health and the amount of data available. Traditional dental information systems were mostly made up of a single-source, structured data set, such as clinical measurements, diagnostic codes, treatment scores and numerical laboratory results. By contrast, modern oral health environments produce massive amounts of multi-modal and heterogenous data from electronic dental records, radiographic imaging, intraoral photographs, three-dimensional scans, salivary analyses, wearable sensors, smartphones and patient-operated sensors. In addition to structured data, modern datasets contain unstructured data like clinical notes, text messages, voice recordings, videos, social-media conversations, and patient-reported symptoms (McRae et al., 2021). In this changing landscape, patients are no longer the sole recipients of dental care but become the active producers of data related to health. Mobile apps, smart toothbrushes, oral cameras and questionnaires on the computer can be used to capture hygiene behaviours, symptoms, dietary practices, treatment experiences and changes in oral conditions outside of conventional clinical settings. The fact that these data streams are continuous and real-world allows for a more detailed, comprehensive understanding of oral health compared with a single dental visit, providing opportunities for clinicians and researchers to study behavioural, environmental, biological and clinical aspects.

AI has the power to manage, organize, and interpret these complex oral health data. Machine-learning algorithms can uncover patterns of disease, forecast individual risks, and categorize oral disease based on clinical, behavioural, imaging, and biomarker data. Deep-learning systems, especially CNN, can be used to analyze dental radiographs, intraoral photographs and three-dimensional scans to assist in the diagnosis of caries, periodontal bone loss, periapical lesions, oral malignancy, and developmental abnormalities. NLP can extract clinically relevant information from unstructured oral history, patients' communications, and consultation notes, and predictive analytics can forecast the risk of disease progression, treatment outcomes, and potential complications. A fusion of data from several sources might also be used for personalized, preventive measures, automated follow-up, remote monitoring, and targeted health education. But these applications will be effective only if the data is effectively governed, standardised, interoperable, secure and controlled. Algorithmic performance and clinical generalizability may be diminished due to incomplete and inconsistent records, datasets, imaging protocols, and patient-generated data.

3.1. AI in Oral Health Data Collection and Analysis

Data on oral health comes from a wide range of sources including patient medical records, imaging tests, physiological data, and everyday oral hygiene practices. Clinical medical records, which include the patient's medical history, visit records, diagnostic data, treatment plans, surgery records, and prescriptions, are an essential source of information on oral health. Oral imaging tests, such as dental X-rays, oral Computed Tomography (CT) scans, 3D oral pictures, and models that offer comprehensive imaging information on teeth, gums, periodontal tissues, and other areas, are crucial instruments for assessing oral health. Physiological data includes vital signs, markers of oral function, and information about the patient's general health, allowing medical professionals to perform a thorough evaluation of the patient's state (Viet et al., 2024).

Oral health data can be collected from various sources that consist of both structured data and numbers as well as unstructured data, which are primarily textual in nature. Such diversity poses a number of challenges for data collection and processing, which need to be carefully undertaken to ensure consistent and high-quality data. Such actions may include addressing duplicate data, missing values, as well as data normalization. The development of preventive and curative measures regarding the issues related to oral health will proceed if the integration and expansion of oral health data is employed on a voluntary basis. With its highly advanced computation abilities, automated cleaning and preprocessing capabilities, precise pattern detection and predictive capabilities, as well as cross-domain data integration abilities, AI has numerous benefits within complex data processing (Labus et al., 2021).

Machine Learning (ML) is an important AI technique that is very effective in recognizing patterns in huge amounts of data and making predictions about trends in unknown data sets. Having a high degree of success in such areas as image recognition, deep learning architectures, which involve the use of neural networks having multiple hidden layers, can autonomously detect complicated patterns in data, enabling elective classification and prediction of complex aspects. The integral part of Deep Learning (DL) technique called Convolutional Neural Networks (CNNs) uses convolutional layers for extracting features from input data and utilizes multi-layer network topology for the further analysis and classification of extracted features. AI is capable of improving ancient and ejective decision-making processes, leading to more successful outcomes and reduced costs through the provision of data-based recommendations (Chen et al., 2024). The use of AI for the analysis of oral health data leads to loss of important analytical help in creation of oral health guidelines (Li et al., 2021). Table 1 summarizes the major sources of oral health data, corresponding AI techniques, and their clinical applications in precision oral healthcare.

Table 1. Types of Oral Health Data and AI Techniques Used for Their Analysis

Data type	Examples	AI technique	Clinical application
Clinical records	Medical history, treatment records	Machine Learning	Risk prediction
Dental imaging	X-rays, CBCT, intraoral images	CNN, Deep Learning	Disease detection
Salivary biomarkers	Metabolites, proteins	AI-based biomarker analysis	Early diagnosis
Oral microbiome	Bacterial profiles	Machine Learning	Systemic disease prediction
Wearable/device data	Smart toothbrush, oral sensors	Predictive analytics	Continuous monitoring
Patient-reported data	Symptoms, questionnaires	NLP	Personalized care

Table 1 presents the major categories of oral-health data and the artificial-intelligence techniques used to analyse them. Clinical records, including medical histories and treatment information, are commonly evaluated through machine-learning algorithms to predict individual disease risk. Dental images, such as X-rays, cone-beam computed tomography scans, and intraoral photographs, are analysed using convolutional neural networks and deep-learning models to identify caries, periodontal bone loss, lesions, and other abnormalities. Salivary biomarkers, including proteins and metabolites, can also be processed using AI-based biomarker-analysis methods to support early disease detection. The table also highlights the importance of microbiome, wearable-device, and patient-reported data in personalized oral healthcare. Machine-learning analysis of oral bacterial profiles may help predict associations between oral dysbiosis and systemic diseases (Aydin et al., 2024) . Data collected from smart toothbrushes and oral sensors can be examined using predictive analytics to enable continuous monitoring of hygiene behaviour and oral-health changes. In addition, natural-language-processing techniques can analyse symptoms, questionnaire responses, and other patient-reported information to generate individualized recommendations, improve communication, and support personalized preventive and therapeutic care.

4. MECHANISMS LINKING ORAL AND SYSTEMIC HEALTH

These findings emphasize the importance of oral hygiene and periodontal health for systemic implications, particularly since the oral cavity is an important reservoir for periodontal bacteria under disease conditions. Periodontal inflammation plays a role in systemic diseases by producing acute-phase proteins such as C-Reactive Protein (CRP) and pro-inflammatory cytokines such as and. These inflammatory mediators exacerbate insulin resistance in diabetes, cardiovascular disease and poor pregnancy outcomes. Lipopolysaccharide (LPS), which is a part of the outer membrane of Gram-negative bacteria, is a major regulator of inflammatory responses. The immunostimulatory properties of LPS are, however, strongly dependent on the LPS structure, such as the lipid A portion which interacts with the host Toll-Like Receptor (TLR4 / MD-2) complex. Bacterial LPS (*E. coli*) has a hexa-acylated lipid A structure which is highly pro-inflammatory.

Unlike periodontal pathogens like *P. gingivalis*, which produce structurally heterogeneous lipid A forms, mostly tetra- and penta-acylated, the latter has differential effects on host immune signaling and plays a role in immune evasion and chronic periodontal inflammation. This is the reason that *P. gingivalis* LPS is either a mild human agonist or an antagonist (Hu et al., 2021). Because of this special trait, *P. gingivalis* may be able to modify or subvert the first strong inflammatory response that is usually brought on by LPS, which could lead to immune evasion and the development of chronic, persistent inflammation as opposed to acute clearance. The Gram-negative periodontal bacteria such as *P. gingivalis* induce endothelial dysfunction, one of the key steps in atherogenesis, through the production of LPS, a bacterial endotoxin. LPS triggers endothelial cells to express adhesion molecules like E-selectin and intercellular adhesion that promote the adherence and migration of leukocytes. This results in inflammation of the blood vessels and development of plaques. LPS can also disrupt the placental barrier, potentially leading to early delivery and adverse birth outcomes (Labko et al., 2024).

The pro-inflammatory cytokines secreted in periodontal inflammation play an important role in systemic metabolic dysregulation by causing insulin resistance via various processes. The pro-inflammatory cytokines reduce insulin action by increasing serine phosphorylation of Insulin Receptor Substrates (IRS), which leads to reduction of insulin receptor signaling and decreased glucose uptake by peripheral tissues. Pro-inflammatory cytokines increase gluconeogenesis in the liver while decreasing adiponectin secretion, an anti-inflammatory hormone crucial for proper insulin action . Overall, these processes interfere with glucose regulation leading to systemic insulin resistance. Some of the systemic diseases such as diabetes and heart diseases are connected with periodontal inflammation by these interconnected processes. These connections are influenced by confounders such as smoking, social class and associated diseases. On the other hand, there is reverse causality because diabetes itself influences periodontal inflammation through the impaired immunity systems.

To address these issues and determine whether effective periodontal treatment can reduce the risks of systemic diseases and vice versa, interventional studies are crucial to fight against periodontal bacterial infection (Wuw et al., 2022). Periodontal inflammation is exacerbated by elevated glucose levels in Gingival Crevicular Fluid (GCF), which foster the growth of harmful microorganisms. Similar to this, the inflammatory disease rheumatoid arthritis causes systemic inflammation that weakens the gingival connective tissues and makes bacteria colonization easier. Chronic low-grade inflammation is a hallmark of cardiovascular illnesses, which may contribute to an inflammatory milieu that speeds up the breakdown of periodontal tissue. Additionally, by inducing gingival overgrowth or suppressing immunological responses, drugs for systemic disorders such calcium channel blockers or immunosuppressants raise the risk of periodontal disease (Deng et al., 2025).

The host's immune response is yet another aspect of the systemic effects of periodontal disease. The immune cells, such as neutrophils, macrophages, and dendritic cells, recognize the periodontal pathogens with the aid of their Pattern Recognition Receptors (PRRs), like Toll-Like Receptors (TLRs). This leads to pro-inflammatory cytokines being released, which subsequently attract the adaptive immune cells, such as B-lymphocytes and T-helper cells (Li et al., 2024). One of the examples of that would be production of the bacterial Heat Shock Proteins (HSPs), such as HSP60 (GroEL) with sequence homology to the human HSP60 (Zolfaghari et al., 2021) during stress. Human HSPs expressed on host cells, such as endothelial cells in blood vessels (implicated in atherosclerosis) or synovial cells in joints (implicated in rheumatoid arthritis), may cross-react with an immune response that was first triggered against these bacterial HSPs, causing inflammation and tissue damage in these systemic conditions. Furthermore, *P. gingivalis* virulence factors, including as gingipains, can weaken immune clearance systems, degrade complement factors, and prolong chronic inflammation, which accelerate the development of systemic diseases. Even while there is mounting evidence between systemic illnesses and periodontal disease, proving causation is still difficult (Hunsrisakhun et al., 2025).

5. PREDICTED FUNCTIONAL PATHWAYS OF ORAL MICROBIOTA IN ACUTE MYOCARDIAL INFARCTION (AMI)

The functional and biological characteristics of the oral microbiota were determined by analyzing them based on their Clusters of Orthologous Groups (COG) annotations, which categorize microbial genes into different groups based on the predicted evolutionary relationships and roles of their encoded proteins (Jeong et al., 2025). This strategy can help identify metabolic, cellular and molecular functions that could be different in people with Acute Myocardial Infarction (AMI) compared to healthy controls. Comparative analysis showed major changes in two functional categories. AMI, which denotes microorganisms or other biological activities that have not yet been completely identified. This enrichment suggests that unrecognized functions of microorganisms are involved in the development or progression of cardiovascular disease. The higher number of unclassified functional pathways also notes the complexity of the oral microbiome, and indicates that the existing genomic databases might not fully capture all microbial mechanisms involved in AMI. Thus, additional metagenomic, transcriptomic, and metabolomic analyses are needed to elucidate the gene-by-gene, protein-by-protein, and microbial product-by-microbial product relationships in these poorly understood pathways.

The functional category of coenzyme transport and metabolism, however, was significantly decreased in patients with AMI compared to control. Coenzymes play a vital role in many microbial biochemical functions such as energy production, redox control, biosynthesis and nutrient metabolism. A decrease in genes related to coenzyme transport and metabolism could thus be a sign of a decrease in the metabolic capacity of microbes and the way they generate energy in the oral microbial community. These known functional abnormalities could alter the levels of microbial metabolites, inflammatory mediators, and signaling molecules that can be distributed to the systemic circulation and alter cardiovascular physiology. Enrichment of unknown function and suppression of the metabolism related to coenzymes indicate that the AMI is correlated not only with changes in the oral microbiome composition but also with a significant reorganization of the functions of the microbial community. The results presented in this study indicate that oral microbial dysbiosis, which is manifested by changes in metabolic activity and host–microbe interactions, plays a role in the pathogenesis of AMI. These microbial changes, however, need to be further validated for function and investigated over time to see if they are causal, part of the AMI process, or a reaction to clinical factors and therapy (Liu et al., 2025).

6. DISCOVERY AND VALIDATION BIOMARKER

AI facilitates discovery through the mining of multimodal, high-dimensional datasets. AI has used imaging, histology, and multimers in biomedical research to find prognostic and predictive signs. AI has been used in gastrointestinal contexts to distinguish between illness subtypes and functional states using metabolomic profiles and microbiome profiles to find microbial biomarkers associated with intestinal ailments (Wang et al., 2025). Bowel sound analysis has been suggested as a non-invasive physiological source for tracking Inflammatory Bowel Disease (IBD) related activity. In Gastrointestinal (GI) oncology, digital pathology also helps with tumor categorization and prognosis prediction. Cohort variety and study design should be taken into consideration when interpreting reported performance because validation depth varies among various modalities. Digital biomarkers driven by AI are developing quickly, particularly when it comes to GI functional diseases.

Vision Transformer (ViT) and other deep learning models are transforming the classification and analysis of intestinal organoid phenotypes, enabling more accurate and automated characterization of organoid morphology and development. Their high image classification performance facilitates the investigation of disease-specific organoid features, particularly in colorectal cancer, supporting early disease detection, therapeutic response assessment, and the advancement of precision medicine (Mallineni et al., 2024). Evidence of analytical validity, clinical validity, and clinical utility is also necessary for translation into practice; these should preferably be shown by prospective multicenter studies and assessment systems that meet regulatory requirements. Instead of concentrating only on biomarker discovery, the story should highlight the entire validation process needed for clinical application, which includes standardized data collection and labeling, modeling techniques with suitable feature selection under collinearity and low signal-to-noise conditions, internal validation with calibration evaluation, and external validation in separate cohorts to establish generalizability.

7. FUTURE PERSPECTIVES

The implementation of robust multimodal platforms that can embed dental images, electronic health records, salivary biomarkers, oral microbiome profiles, wearable-sensor outputs, genomic data and patient-reported information into a single analytical framework will be essential for future advances to be made in AI-supported oral–systemic healthcare. These platforms should advance beyond mere disease classification to the prediction of disease onset, progression, therapeutic response and recurrence along a disease trajectory. Advanced deep-learning and transformer-based architectures could potentially uncover the intricate relationships between microbial dysbiosis, inflammatory mediators, metabolic abnormalities, and structural oral modifications that are currently hard to detect using traditional statistical models (Cao et al., 2025). Future systems need to be trained with large, diverse and clinically representative datasets, however, to minimize algorithmic bias and to maximize generalizability across age groups, ethnic populations, geographic regions and socioeconomic settings. Standardized protocol for sample collection, imaging, biomarker measurement, labeling of data and defining clinical outcome will therefore be critical. Future multi-center trials should assess the accuracy of AI predictions against established clinical guidelines and not only diagnostic accuracy, but also calibration, interpretability, clinical utility, and cost-effectiveness. Finally, the harmonization of trusted multimodal biomarkers with early intervention, personalized prevention and ongoing risk assessment could help to move towards predictive and preventive approaches in integrated patient-centred health care systems from episodic care to dental care.

A second major direction will be towards the development of explainable, interoperable and privacy-preserving AI systems that can be safely integrated into everyday dental and medical practice. Future algorithms need to be transparent, incorporate the most influential biomarkers or image features, communicate uncertainty, and enable clinicians to review or override automated recommendations. Explainability will be especially significant in the scenarios where the use of AI to predict systemic risks like cardiovascular disease, diabetes, inflammatory disorders or oral cancer, from oral-health data. Furthermore, there is a need for better interoperability between dental records, hospital information systems, laboratory databases, imaging archives, and mobile-health platforms, which can be achieved by using standard data formats and common clinical terminologies. Collaborative training of algorithms without sharing sensitive patient data might be possible with federated learning, secure multiparty computation, and privacy-preserving data-sharing models. The methods might increase the variety of the datasets, but also lower privacy and cybersecurity risks (Borges do Nascimento et al., 2021). There will be algorithm updates to address, accountability, validation thresholds, post-deployment monitoring, and handling of performance drift in regulatory frameworks. As a parallel process, the clinicians, data scientists, patient representatives, ethicists, and regulators should be involved in the design and evaluation of the models. This will require an interprofessional approach to governance to ensure that the use of AI for oral–systemic evaluation is clinically responsible, ethically acceptable, respects autonomy, informed consent and equitable access to health care (Chen et al., 2025).

AI could revolutionize oral health in the long term as a constantly integrated aspect of precision medicine and population health. Smart toothbrushes, intraoral cameras, salivary biosensors, wearable devices and mobile applications could provide information on hygiene habits, inflammation, microbial shifts, diet habits and adherence to treatment. With the integration of clinical and systemic health records, these data can enable dynamic digital biomarkers that aren't taken at one point in time but are continually updated. AI-powered virtual assistants could then provide individualised preventive advice, reminders to change behaviour, referrals and follow-up support, while clinicians are alerted when a change in risk is identified. Longitudinal cohorts, intervention trials and multi-omics analyses combining metagenomics, transcriptomics, proteomics and metabolomics (Weingart et al., 2023) should also be studied to examine causal links between oral dysbiosis and systemic disease. This will assist in the identification of whether oral biomarkers are early indicators, contributing mechanisms or consequences of systemic pathologies. On the public health level, anonymized data might help in the surveillance, allocation of resources and identification of high-risk communities. However, technological advances should not contribute to the growing gap. To achieve global impact, future initiatives must prioritize the development of low-cost, offline-capable AI tools that function in resource-constrained environments, alongside culturally and linguistically adapted interfaces for diverse populations (Lan et al., 2024). Public health policies must mandate transparent reporting of algorithmic performance across different demographic subgroups to detect and mitigate bias before deployment. Furthermore, collaborative frameworks involving ministries of health, academic institutions, and private technology partners are essential to build the necessary digital infrastructure, train the dental workforce in AI literacy, and establish sustainable funding models. Without these deliberate health-equity strategies, AI will remain a privilege of the affluent, failing to address the global burden of oral diseases that disproportionately affects marginalized communities. The vision should be an equitable, participatory, and preventive environment where AI adds to the professional judgment and enhances health results (Morze et al., 2022).

7.1. Critical Appraisal of Current AI Limitations and Translational Hurdles

However, despite its potential, the implementation of AI into the domain of oral-systemic healthcare faces a series of essential problems that need to be addressed. One of them is the absence of external validation in a clinical setting. It turns out that most of the papers dealing with AI in medicine use only retrospective, single-center, or open-source databases, which are far from being representative of the diversity of real-world patients' populations. Moreover, there is the problem of overfitting associated with high-dimensional nature of biomarker data that includes genomics, proteomics, and metabolomics (Cao et al., 2025).

Thirdly, there is the problem of the black box nature of algorithms, which poses a serious barrier on medico-legal grounds. Algorithms such as deep learning models, CNNs, and transformers, are like black boxes since doctors cannot determine the reasoning behind the specific risk score or diagnosis provided, hence, posing problems with regard to accountability in cases of misdiagnosis. Fourth, there is poor interoperability between dental proprietary software, hospital EHRs, and wearable devices due to poor data format standardization such as DICOM versus HL7 FHIR (Zolfaghari et al., 2021).

Finally, the digital divide is not merely an ethical footnote but a practical limitation; AI models trained primarily on high-resolution intraoral scans and high-quality radiographs are unusable in clinics lacking such equipment. The pervasive risk of algorithmic bias—where models underperform for specific racial or age groups due to underrepresentation in training data—mandates that regulatory bodies demand stringent bias audits before clinical deployment. Addressing these limitations requires a paradigm shift from retrospective convenience sampling to prospective, multi-center, pragmatic clinical trials that prioritize generalizability, interpretability, and cost-effectiveness over mere diagnostic accuracy (Jeong et al., 2025).

8. CONCLUSION

The integration of oral health biomarkers with systemic health data through Artificial Intelligence (AI) represents a transformative step toward precision and preventive healthcare. AI models can fuse multimodal data from several sources including clinical data, dental imaging, saliva analysis, oral microbial data, wearable technology data and patient reported information to provide a comprehensive perspective on the complicated interplay between oral and systemic health. Such a comprehensive solution will enable early detection of certain diseases including cardiovascular disease, diabetes mellitus, inflammatory disorders and oral cancer, and even individualized risk prediction and treatment plan. In addition, solutions enabled by AI technology such as machine learning, deep learning, natural language processing, virtual health assistants, and predictive analytics will improve diagnostics, education, monitoring, and personalization of oral health care. Biomarker discovery and validation pipelines based on AI technology will facilitate the development of new clinically relevant biomarkers which can be used for evidence-based decision-making and precision dentistry. Implementation of such a system in the clinic will require a standardized data collection approach, interoperability of healthcare systems, explainability of the algorithm and external validation of the algorithms used, regulatory approval, and robust data privacy and ethical guidelines. Future research should be aimed at prospective multicenter research, multimodal data fusion, federated learning approaches and developing clinically relevant AI models. AI can transform the oral health landscape, patients and moving towards an integrated and precision medicine approach to healthcare.

REFERENCES

Aydin, S., Karabacak, M., Vlachos, V., & Margetis, K. (2024). Large language models in patient education: A scoping review of applications in medicine. *Frontiers in Medicine*, *11*, 1477898. DOI: 10.3389/fmed.2024.1477898 PMID: 39534227

Borges do Nascimento, I. J., Marcolino, M. S., Abdulazeem, H. M., Weerasekara, I., Azzopardi-Muscat, N., Gonçalves, M. A., & Novillo-Ortiz, D. (2021). Impact of big data analytics on people's health: Overview of systematic reviews and recommendations for future studies. *Journal of Medical Internet Research*, *23*(4), e27275. DOI: 10.2196/27275 PMID: 33847586

Cao, L., van Nistelrooij, N., Chaves, E., Bergé, S., Cenci, M., Xi, T., Loomans, B., & Vinayahalingam, S. (2025). Automated chart filing on bitewings using deep learning: Enhancing clinical diagnosis in a multi-center study. *Journal of Dentistry*, *161*, 105919. DOI: 10.1016/j.jdent.2025.105919 PMID: 40550354

Chen, J., Ge, X., Yuan, C., Chen, Y., Li, X., Zhang, X., Chen, S., Zheng, W. Y., & Miao, C. (2025). Comparing orthodontic pretreatment information provided by large language models. *BMC Oral Health*, *25*(1), 838. DOI: 10.1186/s12903-025-06246-1 PMID: 40437500

Chen, W., Lin, G., Chen, Y., Cheng, F., Li, X., Ding, J., Zhong, Y., Kong, C., Chen, M., Xia, S., Lu, C., & Ji, J. (2024). Prediction of the Ki-67 expression level in head and neck squamous cell carcinoma with machine learning-based multiparametric MRI radiomics: A multicenter study. *BMC Cancer*, *24*(1), 418. DOI: 10.1186/s12885-024-12026-x PMID: 38580939

Deng, K., Zonta, F., Yang, H., Pelekos, G., & Tonetti, M. S. (2024). Development of a machine learning multiclass screening tool for periodontal health status based on non-clinical parameters and salivary biomarkers. *Journal of Clinical Periodontology*, *51*(12), 1547–1560. DOI: 10.1111/jcpe.13856 PMID: 37697491

Fanelli, F., Saleh, M., Santamaria, P., Zhurakivska, K., Nibali, L., & Troiano, G. (2025). Development and comparative evaluation of a reinstructed GPT-4o model specialized in periodontology. *Journal of Clinical Periodontology*, *52*(5), 707–716. DOI: 10.1111/jcpe.14101 PMID: 39723544

Gottlieb, S., & Silvis, L. (2023). Regulators face novel challenges as artificial intelligence tools enter medical practice. *JAMA Health Forum*, *4*(6), e232300. DOI: 10.1001/jamahealthforum.2023.2300 PMID: 37289461

Hu, M., Shu, X., Yu, G., Wu, X., Välimäki, M., & Feng, H. (2021). A risk prediction model based on machine learning for cognitive impairment among Chinese community-dwelling elderly people with normal cognition: Development and validation study. *Journal of Medical Internet Research, 23*(2), e20298. DOI: 10.2196/20298 PMID: 33625369

Hung, M., Voss, M., Rosales, M., Li, W., Su, W., Xu, J., Bounsanga, J., Ruiz-Negrón, B., Lauren, E., & Licari, F. W. (2019). Application of machine learning for diagnostic prediction of root caries. *Gerodontology, 36*(4), 395–404. DOI: 10.1111/ger.12432 PMID: 31274221

Hunsrisakhun, J., Naorungroj, S., Tangkuptanon, W., Wattanasit, P., Pupong, K., & Pithpornchaiyakul, S. (2025). Impact of oral health chatbot with and without toothbrushing training on childhood caries. *International Dental Journal, 75*(2), 1348–1359. DOI: 10.1016/j.identj.2024.09.028 PMID: 39443262

Islam, S. (2025). Evaluating the impact of AI-generated educational content on patient understanding and anxiety in endodontics and restorative dentistry: A comparative study. *BMC Oral Health, 25*(1), 689. DOI: 10.1186/s12903-025-06069-0 PMID: 40335999

Jeong, J., Kim, K., Gu, Y., Yoon, D., Zhang, M., Wang, L., & Kim, J.-H. (2025). Deep learning for automated dental plaque index assessment: Validation against expert evaluations. *BMC Oral Health, 25*(1), 1000. DOI: 10.1186/s12903-025-06350-2 PMID: 40604649

Labus, A., Radenković, B., Rodić, B., Barać, D., & Malešević, A. (2021). Enhancing smart healthcare in dentistry: An approach to managing patients' stress. *Informatics for Health & Social Care, 46*(3), 306–319. DOI: 10.1080/17538157.2021.1893322 PMID: 33784958

Lan, R., Zhang, M.-J., Liu, K., Meng, F.-F., Xu, X.-H., & Wang, C.-C.. (2024). Cytochrome P450-derived epoxyeicosatrienoic acid, the regulation of cardiovascular-related diseases, and the implication for pulmonary hypertension. *Cardiovascular Drugs and Therapy*, •••, 1–17. DOI: 10.1007/s10557-024-07655-0 PMID: 39652233

Lei, Y., Li, M., Zhang, H., Deng, Y., Dong, X., Chen, P., Li, Y., Zhang, S., Li, C., Wang, S., & Tao, R. (2025). Comparative analysis of the human microbiome from four different regions of China and machine learning-based geographical inference. *MSphere, 10*(1), e00672–e24. DOI: 10.1128/msphere.00672-24 PMID: 39699186

Li, L., Novillo-Ortiz, D., Azzopardi-Muscat, N., & Kostkova, P. (2021). Digital data sources and their impact on people's health: A systematic review of systematic reviews. *Frontiers in Public Health, 9*, 645260. DOI: 10.3389/fpubh.2021.645260 PMID: 34026711

Li, Y., Wu, X., Liu, M., Deng, K., Tullini, A., Zhang, X., Shi, J., Lai, H., & Tonetti, M. S. (2024). Enhanced control of periodontitis by an artificial intelligence-enabled multimodal-sensing toothbrush and targeted mHealth micromessages: A randomized trial. *Journal of Clinical Periodontology, 51*(12), 1632–1643. DOI: 10.1111/jcpe.13987 PMID: 38631679

Li, Y., Ye, H., Wu, W., Li, J., Zhao, X., Liu, Y., & Zhou, Y. (2025). Effectiveness and methodologies of virtual reality dental simulators for veneer tooth preparation training: Randomized controlled trial. *Journal of Medical Internet Research, 27*, e63961. DOI: 10.2196/63961 PMID: 40402564

Liu, J., Zhang, M., Zhu, M., Tan, S., Luo, X., Liu, J., & Zeng, H. (2025). Comparative analysis of diagnostic techniques and treatment modalities for early-stage esophageal carcinoma: A comprehensive review. *Frontiers in Oncology, 15*, 1650965. DOI: 10.3389/fonc.2025.1650965 PMID: 40963869

Liu, T., Lee, K., Mukundan, A., Karmakar, R., Dhiman, H., & Wang, H.-C. (2025). AI in dentistry: Innovations, ethical considerations, and integration barriers. *Bioengineering (Basel, Switzerland), 12*(9), 928. DOI: 10.3390/bioengineering12090928 PMID: 41007172

Lv, X., Zhang, X., Li, Y., Ding, X., Lai, H., & Shi, J. (2024). Leveraging large language models for improved patient access and self-management: Assessor-blinded comparison between expert- and AI-generated content. *Journal of Medical Internet Research, 26*, e55847. DOI: 10.2196/55847 PMID: 38663010

Mallineni, S., Sethi, M., Punugoti, D., Kotha, S., Alkhayal, Z., Mubaraki, S., Almotawah, F. N., Kotha, S. L., Sajja, R., Nettam, V., Thakare, A. A., & Sakhamuri, S. (2024). Artificial intelligence in dentistry: A descriptive review. *Bioengineering (Basel, Switzerland), 11*(12), 1267. DOI: 10.3390/bioengineering11121267 PMID: 39768085

Marashi, S., Hidarnia, A., Kazemi, S., & Shakerinejad, G. (2024). The effect of educational intervention based on self-efficacy theory on promoting adolescent oral health behaviors through mobile application: A randomized controlled trial study. *BMC Oral Health, 24*(1), 1283. DOI: 10.1186/s12903-024-04970-8 PMID: 39448943

McRae, M. P., Kerr, A. R., Janal, M. N., Thornhill, M. H., Redding, S. W., Vigneswaran, N., Kang, S. K., Niederman, R., Christodoulides, N. J., Trochesset, D. A., Murdoch, C., Dapkins, I., Bouquot, J., Modak, S. S., Simmons, G. W., & McDevitt, J. T. (2021). Nuclear F-actin cytology in oral epithelial dysplasia and oral squamous cell carcinoma. *Journal of Dental Research, 100*(5), 479–486. DOI: 10.1177/0022034520973162 PMID: 33179547

Menon, T., Gopalakrishnan, S. N., Balasubramanian, R., & Justin, S. R. (2017). Characterisation of the human oral microbiome in patients with coronary artery disease using next-generation sequencing of 16S rRNA amplicons. *Indian Journal of Medical Microbiology*, *35*(1), 101–104. DOI: 10.4103/ijmm.IJMM_16_370 PMID: 28303827

Morze, J., Wittenbecher, C., Schwingshackl, L., Danielewicz, A., Rynkiewicz, A., Hu, F. B., & Guasch-Ferré, M. (2022). Metabolomics and type 2 diabetes risk: An updated systematic review and meta-analysis of prospective cohort studies. *Diabetes Care*, *45*(4), 1013–1024. DOI: 10.2337/dc21-1705 PMID: 35349649

Murray, P. E., Coffman, J. A., & Garcia-Godoy, F. (2024). Oral pathogens' substantial burden on cancer, cardiovascular diseases, Alzheimer's, diabetes, and other systemic diseases: A public health crisis—A comprehensive review. *Pathogens (Basel, Switzerland)*, *13*(12), 1084. DOI: 10.3390/pathogens13121084 PMID: 39770344

Stephan, D., Bertsch, A., Burwinkel, M., Vinayahalingam, S., Al-Nawas, B., Kämmerer, P., & Thiem, D. G. E. (2024). AI in dental radiology—improving the efficiency of reporting with ChatGPT: Comparative study. *Journal of Medical Internet Research*, *26*, e60684. DOI: 10.2196/60684 PMID: 39714078

Sun, X., Hu, C., & Gong, W. (2025). Follicular dendritic cell sarcoma of the stomach in a young male: A rare case report and literature review. *Medicine*, *104*(27), e43004. DOI: 10.1097/MD.0000000000043004 PMID: 40629639

Szabó, V., Szabó, B., Orhan, K., Veres, D., Manulis, D., Ezhov, M., & Sanders, A. (2024). Validation of artificial intelligence application for dental caries diagnosis on intraoral bitewing and periapical radiographs. *Journal of Dentistry*, *147*, 105105. DOI: 10.1016/j.jdent.2024.105105 PMID: 38821394

Uribe, S., Issa, J., Sohrabniya, F., Denny, A., Kim, N., Dayo, A., Chaurasia, A., Sofi-Mahmudi, A., Büttner, M., & Schwendicke, F. (2024). Publicly available dental image datasets for artificial intelligence. *Journal of Dental Research*, *103*(13), 1365–1374. DOI: 10.1177/00220345241272052 PMID: 39422586

Viet, C. T., Asam, K. R., Yu, G., Dyer, E. C., Kochanny, S., Thomas, C. M., et al. (2024). Artificial intelligence-based epigenomic, transcriptomic, and histologic signatures of tobacco use in oral squamous cell carcinoma. npj Precision Oncology, 8, 130. https://doi.org/DOI: 10.1038/s41698-024-00605-x

Wang, H., Li, J., Lin, Y., Lin, C., Liu, C., Lin, T., Chan, C.-T., & Hsieh, C.-Y. (2025). Machine learning-based toothbrushing region recognition using smart toothbrush holder and wearable sensors. *Biosensors (Basel)*, *15*(12), 798. DOI: 10.3390/bios15120798 PMID: 41440279

Weingart, J., Schlager, S., Metzger, M., Brandenburg, L., Hein, A., Schmelzeisen, R., Bamberg, F., Kim, S., Kellner, E., Reisert, M., & Russe, M. F. (2023). Automated detection of cephalometric landmarks using deep neural patchworks. *Dento Maxillo Facial Radiology*, *52*(6), 20230059. DOI: 10.1259/dmfr.20230059 PMID: 37427585

Wu, W., Hu, L., Chen, Y., Cao, F., Ding, S., Wu, T., & Xu, J. (2022). Effectiveness of an online application of the health action process approach (HAPA) theory on oral hygiene intervention in young adults with fixed orthodontic appliances: A randomized controlled trial. *BMC Oral Health*, *22*(1), 192. DOI: 10.1186/s12903-022-02219-w PMID: 35590291

Zhang, Z., Dou, Z., Zhang, X., Wang, D., Abudoureheman, K., Yan, Y., Kang, F., Zhang, W., Meng, W., Zhang, K., Li, Z., Zhang, J., Liu, B., & Zhang, B. (2025). Development and validation of a novel public prediction platform for deciduous caries in preschool children: An observational study from Northwest China. *BMC Pediatrics*, *25*(1), 600. DOI: 10.1186/s12887-025-05763-w PMID: 40764955

Zolfaghari, M., Shirmohammadi, M., Shahhosseini, H., Mokhtaran, M., & Mohebbi, S. (2021). Development and evaluation of a gamified smart phone mobile health application for oral health promotion in early childhood: A randomized controlled trial. *BMC Oral Health*, *21*(1), 18. DOI: 10.1186/s12903-020-01374-2 PMID: 33413304

Chapter 12
Artificial Intelligence in Dental Radiographic and Clinical Epidemiology:
Deep Learning, Image-Based Diagnostics, CBCT, and Cephalometric Epidemiology

Waseela Ashraf
http://orcid.org/0000-0002-2236-8581
University of Europe for Applied Sciences, UAE

Muhammad Arshed
http://orcid.org/0009-0005-0683-9610
Baqai Medical University, Karachi, Pakistan & College of Public Health, Ziauddin University, Karachi, Pakistan

Muhammad Rehan
Baqai Medical University, Karachi, Pakistan

Syed Muhammad Fauzan Ali
http://orcid.org/0000-0002-7838-2622
Baqai Medical University, Karachi, Pakistan

ABSTRACT

Studies on oral health at the population level are changing through artificial intelligence and data science. This chapter argues that integrating dental imaging data, electronic health records, and systemic outcome registries creates new opportunities for epidemiological research through the EpiDentomics framework. These advances

DOI: 10.4018/979-8-3373-8402-3.ch012

move beyond minor adjustments to current survey techniques and may lead to a structural shift in the measurement, tracking, and correlation of oral disorders with broader health outcomes. The chapter reviews recent research on deep learning in dental radiographic image analysis, including oral cancer screening, caries detection, periapical disease, and periodontal bone loss. It also highlights the role of cephalometric analysis and AI-assisted CBCT in population-level studies of craniofacial morphology, airway dimensions, and links with systemic disorders. The chapter further discusses XAI techniques and the integration of imaging phenotypes with electronic health records to investigate oral–systemic interactions at scale across diverse global populations.

1. INTRODUCTION

Even if it was not always described in this way, dentistry has always been a data-rich field. Radiographs have been used primarily as diagnostic tools for almost a century, but the information they contain goes beyond what is needed for any given clinical encounter. Patterns of caries burden, the degree of periodontal bone loss, the existence of periapical pathology, developmental abnormalities of tooth number and form, cortical bone quality, and early radiographic indicators of systemic conditions, such as osteoporosis and atheromatous calcification, can all be seen on a meticulously taken panoramic image and interpreted by a qualified clinician. The same image, when processed computationally across thousands of patients, becomes qualitatively different: a substrate for population inference.

What has changed in recent years is not the richness of the data but the capacity to extract, standardize, and analyze it on a large scale. Traditional estimates of oral disease burden have depended on cross-sectional population surveys, which are resource-intensive exercises that are conducted infrequently, are vulnerable to inter-examiner variability, and are logistically constrained in lower-income settings. The time between national oral health surveys is frequently 10 years or more, leading to long intervals between surveys and making it hard to identify secular trends or to assess the effectiveness of preventive interventions. The amount of routine dental care, on the other hand, produces millions of radiographic and clinical data points annually, each time a patient gets care. The key idea behind EpiDentomics is that if this information could be accessed and harmonized, and analyzed responsibly, it could provide more continuous, more granular, and more geographically expansive oral health surveillance than current survey methods can offer (Listl & Filho, 2020; Tiwari et al., 2025).

It's possible only due to artificial intelligence, particularly deep learning. Deep learning algorithms are more consistent and faster than human examiners at processing radiographic images. These systems can be used to extract features that are legitimate and repeatable to indicate the presence and severity of the disease and structural variation of the disease under the right circumstances. These properties are important for epidemiology, where measurement inconsistency is a source of outcome misclassification and where the ability to apply the same analytical procedure to data collected years apart or at different institutions is a prerequisite for longitudinal and comparative research.

It is important to be precise about terminology, since these terms are frequently used interchangeably in ways that obscure meaningful distinctions. Artificial intelligence refers to computational systems designed to perform tasks that ordinarily require human cognitive effort. Machine learning is a subset of AI in which algorithms are trained on data to identify patterns and make predictions rather than following explicitly programmed rules. Deep learning is a further specialization built on artificial neural networks with many layers, each learning increasingly abstract representations of the input data. convolutional neural networks (CNNs), the architecture that has most transformed medical imaging research, are particularly effective at identifying spatial patterns in pixel-level data, making them well-suited for the classification, detection, and segmentation tasks that dominate dental radiographic analysis (Huang et al., 2023; Singh & Raza, 2022).

This chapter is organized around three core themes: The first is the current state of deep learning applied to dental radiographic diagnostics, with attention to performance evidence, methodological limitations, and the specific implications for epidemiologic measurement. The second is the contribution of AI to CBCT and cephalometric analysis as tools for population-level research on craniofacial morphology and its association with systemic health. Third, the ethical and legal landscape within which all of this work must be situated. A central argument running through all three themes is that AI must complement, rather than displace, rigorous epidemiologic reasoning, the careful attention to causal inference, confounding, study design, and the evaluation of bias and measurement error that distinguish epidemiology from purely predictive analytics (Chen et al., 2024; Listl & Filho, 2020). (Figure 1)

Figure 1. The EpiDentomics Framework

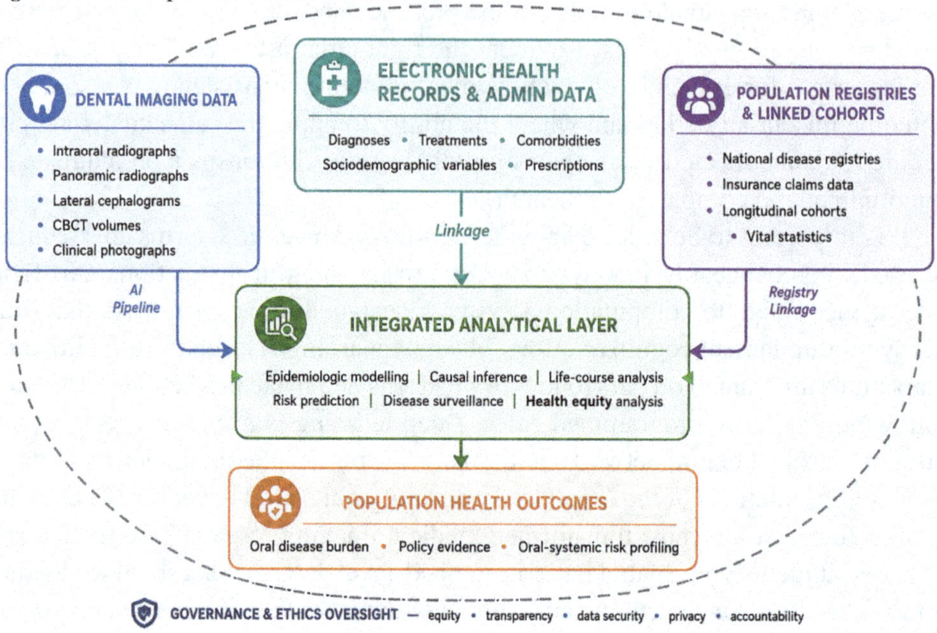

The three convergent inputs to EpiDentomics are depicted in a schematic diagram: (1) dental imaging data (radiographs, CBCT, and photos), which are processed by AI pipelines to produce standardized phenotype variables; (2) administrative databases and electronic health records, which provide clinical, sociodemographic, and systemic outcome data; and (3) population registries and linked cohort datasets. These three streams are fed into an integrated analytical layer that performs health equity analysis, causal inference, and epidemiological modeling. Bidirectional feedback between the analytical layer and governance/ethics oversight is indicated by arrows.

2. DEEP LEARNING AND IMAGE-BASED DIAGNOSTICS IN DENTAL EPIDEMIOLOGY

2.1. How Deep Learning Interprets Dental Images

There are multiple forms of dental imaging, with each offering different information and different radiation dose, field of view, and diagnostic capabilities. Intraoral, periapical, and bitewing radiographs are the mainstays of traditional clinical practice for caries diagnosis and periodontal bone level assessment and provide high-resolution images of the individual tooth and supporting tissues. For surveys, and because a wide field view of the entire dentition and supporting bone is captured in one shot, panoramic radiographs are useful when searching for diseases that span both jaws. Lateral Cephalograms provide a uniform skull profile for diagnostic and growth studies in orthodontics, and are used for skeletal and dental correlations. Cone-beam computed tomography extends the evaluation of structures, which are inevitably compressed and overlapped in 2D projection pictures, to a third dimension.

These photos are used to train AI models that are able to perform one or more of the three main analytical tasks. Classification assigns a picture, or a particular area of interest, to a category, for example, malocclusion class, periapical disease present or absent, carious or noncarious. Detection finds and recognizes items in the picture space, including diseased lesions, individual teeth, and particular anatomical landmarks. Structures with well-defined spatial boundaries, such as teeth, alveolar bone, cysts, and airway volumes, are examples of structures that can be segmented. These three objectives exactly correspond to the measurements required by epidemiologists: they identify the disease's prevalence, location, and severity, as well as how these patterns change over time and between populations. (Huang et al., 2023; Singh & Raza, 2022).

These are the most common uses of convolutional neural networks. The CNNs learn hierarchical feature representations by using consecutive convolutional layers. Deeper layers capture details of the image that are relevant to the disease, the intermediate layers combine low-level image features such as edges and intensity gradients into patterns, such as outlines of teeth and the texture of trabecular bone. Importantly, this learning does not take place through explicit rule descriptions but through training data annotated with rules. The network gradually tweaks its millions of internal parameters until the network outputs begin to match the expert annotations on the training set. Architectures have been modified for particular tasks: YOLO (You Only Look Once) and related single-stage detection frameworks enable the quick localization of multiple objects within a single image, allowing real-time multi-tooth analysis on panoramic radiographs; U-Net, which uses skip connections between encoder and decoder pathways, has become a standard choice for segmentation tasks in dental imaging (Sivari et al., 2023; Katsumata, 2023).

This is information that should be shared with epidemiologists who will use AI-derived metrics as variables in their study. A type of dichotomization of what might be a continuous disease process is introduced when a model trained for classification generates categorical outputs. A segmentation model generates continuous measurements of area or volume; however, the accuracy of these measurements relies on the quality of the segmentation boundary, which is dependent on the attributes of the training data, the image quality, and the anatomical ambiguity for the structure being segmented. As with any epidemiologic exposure or outcome measure, the measuring properties of AI-derived variables (including validity, reliability, and sensitivity to differential misclassification by subgroups) need to be evaluated and tested with the same rigor. (Figure 2).

Figure 2. Dental Radiographic Epidemiology AI Diagnostic Pipeline

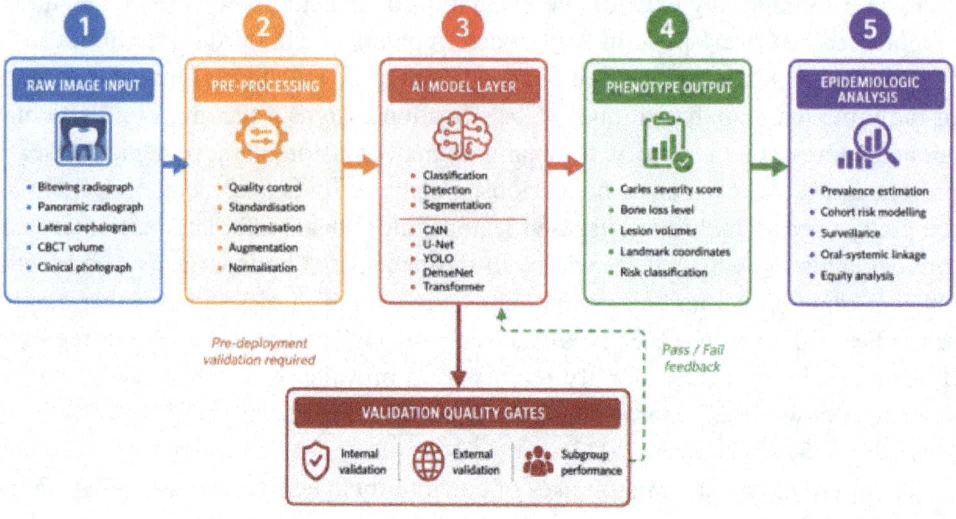

An illustration of the process from unprocessed radiography data to epidemiological results. A structured output of phenotype variables (caries presence/severity, bone loss level, and lesion volume) is produced by the pipeline, which starts with raw image input (bitewing, panoramic, or CBCT), proceeds through a preprocessing stage (image quality control, standardization, and anonymization), and then enters the AI model layer (classification/detection/segmentation). An epidemiological analysis layer (cohort study, prevalence estimation, and risk modeling) on the right received these outputs. Before the outputs reach the epidemiology layer, a validation branch descends from the model layer and displays subgroup performance evaluation, external validation, and internal validation as quality gates.

2.2. Applications and Performance: What the Evidence Shows

The number of studies on the use of deep learning in dental radiography has increased substantially over the last decade. A number of diagnostic domains are now the subject of systematic reviews and meta-analyses, and the overall finding is the same: in some domains, deep learning models perform diagnostic tasks at or above the level of a specialist physician who is well-trained. The finding, however, needs to be put into context, as the conditions under which it applies are not always those found in epidemiological studies or population-level implementation (Table 1).

2.2.1 Dental Caries Detection

Dental caries is the most prevalent non-communicable disease in dentistry, and one of the most studied aims of AI. In a previous umbrella review, Dashti et al. (2024) demonstrated that accuracy levels were between 0.73 and 0.99 for the 7 systematic reviews that combined 24 primary investigations that assessed 2D radiographic images for caries detection. Deep learning models can outperform human examiners, particularly for early subclinical lesions, which are frequently not detected by clinicians. A more in-depth meta-analysis of twenty-one AI platforms for caries detection found that the platforms and the imaging modalities were heterogeneous, with a pooled mean sensitivity of 76% (95% CI: 65–85%) and specificity of 91% (95% CI: 86–95%) and an area under the ROC curve of 92%. More recent single study evidence shows that a DenseNet-121-based model was found to have 93.2% accuracy when tested on over 14,000 tooth images cropped from panoramic radiographs, while a multi-stage segmentation model trained on 500 panoramic radiographs was found to have an overall accuracy of 0.93 to 0.94, with a specificity of the same order for non-carious classification.

These results have important but complex epidemiological implications. An ideal caries AI system would be able to identify early caries on bitewing radiographs, allowing for the application of this AI to existing decades of institutional radiographs in order to generate caries burden estimates across the patient cohort without the inter-examiner variability that limits the use of traditional survey data. This would be particularly useful for the earliest lesions, as these would be the most teachable from a preventative perspective, and most likely to be missed by human inspectors. There are important methodological cautions in the literature, however. Most of the successful models have been developed and tested with data from a single institution, often with the same imaging equipment and processed to the same standard. The performance typically goes downhill, often a lot, when models are applied to images from a variety of sites, on various equipment, and in different ways. The majority of published research has not been comprehensive enough to address this domain shift problem, which is perhaps the most important methodological bias in using AI-generated caries measures as epidemiological variables. (Schwendicke et al., 2019).

2.2.2 Periapical Pathology

One of the challenges is the recognition of periapical lesions (areas of bone loss at the root apices resulting from pulpal infection). These lesions manifest on radiographs differently depending on lesion type, size, stage, and imaging technique. CBCT is more sensitive than 2D radiography, due to the 3D resolution, which could be problematic for early lesions to be distinguished from normal anatomical changes. In a groundbreaking study, Orhan et al. (2020) evaluated a CNN system on CBCT images and concluded that it could successfully identify approximately 93% of lesions, with volumetric accuracy similar to the manual segmentation performed by oral radiologists. The value of using CBCT for epidemiology goes beyond just the accuracy of the figure. It enables three-dimensional measurement of the volume of the lesions, and can track this over time with greater precision than 2D radiographs. This provides opportunities for longitudinal investigations of lesion development, healing, following treatment, or with systemic infection outcome.

2.2.3 Periodontal Bone Loss Assessment

Periodontal disease is a significant cause of the worldwide oral disease burden and is linked to problems with cardiovascular disease, diabetes, and adverse pregnancy outcomes. The subjective and time-consuming nature of manually assessing the severity of attachment loss (AL), the hallmark of periodontitis, has been the traditional approach, and this assessment has been done on panoramic or bitewing radiographs. The potential of deep learning models trained to accurately measure alveolar bone height from panoramic images is the promise of objective, reproducible and scalable estimates of disease severity. The HC Net+ model was validated in a multicenter study that was trained with over 10,800 panoramic radiographs and tested in four centers worldwide, showing an AUROC of 94.2% compared to 85.6% for the periodontal specialists (van Nistelrooij et al., 2025). A second direct equity-related finding was that the model supported junior dentists performing at a level similar to that of specialist dentists, indicating that the use of the model could help alleviate the shortage of specialists in resource-limited areas. But, because all four evaluation centers were in high-income countries, and performance hasn't been tested in other settings that may have fewer resources, patient populations, disease distributions, or image quality may vary significantly, this result should be viewed with caution.

2.2.4 Oral Cancer and Oral Potentially Malignant Disorders

Oral squamous cell carcinoma is one of the most fatal diseases with epidemiological significance for which image-based AI analysis can be useful. There are ~178,000 deaths and 377,000 new cases reported by the WHO in a year worldwide, and often these diseases occur together, with tobacco use, chewing betel quid, and a lack of specialists in South and Southeast Asia (World Health Organization [WHO], 2023). The problem with late diagnosis is that it is a big problem. The majority of patients are found at an advanced stage when the 5-year survival rate is less than 50%. Recognizing this, early detection is most effective as a point of intervention, particularly in a setting where access to trained specialists may be limited (National Cancer Institute, 2026).

Sahoo et al. (2024) found a pooled sensitivity of 0.87 and specificity of 0.81 with an area under the summary ROC curve of 0.98 in a systematic review and meta-analysis of 55 studies evaluating image-based computational methods for detecting potentially malignant oral disorders and oral cancer. The use of clinical photos instead of radiography in several of these investigations is methodologically significant since it increases the possibility of community-based screening with intraoral cameras and cellphones. Using topologies like DenseNet121 and EfficientNetB0, some individual investigations obtained specificity as high as 99% and accuracy of roughly 97.5%. At this point, population-level applications are still mainly aspirational and use clinical photo collections to analyze trends, estimate the incidence of potentially malignant oral illnesses, or connect findings to risk factor information in medical records. However, this path becomes more feasible as imaging infrastructure and validation evidence advance.

Table 1 summarizes deep learning results for diagnostic tasks involving dental radiography. Dice similarity coefficient (DSC); area under the ROC curve (AUC); area under the receiver operating characteristic curve (AUROC); oral potentially malignant disorder (OPMD); and summary ROC (SROC).

Table 1. Learning results for diagnostic tasks

Diagnostic Task	Imaging Modality	Architecture (examples)	Key Performance (from cited sources)	Reference
Caries detection	Bitewing / Panoramic	CNN, U-Net, DenseNet and other DL models	Accuracy across primary studies is approximately 0.73–0.99; most studies report AUC values in the high 0.8s to 0.9s range, with sensitivities and specificities often ≥0.80	Dashti et al., 2024
Caries segmentation	Panoramic / Bitewing	U-Net variants, YOLO-based detectors, "CariesNet"-type models	Typical Dice similarity coefficients reported for caries segmentation are in the range 0.80–0.95, with specificities frequently above 0.90 in recent DL studies	Dashti et al., 2024; Huang et al., 2023; Singh & Raza, 2022; Sivari et al., 2023
Periapical lesion detection	CBCT	CNN, 3D CNN	AI model shows high diagnostic accuracy; in Orhan et al. the deep learning approach achieved performance comparable to expert readers in detecting periapical pathosis	Orhan et al., 2020
Periodontal bone loss / staging	Panoramic	Ensemble CNN, regression	Total diagnostic accuracy about 89%; Pearson correlation with experts 0.83; intraclass correlation 0.81; mean deviation in bone loss degree ≈5%	Xue et al., 2024
Periodontitis (stage II–IV)	Panoramic / Bitewing	Proprietary AI radiographic analysis	AUROC ≈0.94 for stage II–IV periodontitis; AI system significantly outperforms periodontists in correctly staging disease in a multicenter diagnostic study	van Nistelrooij et al., 2025
Oral cancer / OPMD screening	Clinical photographs, radiographs, histopathology	CNN, DenseNet, EfficientNet	Pooled sensitivity 0.87; specificity 0.81; SROC AUC ≈0.98 for AI models detecting OPMDs and oral cancer across 18 studies	Sahoo et al., 2024

continued on following page

Table 1. Continued

Diagnostic Task	Imaging Modality	Architecture (examples)	Key Performance (from cited sources)	Reference
Tooth/structure localisation & numbering	Panoramic / CBCT	Detection and segmentation CNNs	High accuracy for anatomical localisation and tooth detection reported across multiple CNN-based systems, with many studies reporting accuracy or F1-scores >0.90	Huang et al., 2023; Katsumata, 2023; Schwendicke et al., 2019; Singh & Raza, 2022
Age/sex estimation	Panoramic	CNN, regression	In many age-estimation models on dental panoramics, mean absolute errors for age prediction typically fall in the 2–5-year range, with high classification accuracy for sex	Huang et al., 2023

2.3. Methodological and Implementation Challenges

If anyone is thinking of using AI-generated dental measurements in epidemiological studies, the performance numbers published are always misleading. Some common methodology concerns are of particular interest and need further discussion, not as a criticism of individual studies, but as a methodological structure that affects the knowledge that can be gained from this set of studies.

The basic problems are the amount of data and the quality of the annotations. Many published models have been trained with a few hundred images annotated by a single clinician or a handful of clinicians from the same institution. Many published models have been trained using a few hundred photos annotated by a single clinician or a small group from the same clinic or institution. First, the model may not apply to images annotated by different physicians (or using different conventions), as it learns the annotators' interpretive style as well as the underlying pathology. Second, the model cannot be trained from the full spectrum of anatomical variation, pathological appearances and imaging artifacts it would see in real deployment. The resulting overfitting to the training set leads to overestimation of performance on held-out test sets from the same institution and results in suboptimal performance on data that is truly new. Overfitting the training environment can lead to overestimation of performance on held-out test sets from the same institution, and suboptimal performance on data that is truly new (Katsumata, 2023; Sivari et al., 2023).

In the dental AI literature, there is limited evidence for external testing with data from other institutions with different imaging modalities and patient cohorts. This is the methodological gap that is most relevant for epidemiological use since population-level deployment cannot be considered, by definition, internal validation. The domain-shift problem happens whenever the statistical distribution of the test data deviates from the training data, which is typically the situation when models span institutions and/or regions. The radiographic appearance depends systematically on the imaging equipment used, exposure, patient position, patient anatomy and differs from setting to setting and group to group. The model is validated only in one institution, and gives virtually no information to the epidemiologist about its performance in the populations that he or she wants to use it in.

The third problem is which metric to use. In dental AI research studies, the percentage of correct classifications across the entire data set is often reported and is one of the least informative statistics for epidemiologic purposes. A classifier that produces a single negative result for all instances would achieve high accuracy, but have no clinical or epidemiological usefulness, particularly when the prevalence of the condition under study is low, as with oral cancer or periapical pathology, if such data were available. More informative, sensitivity and specificity are dependent on the operating threshold chosen, which is typically optimized on test sets, but may not be optimal for screening and surveillance. Furthermore, subgroup performance analyses are needed to determine whether performance is similar across subgroups, such as across sex, disease severity, and imaging condition, and calibration to establish that the probabilities predicted by the model are true in the populations on which it is applied. Seldom have these analyses been published. (Dashti et al., 2024; Tyagi et al., 2025).

Finally, the concept and appropriateness of the "ground truth" used for the training and evaluation of the models should be explored. In most dental AI studies, the ground truth is created by a radiologist or a specialist clinician who categorizes each image according to their clinical findings. This introduces into the model a set of assumptions by the annotator, which is not an objective biological condition, but how the annotator judged it. For a variety of dental diseases, inter-annotator agreement is not universal, even among the experts, such as those with experience in early caries, modest periodontal bone loss, and subtle mucosal changes. A consensus standard is not apparent in the models that are generated when a few clinicians in a certain setting annotate the same data sets. Reliable techniques such as several annotators' formal agreement assessment, consensus-based labeling, and validation with independent clinical criteria (such as histological testing) should be used in addition to radiographical interpretation.

2.4. Explainable AI and Interpretability in Dental Epidemiology

A major critique of the use of deep learning in clinical and epidemiological contexts is that the models are 'black boxes' and give predictions that are not explainable. This means it is difficult to assess what features of the data resulted in a particular risk estimate, or why a specific image was classified as such. There are several reasons for this opacity to be important. Clinically, this limits the ability of practitioners to critically evaluate AI recommendations before putting them into practice. It is difficult to see if the model in epidemiology reflects physiological differences or makes use of spurious correlations in the training data. When outputs are unexplained and have an impact on screening guidelines, resource allocation, or other population-level decisions that impact distribution, it can be difficult to defend such outputs in public health governance.

Explainable Artificial Intelligence (XAI) is a set of techniques designed to make models more interpretable. In the field of image-based applications, the most popular approaches are variations of the gradient-weighted class activation mapping (Grad-CAM) that produce heatmaps highlighting the parts of the image that are most relevant to a specific prediction. For a dental radiograph, this heatmap could reveal that a caries detection model is focusing on the 'proximal surface of a molar, where there is a subtle density change', or, less encouragingly, it could be focused on an imaging artefact that is not related to tooth structure. In the case of tabular or structured data, approaches like SHAP (SHapley Additive exPlanations) values are able to explain the contribution of each input feature to each prediction, offering a local interpretation of the model's outputs.

In the context of dental epidemiology, interpretability is particularly valuable because it bridges the gap between predictive modeling and the type of risk factor analysis that epidemiology is primarily concerned with. If an AI model identifies a patient as high-risk for periodontitis, it is epidemiologically meaningful to ask whether this classification reflects bone loss severity, tooth loss pattern, sociodemographic variables entered as covariates, or a combination thereof. A model that cannot answer this question in an intelligible manner is of limited use for hypothesis generation or causal inference. By providing such explanations, XAI techniques can direct researchers toward the variables or picture characteristics that influence risk patterns at the population level, generating hypotheses that can subsequently be investigated in suitably planned investigations.

However, there are a few significant limitations. First of all, XAI explanations are approximations of model behavior rather than windows into the real world; different XAI techniques may explain the same prediction in different ways, and explanations are dependent on the reference distribution selection and other technical factors. Second, a model may learn to attend to a feature that is statistically associated with the outcome in the training data but is causally irrelevant, for example, an imaging artifact that happens to co-occur with disease in a particular dataset. XAI methods will faithfully report this feature as influential without flagging its spurious nature. Third, the quality of explanations is constrained by the quality of the underlying model; an explanation of a poorly calibrated or biased model is itself biased. These limitations mean that XAI outputs should be treated as sources of hypotheses rather than evidence and should be scrutinized within the same analytical framework that governs the interpretation of any observational epidemiologic finding.

2.5. Oral Cancer and Oral Potentially Malignant Disorders: Expanded Epidemiologic Considerations

AI in oral cancer detection is a perfect example of the current capabilities and potential of image-based surveillance tools in epidemiology. As mentioned earlier, the results of the metrics in the systematic review are positive. However, there are several attributes of the current evidence base that require some caution before their use in population surveillance systems.

Most research in this field has been performed in research laboratories in the specialized clinical environment with high-quality and curated sets of images. The context that early detection would have the highest population-level impact, community-based screening, is a very different imaging environment. The image quality, angle, and illumination in photos taken by users with a marginal level of training and expertise at the operator level will have much greater variability than those images used to train and evaluate published models. In this context, performance will likely be significantly lower than the published statistics indicate, and the extent of degradation, and how a higher false positive rate and sensitivity for early lesions, can depend on the training method and the main sources of failure of the model. There is a need for empirical research in community settings to inform screening recommendations and require prospective study designs.

A related problem is the difference between the surveillance and the diagnostic instruments. The design criteria for a model that predicts the prevalence of potentially malignant oral diseases within a population are very different from the design criteria for a model designed to help make diagnostic decisions for an individual patient, e.g., should this lesion be biopsied? The latter needs calibrated prevalence estimates and even performance in the different age groups and demographic groups included in the archive, whereas the former needs a high level of sensitivity to avoid the loss of cases in individual patients. These specifications might imply a range of model designs, training approaches, and ways to measure performance. The dental AI literature, which frequently concentrates on individual diagnostic performance without taking the surveillance application into account, hardly ever makes this distinction (Sahoo et al., 2024).

3. AI-ASSISTED CBCT AND CEPHALOMETRIC EPIDEMIOLOGY

3.1. CBCT and Cephalometry as Tools for Population Science

Cone-beam computed tomography can provide high-resolution 3-D images of hard-tissue features in the craniofacial region and is ideally suited to outpatient (dental) settings due to relatively low radiation doses and reduced space requirements compared with medical computed tomography. It has a number of other aspects that make it of great epidemiologic interest, including the three-dimensional morphologic information it contains, including skeletal class and jaw proportions, alveolar bone architecture, root morphology, tooth angulation and position, temporomandibular joint anatomy, airway dimensions, and estimates of bone density. In 2D radiography projections, these quantities can only be estimated as a result of the unavoidable overlapping and geometric distortion from projections. The application of CBCT to develop a much more comprehensive structural framework for a science that seeks to relate oral characteristics to systemic consequences.

Until recently, the most commonly used method to measure skeletal and dental relationships in orthodontics and craniofacial research has been traditional cephalometric analysis of lateral skull radiograph images taken from standard cephalometric cephalographs since the 1930s. The identification of anatomical landmarks (points determined by bony or dental features), measurement of the angular and linear features and comparison to norms (mean values from reference populations). The manual cephalometric tracing is labour-intensive, requires training and has inter-operator variability, which makes it difficult to pool the results across different operators, institutions or centers. These features have limited the use of cephalometric epidemiology to small-scale studies (usually single institution) with limited generalizability. AI landmark detection removes these limitations and allows thousands of photos to be analyzed in the same way without requiring a lot of operator time, through an automated identification and measurement procedure.

Two important selection biases are to be noted when using CBCT and cephalometric data in population-level studies. CBCT is not routinely ordered for all patients but is generally ordered for specific clinical situations such as: difficult orthodontics, planning for implants, evaluation of orthognathic surgery, and specific endodontic or pathological investigation. This means there are clinically relevant differences between the population of patients who have access to CBCT and the population of general dentists (more severe malocclusion, more complicated treatment demands and more likely to have access to specialist care due to their socioeconomic status). Likewise, the percentage of cephalograms in the orthodontic settings is higher. As with all epidemiologic studies based on clinic data, the results that are obtained from an AI-processed CBCT or cephalometric archives should consider these selection effects (Table 2).

3.2. Automated Landmark Detection: Accuracy and Practical Limitations

The most comprehensive synthesis to date of automated landmark detection on 2D lateral cephalograms is the systematic review and meta-analysis undertaken by Hendrickx et al. (2024), which identified 27 papers that evaluated automated landmark detection in 2D lateral cephalograms. The pooled mean (95% CI: 1.39 mm [0.85–1.92 mm]) of the clinically recognized criterion of 2 mm was surpassed. Both 2D and 3D automated landmarking were regularly completed within a minute, while it typically takes 10–20 minutes for a qualified orthodontist to manually trace the landmarks. The difference in this case is quite drastic; it's a workflow that can process hundreds of images as opposed to tens of thousands.

The image, however, is not as clear when viewed with a 3D CBCT scan. The qualitative synthesis in the same review showed a range of mean landmark recognition errors of 1.0 – 5.8 mm across the studies, and was heterogeneous due to differences in model architecture, field of view, image quality and landmark definition. Although there was an increase in performance with the use of incremental systems, the parallel umbrella review conducted by Polizzi & Leonardi (2024) suggested that 3D landmarking was less accurate than 2D landmarking, and that performance achieved by the AI systems in most cephalometric landmarks had surpassed the recommended margin of error in the majority of experiments. There is still clinical agreement that AI-driven cephalometric analysis needs to be finalized under the supervision of a skilled orthodontist, especially when it comes to treatment planning.

An epidemiologic point of view extends beyond mean errors being above or below a clinical threshold. The key question is whether the errors are constant across the various categories of the morphology and demography that are to be reported in the population statistics and whether they are random or systematic. In the epidemiologic analysis, non-differential misclassification will be incorporated in a model that has random 3D landmark detection errors, with equal probability in any direction, with no correlation with patient characteristics, and that weakens relationships toward the null. A model with systematic errors will cause differential misclassification, which could be larger among patients with a certain skeletal class, age group, or ethnic group and may affect the direction of the relationship. However, the vast bulk of primary research and published systematic reviews do not provide enough information to tell us which of these situations is more likely to exist. The lack of evidence is a big challenge for anyone interested in using AI-based cephalometric measurements as epidemiologic variables.

3.3. CBCT-Generated Cephalograms and Low-Dose Radiation Strategies

A major use of AI in this field is the ability to make 2D lateral cephalograms from volumetric CBCT data. Being able to get accurate 2D measurements from existing CBCT data suggests that there would be a real savings in radiation dose, since many patients who would have had CBCT for clinical purposes (such as orthodontic and orthognathic) would have also had lateral cephalograms. The measurements of AI analysis of CBCT-derived cephalograms were compared to the lateral cephalogram, and the results were similar. The same group expanded the findings of this study to AI-processed low-dose CBCT, where they found that measurements obtained using the low radiation dose scans were close enough to the standard radiation dose scans for clinical use (Chung et al., 2024). The results revealed that a population cephalometric profile was possible using historical scans and that potentially an existing CBCT database could be used to produce a population cephalometric profile for population studies. This would be an ideal way to increase the analytical usefulness of the data that has already been collected without having to collect additional data or expose them to further radiation.

3.4. Population-Level Applications: Life-Course Research.

The potential of automated CBCT and cephalometric analysis for epidemiology is most evident on the scale. An AI pipeline that processes the same number of cephalograms as a single orthodontist in a year, but in hours, is working on an institutional database. When scaled up to the large teaching hospital with decades of archived scans, it becomes possible to have longitudinal craniofacial morphometric databases of size and time span never before possible by manual analysis.

Research on a variety of topics could be aided by such databases. Growth trajectory studies examining the alterations of the skeletal and dental connections of community samples during the adolescent period and not clinical samples could be beneficial in distinguishing the other factors that influence craniofacial development, such as environment, dietary factors, and genetic factors. Secular trend analysis can be used to examine whether bone size or airway dimensions are changing at the population level over decades, which may affect nutrition, posture, and breathing patterns. The normative norms used in clinical treatment planning may be influenced in cross-population comparison studies that examine the generalizability of the norms across ethnic groups. These are not simple scientific questions, but have implications for the design of orthodontic and surgical intervention programs, for identifying populations at higher risk for sleep-disordered breathing, and for understanding the developmental origins of oral and systemic conditions (Huang et al., 2023; Singh & Raza, 2022).

One area of AI-CBCT epidemiology that is of great interest is the upper airway morphology. Obstructive sleep apnea (OSA) is an established condition with systemic effects such as increased cardiovascular and metabolic risk, caused by narrowing of the upper airways in sleep. The upper airway can be automatically and consistently segmented by AI, and airway dimensions can be automatically measured with three-dimensional precision using CBCT. If respiratory function data or the outcomes of sleep studies were shared with the existing CBCT archives in orthodontic and oral surgery clinics in the same patients, it would be possible to examine correlations between anatomic predictors of airway narrowing and clinical sleep apnea parameters that would be difficult to achieve in prospective studies. In the field of osteoporosis research, the measurement of the cortical index and other bone texture features, accessible from panoramic or CBCT images, are analogous: they are suggested to reflect skeletal bone mineral density, and thus, dental imaging databases can be used as population-level screens for fracture risk in older persons.

Overall, machine learning applied to longitudinal health data can model a person's health trajectory throughout their life, identify vulnerable time periods for interventions to be most effective, and integrate data from different data streams, including clinical, social, environmental, and imaging data, in a single analytical framework (Chen et al., 2024). In the field of oral health, these methods allow for the prediction of the course of periodontal disease and caries from childhood to adulthood, identification of the best window of opportunity to intervene and improve oral health outcomes, and the ability to assess if oral health improvement in one period is associated with reduced systemic disease risk in a different period. In the majority of settings, the data infrastructure needed for this type of research isn't in place yet, and AI automation of image analysis is a prerequisite for developing it.

Table 2. AI applications in CBCT and cephalometric epidemiology, with associated epidemiologic potential and current state of evidence.

Application Area	AI Task	Epidemiologic Potential	Current Evidence Level
2D cephalometric landmarking	Landmark detection (CNN)	Population morphometric surveys; growth trajectory studies; secular trend analysis	Systematic review and meta-analysis; mean error <2 mm (Hendrickx et al., 2024)
3D CBCT landmarking	Volumetric landmark detection	Orthognathic surgery populations; 3D morphometrics at scale; cross-ethnic comparisons	Qualitative synthesis; error 1.0–5.8 mm; high heterogeneity; variable
CBCT-derived cephalograms	Image synthesis + landmarking	Retrospective cohort studies from CBCT archives; dose reduction strategies	Clinical validation (Chung et al., 2022, 2024)
Airway volume segmentation	Volumetric segmentation	Sleep apnea–oral health links: upper airway epidemiology in large clinic cohorts	Emerging, proof-of-concept; no large population cohort studies yet.
Alveolar bone / cortical density	3D segmentation, texture analysis	Osteoporosis screening; implant epidemiology; fracture risk prediction	Proof-of-concept; limited external validation
Malocclusion classification	Classification (skeletal class)	Prevalence surveys; secular trends; treatment need estimates at the population level	Limited population-scale validation outside high-income settings

4. AI IN CLINICAL AND LIFE-COURSE ORAL–SYSTEMIC EPIDEMIOLOGY

4.1. Electronic Health Records, Big Data, and ML-Driven Surveillance

In addition to imaging, structured data from electronic health records, dental insurance claims, national disease registers, and clinical audit databases are increasingly important sources of information for AI applications in oral epidemiology. They are valuable data sources to feed into machine learning algorithms developed for risk prediction, surveillance, and identification of population segments with unmet needs due to their content of diagnostic codes, treatment records, prescription information, comorbidity data, sociodemographic data, and outcome data. Realizing this integration at scale requires adherence to established data interoperability standards, particularly DICOM (Digital Imaging and Communications in Medicine) for radiographic and imaging data, and HL7 FHIR (Fast Healthcare Interoperability Resources) for structured clinical records, both of which remain inconsistently implemented across dental practice settings internationally, representing a foundational infrastructure gap for EpiDentomics.

Listl & Filho (2020) have argued that big data and machine learning can generate testable causal hypotheses that traditional epidemiologic tools are unable to generate, can map the social determinants of oral disease, and can predict the risks of oral diseases, such as periodontal disease and caries, at the individual and population level.

As Tiwari et al. (2025) noted in their critical appraisal on big data and oral health disparities, there is already growing evidence from the analysis of large administrative and EHR data sets that significant oral health inequalities exist by race, socioeconomic status, geographic location and insurance status across several high-income country contexts. Untreated disease burden is higher, preventive care attendance is lower and tooth loss is higher at older ages among populations with fewer socioeconomic resources, rural populations, and members of racial or ethnic minority groups, with all of these trends being pretty consistent. These analyses are not yet reliable to provide a causal explanation of the inequalities; they only identify inequalities and do not account for differences in exposure to risk factors, access to care, or how care is delivered once it is received. These most at-risk patients can be identified from machine learning models, which have been trained using EHR data; however, study designs to transform this predictive power into causal inference, such as natural experiments, instrumental variable analysis, suitably designed interventional studies, etc., and must further be developed. Large national datasets enable AI to identify behavioral and socioeconomic determinants, supporting targeted public health interventions and surveillance (M et al., 2025).

4.2. Linking Oral Imaging Phenotypes to Systemic Outcomes.

EpiDentomics' most advanced, science-focused dimension is the integration of AI-based oral imaging metrics to actual systemic health outcomes. Biological links between periodontitis and cardiovascular disease via systemic inflammatory response, oral bacterial translocation to poor pregnancy outcomes, and poor glycemic control to rapid periodontitis tissue loss have been documented. The biological rationale is in place: There are risk factors upstream of oral disease and risk factors upstream of systemic disease, and they are similar. The relationships between these have been explored for decades in clinical and epidemiologic studies. AI can be used to measure the extent of oral exposures, bone loss, burden of periapical pathology, and the pattern of tooth loss, with a sufficiently high level of accuracy and scale to allow investigation of mediation pathways, testing of dose-response relationships, and analyses of clinically significant subgroups.

A reasonable study design to illustrate this potential is to link the cardiology, endocrinology, and respiratory records of the same patients with the accumulated

CBCT records stored in a large hospital that has been collecting data in a multi-decade time series. The AI pipeline will automatically analyze CBCT data to classify the quality of mandibular cortical bone, classify the presence of periapical disease and its quantity, segment alveolar bone and estimate the degree of bone loss, and quantify the upper airway dimensions. In all patients, these would be a set of time-varying oral phenotypic exposures. In future survival analyses, where potential confounders are extracted from the clinical record, an association between oral disease burden at baseline and the risk of cardiovascular events, incident diabetes, or diagnosis of sleep apnea could be explored. Though the methodological aspects of this design are present, the challenges are in the infrastructure, governance and analytical capacity, not necessarily in the concept. (Tyagi et al., 2025)

Deriving information from unstructured clinical notes is a related, but under-researched approach that can be achieved using natural language processing (NLP). In dental practices, much of the data is not easily accessible through the regular database queries—they are free text data. This involves any symptoms that the patient has reported, reason for presentation, description of type and duration of pain and details of previous treatment. With the assistance of large language models or other NLP techniques, these materials can then be used to create the structured data for the variables. Some of the variables might be related to patients' oral health experiences or their access to health care that doesn't fit into a structured field in the record. These NLP variables, combined with imaging phenotypes and structured clinical data in current dental record archives, would greatly increase the number of research questions that can be addressed.

4.3. Treatment Planning and Population Level Implications

Computational Treatment Planning is another promising new area with possible epidemiologic applications in which AI can be used to make structured recommendations based on clinical, imaging, and historical patient data. On a population level, there is an opportunity to explore patterns of treatment decisions within large patient populations to gain a better understanding of care disparities, over- or under-treatment, and to investigate if there are inequities in treatment distribution by sociodemographic groups. While an AI system that recommends a range of interventions for people with the same objective disease from a specific clinical context, for patients who have different sociodemographic characteristics, could further reinforce inequities in the system and not be detected unless explicitly monitored.

Stephan et al. (2024) studied the use of a large language model for creating radiology reports from panoramic images for dentistry students. The reports were prepared in a similar format to the reference reports and no obvious errors were noted, but in some instances were lacking in clinical subtlety, as might be expected by an experienced specialist. The narrow definition of this application will impact the quality and completeness of the structured data that will ultimately support epidemiologic research, but also suggest a future where imaging data can be recorded quickly and accurately. Being consistent in the reporting of radiographs over large patient cohorts would help increase the accuracy of the estimation of disease burden using clinical records, among other things.

4.4. Observational Performance and Real-World Impact: A Necessary Caution

Any discussion of AI in oral epidemiology needs to be frank about the data showing how model performance translates into practical effects. Chen et al. (2024) examined AI prediction tools that had been tested in randomized controlled trials and discovered that, although they had shown good discriminative performance in observational development studies, almost 40% of them did not significantly outperform standard care. Several converging mechanisms are shown in this conclusion that AUC or accuracy in a held-out test dataset is not a good predictor of whether a tool would improve outcomes when implemented. It is possible that patients and clinicians will not react to model-generated predictions in the ways that model researchers anticipated. Implementation context is important: a tool may not generalize if it is used in a setting with different patient characteristics, clinical workflows, or baseline care quality from those in which it was developed. Furthermore, a model calibrated to one period may become miscalibrated when the population shifts because risk factor distributions change over time.

These findings, especially for oral epidemiology, indicate a rigorous evaluation approach that goes much beyond technical performance. Before being integrated into surveillance systems, screening programs, or resource allocation algorithms, AI-derived measurements should be tested in prospective studies, ideally pragmatic randomized trials or robust natural experiments, that evaluate actual health outcomes rather than proxy measures of model accuracy. This threshold is difficult and will slow down implementation, but it seems sensible given the population-level consequences of acting on consistently erroneous or poorly calibrated estimates.

5. FUTURE DIRECTIONS IN AI-DRIVEN DENTAL EPIDEMIOLOGY

5.1. Federated Learning and Privacy-Preserving Analytics

For the purpose of training an AI model that will be useful for external purposes such as dental epidemiology, a large, diverse, multiethnic data set from multiple clinical settings and imaging technologies is required. Sensitive patient information can only be aggregated at one institution if it is not centralized in a manner that causes significant privacy and governance issues. One possible way forward is Federated learning, which allows each participating institution to train a local model but only sends model parameters rather than raw information to a central point of control. This helps ensure data sovereignty and minimizes re-identification risks, while allowing the model to be trained on the entire diversity of data from the multi-site data set. In the field of dental imaging, feasibility studies have already been conducted with federated learning, and it has been formally suggested as a means to overcome the current limitations of models due to data diversity and data governance (Rädsch et al., 2022).

But, in the dental context, there are indeed substantial practical challenges with federated learning. For successful federation, consistent data labelling across sites, appropriate imaging techniques and equipment configurations, and adequate technical infrastructure to participate in iterative model training are required. The standards are much harder to satisfy across national boundaries or in areas where there is less resource and are not always met even within institutions in a single country. The field focuses on the development of strong federation techniques that can deal with inconsistently labeled data and diverse data quality.

5.2. Multimodal and Integrated Data Models

The next generation of EpiDentomics research is likely to be based on AI models that integrate data from different imaging sources, structured clinical records, patient-reported data, genomic/microbiome data, and environmental exposures, all using a single analytical framework. The idea for this conceptual goal is to integrate the risk scores from these other streams of data with oral imaging phenotypes to produce overall risk scores for diseases such as type 2 diabetes, cardiovascular disease, and osteoporosis. This may provide an opportunity to make dental care a gateway for additional health risk assessment. Vision-language foundation models, including large multimodal architectures capable of jointly processing images and clinical text, represent a further frontier. Their capacity to interpret radiographic findings alongside patient history and contextual clinical notes may enable more integrated diagnostic reasoning than single-modality systems can achieve.

The challenges to achieving this vision are huge. Data multimodality is a prerequisite for data integration, and is not yet fully achieved in many existing data sets, with the need to carefully handle missing data. Also, it poses interpretability challenges, as it is much harder to interpret the relative importance of imaging data, clinical factors, genomic data, and social factors in a specific prediction when compared to single-modality models. Further, the linkage of oral health to genetic and/or metabolomic information intersects with categories of sensitive information that are subject to heightened regulatory scrutiny in most jurisdictions, which boosts expectations regarding governance (Kraemer et al., 2025).

5.3. Build Capacity and Infrastructure in Low-Income Areas.

Perhaps most importantly, investing in the data infrastructure, analytical capabilities, and governance foundations required to make lower-income settings accessible to and able to benefit from this research is the biggest future avenue for equitable AI in dental epidemiology. The vast majority of dental AI research has been conducted in high-income countries, leading to instruments for which generalizability to the countries with the greatest burden of oral disease has yet to be substantiated, both in terms of the model development and its clinical assessment. This is really a research investment and priority problem, not a technical complexity problem.

To do this, continuous funding is required for dental research in LMICs – investing in the digitization of clinical records and imaging infrastructure, training local epidemiologists and data scientists, establishing governance frameworks appropriate to local regulatory contexts, and developing multi-site partnerships that enable LMIC institutions to have real intellectual leadership rather than acting as data contributors to studies that are planned elsewhere. At the same time, equitable implementation of AI may accelerate progress toward universal health coverage (Arshed, Kazi, Kiran, et al., 2025). Open-source model architectures and jointly shared evaluation datasets tailored to different demographics will also help, as they reduce the technical entry barriers to academics who don't have access to huge computational resources. Moreover, digital health interventions are designed and executed in LMIC settings and may serve as implementation models for AI-enabled oral health programs (Arshed, Mahmud, Umer, et al., 2025).

6. ETHICAL AND LEGAL IMPLICATIONS OF AI IN DENTAL EPIDEMIOLOGY

6.1. Core Ethical Principles and Their Application in Dental Epidemiology

Ethical concerns that are prevalent in many medical specialties but take on distinct forms in the setting of dental health are raised by the application of AI in health research and practice. While the general principles of bioethics (autonomy, fairness, beneficence and non-maleficence) may serve as a foundation, they need to be adapted to dental practice and dental data. Social justice (the structural dimensions of oral health inequality that AI can help address or exacerbate); accountability (clear lines of responsibility must exist for AI system behaviour and its outcomes); and transparency (AI systems must be interpretable or at least auditable) are added to these (Al-Hwsali et al., 2023; Mohammed et al., 2025; Huang et al., 2023).

Dentistry has a relatively unique role in health systems because it is typically separated from general health care in regard to financial, governance and data system arrangements. As a result, medical AI governance and ethical standards might not always be transferable at the literal level. Access to and use of dental and general health records is governed by different types of legislation, and many systems store records. Particularly with regard to routine radiography preservation, patients may have different expectations regarding the use of their dental data than they have with general medical data. The basic ethical principles require adaptation to the specific situation, taking into account the contextual peculiarities of the EpiDentomics environment. (Rölsch et al., 2022) (Figure 3).

Figure 3. Ethical Governance Framework for AI in Dental Epidemiology

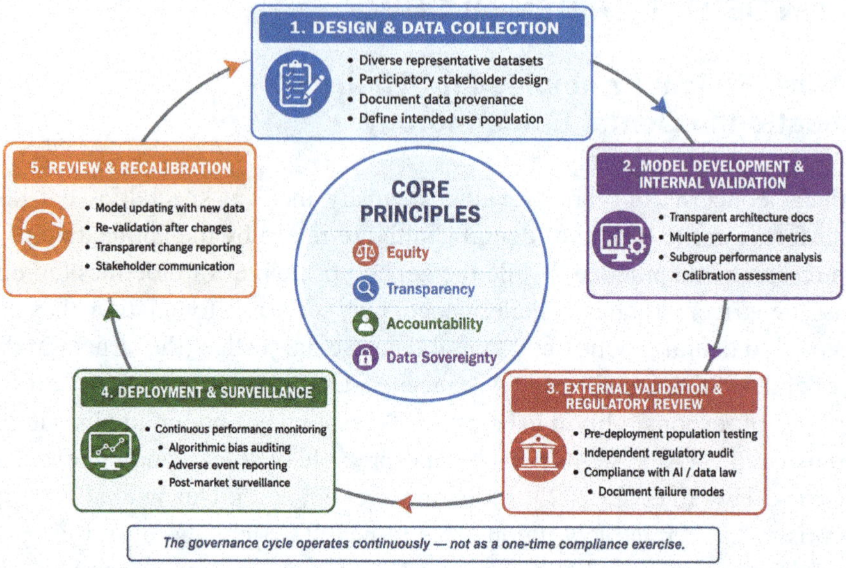

Five interconnected stages make up this circular governance cycle diagram: (1) Design and Data Collection (top), which shows requirements for diverse, representative datasets, participatory stakeholder involvement, and documentation of training data provenance; (2) Model Development and Internal Validation (right), which shows requirements for transparent architecture documentation, multiple performance metrics, and subgroup analysis; (3) External Validation and Regulatory Review (bottom right), which shows pre-deployment testing in deployment populations, regulatory compliance, and independent audit; (4) Deployment and Post-Market Surveillance (bottom left), which shows mechanisms for model updating, re-validation after recalibration, and transparent reporting of changes. Overarching governance values, such as equity, openness, accountability, and data sovereignty, are represented by an outer ring surrounding the cycle.

6.2. Algorithmic Bias, Data Poverty, and the Risk of Entrenching Inequality

Algorithmic bias, stemming from algorithmic processes of spread of dental disease across populations and the methods in which dental datasets are created, is the most pressing equity issue in dental AI. If the training data consistently overrepresents some groups and underrepresents others, the final model will perform well for some patient groups or clinical settings, and not so well for others. This is due to the fact that AI models pick up on trends from their training data. Most dental imaging training data has come from specialized clinics in teaching institutions in highly developed nations (usually in East Asia, North America, and Western Europe). These groups may not represent individuals that live in impoverished communities due to their clustering of disease and relatively accessible health care. (Yu & Zhai, 2024; Li et al., 2024).

The repercussions for epidemiology are important too, although not as widely recognized. If a caries detection algorithm continues to underdetect sickness in certain areas, false low estimates of the disease burden would be obtained for those same towns if this algorithm were incorporated into a surveillance system. If these estimates are believed, policymakers might be able to argue that they should cut preventative services in the areas where they are most needed. This may lead to a vicious circle of unfair policy, based on false assessment. Dankwa-Mullan (2024) refers to the export of AI tools from high-income countries to low-income countries without local adaptation as "technological colonization," which reflects the uneven power dynamics between the exporting and the importing population when an AI tool developed for one population is used by another without any consultation, adaptation, or validation. This requires both technical solutions (e.g. domain adaptation, transfer learning with local data) and explicit efforts to build up annotation infrastructure, local research capacity, and multi-center validation in the settings in which tools will be used (Arshed, Kazi, Ashraf, et al., 2025).

To help alleviate these concerns, as mentioned above, it is possible to train a model using a range of data without it being centralized, via federated learning. On its own, though, it is insufficient. In the deployment context, models should also be evaluated for differential performance by clinical setting and population subgroups due to changing population characteristics and the distribution of illnesses over time. This review must be repeated on a regular basis. An important aspect of responsible deployment of AI that the dentistry industry has not yet put in place is post-deployment monitoring, similar to pharmacovigilance systems for monitoring drug safety after a drug is approved for use.

6.3. Consent, Data Ownership, and the Governance of Secondary Use.

A dental radiograph is a medical record that is used for diagnosis during a visit to the dentist. While using the patient might have been approved by the patient, it may not necessarily be for epidemiologic research or AI training. EpiDentomics imagines the amalgamation of dental and systemic health data allows for re-identification risks that cannot be adequately mitigated with a simple anonymisation. Identification of individuals from dental radiographs is feasible, particularly if they are used in conjunction with other data streams. Governance frameworks, like the GDPR in Europe, affecting the use of secondary data in clinical studies, make multi-site international studies more difficult to conduct. All these frameworks involve the requirement of a documented lawful basis for each use, and the requirement is different in each national context (Al-Hwsali et al., 2023; Li et al., 2024; Yu & Zhai, 2024).

Large language models that can generate clinical text from structured data create novel re-identification threats that current anonymization solutions fail to address. If a model is able to provide patient level summaries or treatment narratives from radiography and health record data, maintaining the separation between identifiable clinical data and de-identified research data can become more difficult. This is a frontier regulatory challenge with implications that are relevant to EpiDentomics, as it strives for the objective of linking dental imaging with other health record streams. It takes more than just technical anonymization to build an appropriate governance infrastructure. It requires open discussion with the public of the potential uses of dental information for research, lay or patient advisory panels, institutional data access committees that have truly independent control, and data sharing agreements that identify permitted uses.

6.4. Regulatory Frameworks and Liability.

Ensuring regulatory compliance is not an option anymore as AI systems evolve from research to clinical decision support and public health surveillance tools. AI software used to support diagnostic decisions is considered a medical device for most jurisdictions and is subject to pre-market validation (including post-market surveillance, training data characteristics documentation, and safety and performance demonstration in the intended use population). This regulatory landscape is changing quickly, driven by key pieces of EU legislation stemming from the AI Act and the US Food and Drug Administration's regulatory strategy for AI and machine learning in software as a medical device, along with a comparable approach in other jurisdictions. To leverage these frameworks, dental AI researchers and developers must be proactively involved in them instead of being forced into them as a compliance measure (Mohammed et al., 2025).

The same is true of obligations distribution. In most countries, questions regarding the legal liability of an AI-assisted diagnosis's error and any resulting harm to a patient remain unanswered. This includes the physician relying on the result of the AI, the health organization where it was used, and the developer who produced it. The lack of clarity raises the issue of governance of the use of AI, resulting in actual resistance from institutions and clinicians. A practical way to mitigate liability risk while building trust in the responsible deployment of AI is to ensure there is clear documentation of the training data, the characteristics of the models, and the scope of intended uses, while engaging in open dialogue with clinicians and patients about the role of AI in care decisions.

6.5. Health Equity, Participatory Design, and Global Justice

In the end, the ethical dilemma of AI in dental epidemiology boils down to a distributive question: who gains and who assumes the risks and expenses? The current trajectory of the field, where development and validation are concentrated in high-income settings, tools are then exported to lower-income contexts, and the communities most affected have limited involvement in design, governance, or benefit sharing, is unethical, even if individual studies are conducted to high technical standards. For a more egalitarian option, participatory design must be a structural commitment rather than a tokenistic addition. The specification, development, validation, and continuous governance of AI tools must involve local clinicians, community health workers, patients, and public health policymakers from the outset, with genuine decision-making authority rather than merely advisory roles. (Chen et al., 2024; Mohammed et al., 2025).

The technical tools that make this possible are shared benchmark datasets, open-source model architectures, and federated learning. The institutional will and research funding to give them priority are what is left. The scientific community, funding organizations, and business partners all have a part to play in ensuring that the EpiDentomics agenda advances in a way that benefits the populations most affected by oral disease rather than exacerbating already-existing disparities through technically remarkable but unequally distributed innovation.

Table 3. Ethical dimensions of AI in dental epidemiology and corresponding mitigation strategies. LMIC = low- and middle-income country; LLM = large language model; XAI = explainable artificial intelligence.

Ethical Dimension	Key Concern in Dental AI Epidemiology	Mitigation Strategy
Algorithmic bias	Training data from narrow, high-income populations; systematic underperformance for marginalized or LMIC groups; feedback loop to inequitable policy	Diverse, multi-ethnic training datasets; mandatory subgroup performance reporting; external validation in deployment populations; transfer learning with local data
Data privacy and re-identification	Secondary use of clinical radiographs without specific consent; re-identification risk amplified by data linkage; LLM-generated text bypasses anonymization	Robust data governance frameworks; formal anonymization protocols; consent or public interest justification; GDPR and equivalent compliance
Transparency and explainability	Black-box models used in clinical or population-level decisions; limited interpretability for hypothesis generation or causal inference	XAI methods (Grad-CAM, SHAP values); audit trails; mandatory disclosure of model architecture and training data; human-in-the-loop review for high-stakes decisions
Accountability and liability	Unclear responsibility when AI-assisted diagnosis is wrong; absence of post-deployment monitoring frameworks analogous to pharmacovigilance	Clear documentation of intended use, training data provenance, and performance characteristics; institutional governance policies; regulatory compliance
Health equity and global justice	Technology designed in and for high-resource settings; deployed without adaptation in LMICs; LMIC researchers excluded from leadership roles	Participatory and equity-centered design; federated learning; open-source tools; investment in LMIC research capacity and data infrastructure
Data sovereignty	Cross-border data flows in multi-site studies; national regulatory frameworks are not harmonized.	Data sharing agreements with defined permitted uses; national and institutional ethics review; patient advisory panels; transparent data management documentation

7. SYNTHESIS: TOWARD A RESPONSIBLE EPIDENTOMICS

In this chapter, the contours of a field in formation have been mapped. It is not that AI has transformed the landscape of dental epidemiology; it's just that reliable tools that are incorporated into routine operational surveillance or population health monitoring have not yet come about. Rather, it is claimed that the conditions for such transformation are already present and that the decisions made in the next decade over the future course of this area will decide on the ethical acceptability, scientific viability, and fairness of the transformation that follows.

The evidence presented here demonstrates that deep learning can be used for dental radiographs to achieve diagnostic performance that is comparable to that of a specialist clinician for a variety of conditions, and that AI-driven analysis of cephalometric and CBCT images can help to standardize and scale measurements that could only be done in small clinical samples before. Additionally, it is conceptually and technically feasible to combine information about the oral cavity with information about outcomes for a variety of systems into electronic health records. These are meaningful and verifiable advances. They offer truly innovative options for monitoring oral health, comprehending the impact of the oral system, and, more specifically, focusing preventive efforts.

However, the chapter has also invested significant effort to provide evidence-based support for what has not yet been proven. For many dental AI products, there is insufficient reporting on external validity (performance in populations and contexts other than the training population). The impact of the use of AI tools in the real world, that is, the extent to which they can enhance public health outcomes, as opposed to simply replicating the performance of specialists in a research environment, has been scarcely assessed. Dental AI researchers should not ignore the terrible example of related fields where over 40% of the predictors used in real-world trials that were studied failed to prove superiority over traditional care. Moreover, the ethics of algorithmic bias, data governance and global health equity are structural features of the research enterprise that shape who benefit from EpiDentomics and under what conditions, rather than being appendages to be solved after development of technical solutions.

The four industries need to be invested to prepare for the future. In terms of methodology, the larger and wider variety of training data required, as well as comprehensive external validation studies, uniform reporting systems, and prospective assessments of real-world impact. For dental records, explainability, federated learning, multimodal integration, and natural language processing are required to enable technological advancements. From governance, it requires both a legislative framework appropriate to the new class of diagnostic tools, AI, and data governance infrastructure, which has the capability of safeguarding patients' privacy and enabling access to the data for responsible studies. Research resources should be especially targeted at the populations with highest burden of oral disease and where the greatest benefit can be derived from improved risk assessment and surveillance to ensure equality.

When best implemented, the EpiDentomics paradigm promises a more integrated, comprehensive, and systemic view of oral health research that is more relevant to the systemic health environment where oral disease occurs. To accomplish that goal, it will be crucial to possess not only the technology capabilities that exist today, but also the scientific rigor, ethical accountability and interdisciplinary and geographical collaboration to leverage those capabilities.

REFERENCES

Al-Hwsali, A., Alsaadi, B., Abdi, N., Khatab, S., Alzubaidi, M., Solaiman, B., & Househ, M. (2023). Scoping Review: Legal and Ethical Principles of Artificial Intelligence in Public Health. *Studies in Health Technology and Informatics*, *305*, 640–643. DOI: 10.3233/SHTI230579 PMID: 37387113

Arshed, M., Kazi, A. K., Ashraf, W., Kiran, M., Arshed, M., Kazi, A. K., Ashraf, W., & Kiran, M. (2025). *Universal Health Coverage: Progress Toward Achieving Universal Health Coverage and Lessons Learned* [Chapter]. Innovation and Transformation of Public Health. IGI Global Scientific Publishing. (universal-health-coverage). Https://Services.Igi-Global.Com/Resolvedoi/Resolve.Aspx?Doi=10.4018/979-8-3373-1992-6.Ch002. https://doi.org/DOI: 10.4018/979-8-3373-1992-6.ch002

Arshed, M., Kazi, A. K., Kiran, M., Ali, S. M. F., Arshed, M., Kazi, A. K., Kiran, M., & Ali, S. M. F. (2025). *Challenges in Health Equity: Balancing Innovation With Fairness and Addressing Algorithmic Biases* [Chapter]. Innovation and Transformation of Public Health. IGI Global Scientific Publishing. (challenges-in-health-equity). Https://Services.Igi-Global.Com/Resolvedoi/Resolve.Aspx?Doi=10.4018/979-8-3373-1992-6.Ch004. https://doi.org/DOI: 10.4018/979-8-3373-1992-6.ch004

Arshed, M., Mahmud, A. B., Umer, M. F., Mashhadi, F., & Kawish, A. B. (2025). Study protocol for a randomized control trial investigating the effectiveness of a multifaceted mHealth approach on adherence to antihypertensive treatment among patients in Pakistan. *Pakistan Journal of Medical Sciences*, *41*(1), 1. Advance online publication. DOI: 10.12669/pjms.41.1.9272 PMID: 39867791

Chen, S., Yu, J., Chamouni, S., Wang, Y., & Li, Y. (2024). Integrating machine learning and artificial intelligence in life-course epidemiology: Pathways to innovative public health solutions. *BMC Medicine*, *22*(1), 354. Advance online publication. DOI: 10.1186/s12916-024-03566-x PMID: 39218895

Chung, E., Yang, B., Kang, S., Kim, Y., Na, J., Park, S., On, S., & Byun, S. (2024). Validation of 2D lateral cephalometric analysis using artificial intelligence-processed low-dose cone beam computed tomography. *Heliyon*, *10*(21), e39445. DOI: 10.1016/j.heliyon.2024.e39445 PMID: 39583802

Chung, E., Yang, B., Park, I., Yi, S., On, S., Kim, Y., Kang, S., & Byun, S. (2022). Effectiveness of cone-beam computed tomography-generated cephalograms using artificial intelligence cephalometric analysis. *Scientific Reports*, *12*(1), 20585. Advance online publication. DOI: 10.1038/s41598-022-25215-0 PMID: 36446924

Dankwa-Mullan, I. (2024). Health Equity and Ethical Considerations in Using Artificial Intelligence in Public Health and Medicine. *Preventing Chronic Disease*, *21*, 240245. Advance online publication. DOI: 10.5888/pcd21.240245 PMID: 39173183

Dashti, M., Londono, J., Ghasemi, S., Zare, N., Samman, M., Ashi, H., Amirzade-Iranaq, M., Khosraviani, F., Sabeti, M., & Khurshid, Z. (2024). Comparative analysis of deep learning algorithms for dental caries detection and prediction from radiographic images: A comprehensive umbrella review. *PeerJ. Computer Science*, *10*, e2371. DOI: 10.7717/peerj-cs.2371 PMID: 39650341

Hendrickx, J., Gracea, R., Vanheers, M., Winderickx, N., Preda, F., Shujaat, S., & Jacobs, R. (2024). Can artificial intelligence-driven cephalometric analysis replace manual tracing? A systematic review and meta-analysis. *European Journal of Orthodontics*, *46*(5), cjae029. Advance online publication. DOI: 10.1093/ejo/cjae029 PMID: 38895901

Huang, C., Wang, J., Wang, S., & Zhang, Y. (2023). A review of deep learning in dentistry. *Neurocomputing*, *554*, 126629. DOI: 10.1016/j.neucom.2023.126629

Katsumata, A. (2023). Deep learning and artificial intelligence in dental diagnostic imaging. *Japanese Dental Science Review*, *59*, 329–333. DOI: 10.1016/j.jdsr.2023.09.004 PMID: 37811196

Kraemer, M., Tsui, J. L.-H., Chang, S. Y., Lytras, S., Khurana, M. P., Vanderslott, S., Bajaj, S., Scheidwasser, N., Curran-Sebastian, J. L., Semenova, E., Zhang, M., Unwin, H. J. T., Watson, O. J., Mills, C., Dasgupta, A., Ferretti, L., Scarpino, S. V., Koua, E., Morgan, O., & Bhatt, S. (2025). Artificial intelligence for modelling infectious disease epidemics. *Nature*, *638*(8051), 623–635. DOI: 10.1038/s41586-024-08564-w PMID: 39972226

Li, Y., Zou, Y., & Xu, H. (2024). *From Data to Decisions: The Integration of AI in Epidemiological Research*. Frontiers in Computing and Intelligent Systems., DOI: 10.54097/7jktck77

Listl, S., & Filho, A. (2020). *Big Data and Machine Learning*. Textbooks in Contemporary Dentistry., DOI: 10.1007/978-3-030-50123-5_23

M, A., M, K., Mf, U., Ja, S., Smu, H., S, Q., Ah, G., S, H., W, A., H, M., & Mn, K. (2025). Prevalence and associated factors of adherence to antihypertensive medication: A nationwide cross-sectional study. *BMC Public Health*, *25*(1). https://doi.org/DOI: 10.1186/s12889-025-21456-6

Mohammed, S., Mohammed, N., Balammagary, S., Kolla, S., Ganta, S., & Khader, S. (2025). Harnessing artificial intelligence for public health and epidemiology: Opportunities, barriers, and pathways to equitable global impact. *International Journal of Computer Science and Information Technologies*, *17*(5), 37–52. DOI: 10.5121/ijcsit.2025.17504

National Cancer Institute. (2026). *SEER cancer stat facts: Oral cavity and pharynx cancer*. Surveillance, Epidemiology, and End Results (SEER) Program. https://seer.cancer.gov/statfacts/html/oralcav.html

Orhan, K., Bayrakdar, I., Ezhov, M., Kravtsov, A., & Özyürek, T. (2020). Evaluation of artificial intelligence for detecting periapical pathosis on cone-beam computed tomography scans. *International Endodontic Journal*, *53*(5), 680–689. Advance online publication. DOI: 10.1111/iej.13265 PMID: 31922612

Polizzi, A., & Leonardi, R. (2024). Automatic cephalometric landmark identification with artificial intelligence: An umbrella review of systematic reviews. *Journal of Dentistry*, *146*, 105056. DOI: 10.1016/j.jdent.2024.105056 PMID: 38729291

Rädsch, T., Seidlitz, S., Moosbauer, J., Rasche, L., & Tolios, I. (2022). Federated learning in dentistry: Chances and challenges. *Journal of Dental Research*, *101*(12), 1524–1532. DOI: 10.1177/00220345221108186 PMID: 35912725

Sahoo, R. K., Sahoo, K. C., Dash, G. C., Kumar, G., Baliarsingh, S. K., Panda, B., & Pati, S. (2024). Diagnostic performance of artificial intelligence in detecting oral potentially malignant disorders and oral cancer using medical diagnostic imaging: A systematic review and meta-analysis. *Frontiers in Oral Health*, *5*, 1494867. DOI: 10.3389/froh.2024.1494867 PMID: 39568787

Schwendicke, F., Golla, T., Dreher, M., & Krois, J. (2019). Convolutional neural networks for dental image diagnostics: A scoping review. *Journal of Dentistry*, *91*, 103226. DOI: 10.1016/j.jdent.2019.103226 PMID: 31704386

Singh, N., & Raza, K. (2022). Progress in deep learning-based dental and maxillofacial image analysis: A systematic review. *Expert Systems with Applications*, *199*, 116968. DOI: 10.1016/j.eswa.2022.116968

Sivari, E., Senirkentli, G., Bostanci, E., Guzel, M., Açıcı, K., & Aşuroğlu, T. (2023). Deep Learning in Diagnosis of Dental Anomalies and Diseases: A Systematic Review. *Diagnostics (Basel)*, *13*(15), 2512. Advance online publication. DOI: 10.3390/diagnostics13152512 PMID: 37568875

Stephan, D., Bertsch, A., Burwinkel, M., Vinayahalingam, S., Al-Nawas, B., Kämmerer, P. W., & Thiem, D. G. E. (2024). AI in Dental Radiology, Improving the Efficiency of Reporting With ChatGPT: Comparative Study. *Journal of Medical Internet Research, 26*, e60684. DOI: 10.2196/60684 PMID: 39714078

Tiwari, T., Patel, J., & Nascimento, G. (2025). Big data and oral health disparities: A critical appraisal. *Journal of Dental Research, 104*(2), 119–130. DOI: 10.1177/00220345241285847 PMID: 39629938

Tyagi, P.. (2025). Artificial Intelligence Applications in Dentistry: A Systematic Review. *Cureus*. Advance online publication. DOI: 10.7759/cureus.85062

Tyagi, P., Jain, S., Ranjan, M., Hassan, S., Prakash, N., Kumar, D., Kumar, A., & Singh, S. (2025). Artificial intelligence tools in dentistry: A systematic review on their application and outcomes. *Cureus, 17*(5), e85062. DOI: 10.7759/cureus.85062 PMID: 40585609

van Nistelrooij, N.. (2025). A novel AI-powered radiographic analysis surpasses specialists in stage II–IV periodontitis detection: A multicenter diagnostic study. npj. *Digital Medicine, 8*(1), 691. DOI: 10.1038/s41746-025-02077-0 PMID: 41254181

World Health Organization. (2023, November 29). *Comprehensive assessment of evidence on oral cancer prevention released.* https://www.who.int/news/item/29-11-2023-comprehensive-assessment-of-evidence-on-oral-cancer-prevention-released-29-november-2023

Xue, T., Chen, L., & Sun, Q. (2024). Deep learning method to automatically diagnose periodontal bone loss and periodontitis stage in dental panoramic radiograph. *Journal of Dentistry, 150*, 105373. DOI: 10.1016/j.jdent.2024.105373 PMID: 39332519

Yu, L., & Zhai, X. (2024). Use of artificial intelligence to address health disparities in low- and middle-income countries: A thematic analysis of ethical issues. *Public Health, 234*, 77–83. DOI: 10.1016/j.puhe.2024.05.029 PMID: 38964129

Chapter 13
Artificial Intelligence-Driven Epidemiology of Endodontic and Restorative Diseases:
Linking Oral Infections to Systemic Health Outcomes

Rizwan Jouhar
http://orcid.org/0000-0001-5901-1482
King Faisal University, Saudi Arabia

Muhammad Adeel Ahmed
http://orcid.org/0000-0002-3279-8278
King Faisal University, Saudi Arabia

Mohamad Syahrizal Halim
http://orcid.org/0000-0002-0423-8070
Universiti Sains Malaysia, Malaysia

Fayez Hussain Niazi
http://orcid.org/0000-0003-1602-9740
Dar Al Uloom University, Saudi Arabia

Fahim Vohra
University of Minnesota, USA

DOI: 10.4018/979-8-3373-8402-3.ch013

ABSTRACT

The integration of artificial intelligence (AI) into dental epidemiology has transformed the evaluation, diagnosis, and management of endodontic and restorative treatments, thus presenting a unique opportunity to explore the association between oral infections and systemic health outcomes. Techniques based on AI have been observed to demonstrate high accuracy in the assessment of dental caries, periapical diseases, and periodontal diseases based on the assessment of radiographic images, mining of electronic health records, and predictive modeling of outcomes. In addition to that, AI-based techniques have been effective in the integration of oral health with systemic health parameters to understand the relationship between chronic oral health diseases and systemic health conditions like cardiovascular diseases, diabetes, and inflammatory diseases.

1. INTRODUCTION

1.1 Oral-Systemic Interrelationship: A Contemporary Perspective

Traditionally, oral health was considered to be separate from general health, but present research highlights the need to consider a holistic approach towards health by incorporating dental health with general medical health. This has been considered important as oral health is part of the body and is linked to general health and well-being (Prasad et al., 2019; Chan et al., 2023). Around 3.5 billion people worldwide suffer from various oral health problems such as dental caries, periodontitis, or orofacial pain, which are the most common health issues. The impact of these issues is seen mostly in middle- and low-income countries due to a lack of oral healthcare facilities. Thus, the projected rise in these conditions, improving oral health is a critical yet inadequately addressed global health issue (World Health Organization, 2023).

Recent studies have further emphasized the important role of oral health in systemic health outcomes (Prasad et al., 2019; Chan et al., 2023). The key to the oral-systemic health relationship lies in the oral microbiome, which is the second only to the gut in microbial abundance. Up to the present time, over 700 microbial species have been discovered in the oral cavity (Deo & Deshmukh, 2019). In a state of equilibrium, this intricate microbial community plays a role in the activation of the immune system and the prevention of colonization by pathogenic microbes. Nevertheless, an imbalance of this microbial community, or "dysbiosis," has been shown to contribute to the development of both oral and systemic diseases. Recent studies have suggested that an imbalance of the oral microbiome may contribute to the development of systemic inflammation, thereby leading to an increased chance of developing systemic diseases such as cardiovascular disease (Rydén et al., 2016), inflammatory bowel disease (Elzayat, Mesto, & Al-Marzooq, 2023), metabolic disease (Esfanjani et al., 2023), and other chronic diseases.

Systemic disorders can also significantly influence oral health outcomes. For instance, diabetes mellitus has been strongly linked to a greater susceptibility to periodontal disease. Persistent hyperglycemia can lead to an increased risk and severity of gingival inflammation, thus forming a two-way relationship where both conditions can exacerbate each other (Taylor, 2001). Likewise, rheumatic diseases like rheumatoid arthritis and Sjögren's syndrome can also lead to the degeneration of the temporomandibular joint (TMJ), thus causing problems with mastication and changes in facial aesthetics, thus affecting oral health (Collin et al., 2024). Patients with these diseases are also at higher risk of dental caries, partly due to xerostomia, immunosuppression, and poor manual dexterity, all of which make oral hygiene practices difficult (Aloyouny et al., 2022). A two-year prospective longitudinal study by Collin et al. in children and adolescents with juvenile idiopathic arthritis demonstrated involvement of the TMJ due to the underlying inflammatory process. The progression of the deformity in the TMJ was also observed over a period of time through cone beam computed tomography. The study highlights the necessity of involving both medical and dental practitioners in patient management. Accordingly, the importance of integrative practice must be recognized to attain a deeper understanding of the complex relationship between oral health and systemic health.

1.2. Need for Artificial Intelligence in Dental Epidemiology

Artificial intelligence (AI) and machine learning (ML) are some of the emerging technologies in the healthcare industry. It is worth noting that AI refers to computer systems that have the potential to perform tasks that need human intelligence and decision-making. ML refers to a subset of AI that aims to create algorithms with the potential to analyze data, identify patterns, and learn from their experiences. It is also imperative that AI and ML have the potential to perform complex tasks such as diagnostic analysis, treatment plan development, and population health monitoring (Ding et al., 2021).

In the context of dental public health, it is important that AI and ML have tremendous potential in enhancing early disease detection, patient-centered healthcare, and resource allocation in the healthcare industry. For instance, it is worth noting that AI systems have shown tremendous potential in analyzing dental radiographs, thereby enhancing the detection of dental caries and impacted teeth (Zhu, 2021). Moreover, artificial intelligence systems can analyze large data to identify important patterns and predict possible outbreaks, thus informing more strategic public health interventions (Fisher, 2021).

Endodontic and restorative diseases are complex, multifactorial conditions with increasing evidence relating chronic oral disorders to worse systemic health outcomes. Conventional epidemiological techniques are limited in their capacity to assess high-dimensional, heterogeneous data and to capture nonlinear relationships across clinical, radiographic, and longitudinal health datasets. An AI-powered structure offers the ability to execute sophisticated pattern recognition, predictive analytics, and more precise data integration and dynamic observation of disease distribution and progression, and oral-systemic relationships at both the individual status and population levels. This chapter has reviewed the use of AI-driven epidemiologic models for the assessment of endodontic and restorative diseases and their relationship to systemic health outcomes, which have the potential to improve disease surveillance, risk assessment, and evidence-based decision-making.

2. PRINCIPLES OF ARTIFICIAL INTELLIGENCE

Artificial intelligence (AI), a term introduced by John McCarthy, was defined as "the science and engineering of creating intelligent machines." McCarthy and colleagues suggested a "two-month study with ten people" in 1955 based on the assumption that "every aspect of learning or any other feature of intelligence can in principle be so precisely described that a machine can be made to simulate it" (McCarthy et al., 2006). This historic initiative has grown rapidly to influence many aspects of contemporary life. Currently, AI acts as a solution to complex problems, encompassing machine learning, representation learning, and deep learning.

2.1. Machine learning (ML)

A branch of artificial intelligence (AI), ML uses algorithms rather than traditional rule-based programming for data processing, pattern recognition, and decision-making (Choi et al., 2020). In contrast to other kinds of programming that can be clearly programmed for a task, ML programming uses a system that learns from its experience to improve its performance. This process commences with the use of relevant data for training the ML system to recognize patterns or make predictions. Consequently, the model may be adjusted by a human expert to improve its accuracy and efficiency. Eventually, another dataset may be introduced for the assessment of the model's accuracy in making predictions.

2.2. Deep Learning (DL) and Neural Networks

Deep learning (DL), which is a sub-domain of machine learning (ML), involves the development of neural networks to process complex information for prediction (Choi et al., 2020). A number of models of deep learning, for instance deep neural networks, deep perception networks, recurrent neural networks, and convolutional neural networks, have been employed for multiple purposes in different domains (Sarvamangala & Kulkarni, 2022). Among these models, convolutional neural networks (CNNs) are best suited to deal with image-based information, which can be applied in medical diagnostics using image-based diagnostic tools like X-rays and MRIs (Sarvamangala & Kulkarni, 2022).

2.3. Natural Language Processing (NLP)

Natural language processing (NLP) is a set of techniques that permit computers to understand and process human language. NLP is applied in the healthcare industry to obtain significant understandings from unstructured data, including clinical records and scientific literature, to aid diagnostic decisions and knowledge synthesis for predicting patient outcomes (Zhou et al., 2024). However, AI algorithms are a significant shift in understanding and managing health and disease, beyond improving efficiency in diagnosing and predicting diseases.

3. EVOLUTION OF AI IN MEDICINE AND DENTISTRY

Artificial intelligence has made tremendous advancements in the field of medical science, thereby bringing forth a variety of applications. These include aligning patient symptoms with suitable physicians, supporting medical diagnosis and prognosis, facilitating drug discovery, enabling automated language translation, and managing clinical notes, medical records, and imaging data (Jing et al., 2018).

3.1. Overview of AI in Dentistry

Artificial intelligence has been recognized as an integral component of dentistry, significantly transforming dental diagnosis, treatment, and management processes. AI utilizes a wide range of algorithms like ML and NN to achieve precision in the process and achieve a better understanding of the dental treatments performed (Tyagi et al., 2025). It has been found that one of the most promising areas for the use of AI in dentistry is in diagnostic procedures. Particularly, DL algorithms, including CNNs which can be applied in evaluating dental images such as X-rays and CT scans, which may help in the early diagnosis of dental problems such as cavities, periodontal disease, and oral cancer (Rahim et al., 2024).

The inclusion of artificial intelligence in dental treatments has revolutionized dental workflow management, patient handling, and decision-making processes. AI tools are now recognized for enhancing the timeliness and accuracy of clinical decisions, making advanced decision support systems as important driver of productivity. These systems can handle time-intensive tasks such as appointment planning, record management, and preliminary diagnosis, permitting dental specialists to focus on specialized clinical duties (Faiyazuddin et al., 2025). Consequently, it has a positive impact on administration processes as well as the efficiency of task execution. One of the most prominent uses of this technology in dental clinics is in the analysis of radiographs, where it is capable of identifying caries, bone destruction, and cystic changes with a minimum of time and a maximum of precision compared to humans. It has been proved that this technology is capable of providing diagnostic outcomes with precision similar to a skilled dentist; thus, diagnosis efficiency is promoted (Faiyazuddin et al., 2025). This not only promotes better patient and outpatient services but also enables decisions in real time through radiographic evaluation, thus enabling effective interventions.

3.2. Modernizing endodontics: the impact and innovations of artificial intelligence

Artificial intelligence has driven substantial innovations in various domains of healthcare services, including cardiovascular surgery, radiology, and neurology, etc (Zhu et al. 2022). So far, a total of 171 medical applications using AI technology have been approved by the U.S. FDA (Food and Drug Administration 2023). AI technology is primarily applied to radiologic diagnosis, its application is also extended to clinical decision support and outcome prediction. In endodontic therapy, AI technology is expected to develop diagnosis, treatment, and prevention of periapical and pulpal diseases. Various reviews on AI technology have been conducted to assess its application in endodontic therapy (Boreak 2020; Aminoshariae et al. 2021; Das 2022; Khanagar et al. 2023; Karobari et al. 2023; Patel et al. 2023), including limitations and challenges (Aminoshariae et al. 2021; Das 2022; Patel et al. 2023).

Recent AI innovations in endodontics include the identification and diagnosis of periapical lesions (PLs), root fractures, resorptions, and the anatomy of root canals, along with the prediction of clinical treatment outcomes. Although 3-dimensional (3D) imaging modalities, such as cone beam computed tomography (CBCT), enhance the detection of PLs compared to 2D imaging techniques, substantial inter- and intra-observer variability in CBCT interpretation persists among clinicians, compromising diagnostic sensitivity and specificity (Parker et al., 2017). In this context, the integration of AI in CBCT analysis is increasing important, as it offers a means to standardize interpretation, reduce observer-related discrepancies, and improve diagnostic reliability in endodontic assessment.

4. ARTIFICIAL INTELLIGENCE IN ENDODONTICS AND RESTORATIVE DENTISTRY

4.1. Neural Networks in Endodontics

4.1.1. AI in Endodontic Diagnosis and Periapical Lesion Detection

Artificial intelligence has a progressive role in the field of endodontic therapy, especially in the accuracy of diagnosis and management strategies. Due to the complexity of the endodontic treatment process, the inclusion of AI helps dental practitioners to manage the complexity of the process and reduce the chances of error during the treatment process (Ahmed et al., 2023). One of the most important uses of artificial intelligence is the identification of periapical pathologies. Deep learning models, especially CNNs, have been implemented for the identification of periapical pathologies using periapical and panoramic radiographs, showing sensitivity and specificity compared to skilled clinicians, especially in identification of periapical pathologies at an early stage, which might go unnoticed (Fontenele & Jacobs, 2025).

A study by Setzer *et al.* used DL algorithms to identify periapical radiolucency on CBCT images, achieving 93% accuracy (Setzer et al., 2020). Likewise, Orhan *et al.* used CNN models on CBCT scans and found 92.8% accuracy in detecting periapical pathologies, comparable to those of experienced clinicians (Orhan et al., 2020). This was further supported by an in vitro study where Pauwels et al. used convolutional neural networks (CNNs) to evaluate periapical radiographs of experimentally induced lesions in bovine ribs. It was found that the accuracy of detecting periapical lesions is 87%, which was comparable to the performance of three oral radiologists (Ekert et al., 2019; Pauwels et al., 2021). Similarly, Ekert et al. evaluated panoramic images for the detection of periapical lesions and observed that the accuracy of CNN assessment differed depending on the type of tooth; sensitivity was highest for molar teeth (87%), although specificity was lower compared to other teeth (Ekert et al., 2019). CNNs are specialized neural networks that are effective in extracting features from images using convolution; thus, CNNs are best applied in image assessment for radiographic analysis in endodontic practice (Ekert et al., 2019; Pauwels et al., 2021).

4.1.2. Canal Detection, Segmentation, and Working Length Determination

AI has been utilized to perform automatic root canal detection and segmentation, especially in cases of complex root canal anatomy, such as mandibular molar and maxillary premolar teeth. This helps in accurate visualization of the root canal anatomy through the segmentation of the CBCT image datasets, facilitating minimally invasive access cavity preparation, which is crucial to improving treatment outcomes while keeping the tooth structure intact. In addition, machine learning models have been used to aid in the determination of working length based on the evaluation of electronic apex locator data and radiographic information, improving accuracy and facilitating greater standardization among clinicians (Khanagar et al., 2023).

4.1.3. Prognostic modeling and real-time procedural assistance

In the domain of prognosis, AI has demonstrated tremendous potential, as it can predict the result of the treatment or the probability of retreatment depending on the preoperative pain, pulp vitality, root canal anatomy, age of the patient, and surgical variables by using the algorithm of artificial intelligence (Ourang et al., 2024).

The recent advances also include the creation of AI-assisted endodontic motors, which are able to provide intraoperative feedback. These are expected to identify canal curvatures, binding, and ledge formation, thereby reducing errors and iatrogenic accidents. These innovations are still in the development phase which is a paradigm shift in the role of AI from a diagnostic tool to an active chairside assistant in complex endodontic therapy (Asiri & Altuwalah 2022).

4.2. Neural Networks in Restorative Dentistry

4.2.1. AI in Dental Caries Detection.

In the field of restorative dentistry, AI is used mainly in the early identification of dental caries, evaluation of existing restorations, and formulation of treatment strategies. This is because the field of restorative dentistry highly relies on the assessment of the oral condition through inspection and imaging techniques. In this field, the accuracy of the results can be improved through the assistance of AI technology (Tabatabaian et al., 2023).

Deep learning techniques based on bitewing and periapical radiographs have been reported to yield promising outcomes with regard to the detection of both pre-existing cavitated caries lesions as well as those that are at the initial stage of incipient caries. In some situations, the systems function better compared to even clinicians, especially in the detection of occlusal and approximal caries lesions that often go undetected during routine clinical practice. In addition, AI promotes standardized procedures and minimizes operator variability, thus enhancing the quality of care (Albano et al., 2024).

4.2.2. Restoration Assessment and Classification

AI has demonstrated considerable potential in assessing existing dental restorations, facilitating the detection of marginal leakage, overextended margins, and secondary caries. Furthermore, CNN models enable efficient identification of defective restorations that require follow-up treatment or corrective intervention (Ibraheem et al., 2025).

A study by Abdalla-Aslan R *et al.* demonstrated that AI algorithms could accurately identify 93.6% of dental restorations from 83 panoramic radiographs. with restorations further categorized into 11 groups based on morphological characteristics and grey value distribution (Abdalla-Aslan *et al.*, 2020).

Another remarkable improvement by AI in dentistry is the use of automated cavity classification that uses intraoral camera images and radiographs to identify the classification of caries as Class I, II, III, IV, V, and VI. This helps in selecting the correct design for cavity preparation and minimizing the dependence on subjective clinical assessment, which is beneficial in academic and training settings (Kang et al., 2024).

4.2.3. Material selection, longevity prediction, and digital workflows

AI-based systems can support material selection and restorative treatment planning by integrating patient-specific factors such as occlusal patterns, parafunctional habits, caries susceptibility, and aesthetic demands. Additionally, predictive models may estimate the longevity of direct restorative materials by considering clinical and behavioral factors (Rokaya et al., 2024).

In digital restorative dentistry, AI can aid in automated segmentation and virtual modeling in the production of indirect dental restorations like inlays, onlays, and veneers. Moreover, AI can aid in predicting shade matching and esthetic integration after treatment, which is a crucial factor for anterior restorations because the appearance is a major factor to be considered for dental restorations (Yeslam et al., 2024).

5. AI-DRIVEN EPIDEMIOLOGICAL MODELING

5.1. Risk stratification and early intervention

Prevention is a main principle of public health, and AI-based algorithms offer significant potential to support this aim by analyzing large datasets to recognize individuals who are at a greater risk of developing certain oral diseases, such as dental caries and periodontal diseases. These predictions derived from multiple determinants, including past history of dental problems, socio-economic status, dietary habits, and genetic susceptibility (Reyes et al., 2022). Consequently, this enables public health programs to effectively focus on high-risk groups, therefore allocating more resources to these programs and implementing timely, effective preventive interventions, including awareness and early screening visits (Reyes et al., 2022).

5.2 Improved access to care through teledentistry and remote monitoring

Geographical constraints may hinder access to dental services, especially in rural communities. AI-based platforms may offer the possibility of remote consultation services through teledentistry, where the patient may access the services of dental experts through virtual interaction. These platforms may include AI-based image analysis tools, where the patient's oral health status may be assessed by series of images sent by the patient (Kaushik & Rapaka, 2025).

Although the use of AI-based platforms may not offer the same benefits as the direct examination of the patient, they may serve as effective tools in the early identification of urgent dental conditions, ensuring prompt intervention in such cases. In addition, AI-based wearable technology may offer the possibility of observing the oral health status of the patient through the use of AI-based smartphone applications (Li et al., 2026).

5.3 Personalized education and behavior change

The promotion of appropriate oral hygiene practices remains Central to the prevention of dental disease. In this context, AI-based chatbots can function as virtual dental assistants, delivering patient-tailored oral health education and motivational support tailored to individual risk profiles and patient needs. These virtual assistants use natural language processing to respond to patient queries, offer information regarding appropriate oral hygiene practices, and provide reminders for scheduled dental appointments. In addition, these AI-based technologies can offer patient education according to patient demographics, cultural background, and learning styles, which can maximize patient understanding, retention, and positive behavioral changes (Zhang et al., 2025).

5.4 Data-driven public health strategies

Substantial amounts of data gathered in dental clinics and health facilities are often underutilized. AI systems can utilize these datasets by detecting patterns, identifying at-risk population segments, and predicting future service needs, thereby enabling more precise, evidence-based public health strategies. For instance, AI can evaluate geospatial data to locate regions with high caries prevalence among children, allowing policymakers to focus school-based preventive programs in those high-risk areas (Karamüftüoğlu *et al.*, 2026). In addition, AI can enhance resource allocation in dental public health systems by directing support to areas of greatest need (Panahi 2024).

5.5 Enhanced decision-making and clinical support

Although AI cannot replace the decision-making skills of dental specialists, AI systems can use the information provided by the patient and the images obtained through the use of radiographs to find possible pathologies, thereby assisting the dentist in making precise decisions (Vashisht et al., 2024). In addition, AI can enhance diagnostic accuracy by detecting subtle changes in radiographs that may be overlooked by the human eye, particularly in early-stage lesions such as incipient caries or periapical abnormalities. AI-driven tools also support risk assessment by analyzing large datasets to predict disease progression and treatment outcomes, enabling more proactive and preventive care.

Furthermore, AI can facilitate treatment planning by integrating patient history, clinical findings, and imaging data to suggest optimal treatment options tailored to individual patients. This contributes to improved consistency in clinical decisions and reduces variability among practitioners. AI systems can also provide real-time clinical decision support during procedures, offering guidance based on established protocols and up-to-date evidence.

Another important advantage is the ability of AI to continuously learn and improve through exposure to new data, which enhances its diagnostic and predictive capabilities over time. Additionally, AI can assist in workflow efficiency by prioritizing urgent cases, automating routine diagnostic tasks, and reducing the cognitive burden on clinicians. This allows dental professionals to focus more on complex clinical judgments and patient-centered care.

6. AI IN LINKING ORAL AND SYSTEMIC HEALTH DATA

6.1. Endodontic Infections as Systemic Risk Factors

The field of endodontics has evolved from a discipline focused primarily on pain relief and tooth preservation to one that recognizes the profound impact of oral infections on systemic health. A key example is apical periodontitis; while it leads to tooth removal in 60 to 80% of cases, its effects may extend beyond the oral cavity. As established by Nair, this condition can compromise general health by interfering with the body's immune response to polymicrobial infections (Nair 2004).

Pathogens originating from infected root canals can spread to the bloodstream, causing immune reactions. Apical periodontitis has been related to systemic conditions like diabetes (Rosen et al., 2017), hypertension (Wang et al., 2011), adverse pregnancy outcomes, skeletal infections, and coronary heart disease (CHD) (Aminoshariae et al., 2017) - the most common form of cardiovascular disease (CVD). These associations are thought to result from increased risk of bacteremia (Bender, Seltzer, & Yermish, 2003), the spread of microbial products, inflammatory mediators, and hemostatic factors into circulation (Li et al., 2000), which can lead to metastatic infections, tissue damage, and chronic low-grade systemic inflammation.

Apical periodontitis frequently manifests as an asymptomatic condition, where the lesion is detected only as a periapical radiolucency in the presence of pain, swelling, or the formation of an abscess or sinus tract. This diagnostic ambiguity, particularly in early stages, underscores the critical role of AI in enhancing the detection and interpretation of radiographic changes, thereby facilitating timely diagnosis. Given that both symptomatic and asymptomatic conditions may exist for prolonged periods and contribute to adverse systemic health, the integration of AI-driven diagnosis has become increasingly important to address a significant global health issue.

6.2. Inflammatory Biomarkers and Disease Progression

6.2.1. AI Integration with Immunological and Biomarker Data

Biomarkers, including leukocyte counts and interleukin levels, have been integrated into CNNs, resulting in accurate differentiation between aggressive and chronic periodontitis (Nguyen et al., 2021). Salivary and gingival crevicular fluid cytokines and enzymes allow AI algorithms to detect periodontal inflammation and establish correlations with systemic conditions such as cardiovascular disease and diabetes (Majeed, Jassim, & Kamil, 2023).

Oral pathogens, particularly Porphyromonas gingivalis, are closely linked to systemic inflammation and cardiovascular complications (Mei et al., 2020). Combining microbial profiles with inflammatory biomarkers marks a major advancement in AI-assisted differentiation of periodontal versus other systemic inflammatory conditions and in predicting susceptibility to viral infections.

Moreover, physical characteristics derived from tongue coating-such as thickness, color, and pattern have been utilized to train CNN models. These systems can classify health risks, including heart disorders, gastrointestinal disorders, and viral infections, with remarkable accuracyBottom of Form (Wang et al., 2022).

6.2.2. AI in Salivary Biomarker Research

Currently, artificial intelligence has been increasingly implemented for salivary biomarker research to enhance diagnostic precision and automatically detect significant biomarkers (Garcia-Junior et al., 2025). Machine learning techniques, including Support Vector Machines, Convolutional Neural Networks, and Random Forest classifiers, have been presented to be very effective for complex biomarker data analysis (Guido et al., 2024).

• Support Vector Machines (SVMs):

SVMs are popular for pattern recognition and biomarker classification problems. SVMs are found to perform better in differentiating between disease states on the basis of salivary protein expression profiles, which enhances the accuracy in diagnosis as compared to traditional statistical approaches (Guido et al., 2024).

• Convolutional Neural Networks (CNNs):

CNNs are generally applied to image and spectral data. CNNs are applied to salivary proteomics and mass spectrometry data. The features are automatically extracted from the data by CNNs. It results in accurate classification with low false positive rates (Carrillo-Rodriguez, Selheim, & Hernandez-Valladares, 2023).

• Random Forest Classifiers:

Random Forest Classifiers are a suitable algorithm for dealing with high-dimensional biomarker data. The Random Forest model examines salivary metabolomics and proteomics to detect diseases. The model is effective in detecting diseases by comparing traditional regression techniques (Wang et al., 2018).

Compared to traditional statistical approaches, AI models can handle non-linear relationships, large datasets, and complex multivariable interactions, which are important in personalizing medicine and detecting diseases in early stages using saliva-based diagnostics (Wang et al., 2018).

6.2.3. Future Directions in AI-Driven Salivary Diagnostics

Future prospects of AI and DL are expected to take salivary biomarker analysis to the next level to allow for real-time and fully automated diagnostics. AI can be used in conjunction with biosensors and microfluidic devices to improve point-of-care diagnostics, making salivary diagnostics more accessible and reliable (Guevara-Vega et al., 2024).

The AI and big data analytics have revolutionized the salivary biomarker research domain to an impressive extent by processing biological big data to identify patterns in salivary biomarkers for precise diagnostic capabilities (Adeoye & Su, 2024). It is possible to use ML techniques for the classification of diseases, progression of diseases, and development of personalized treatment plans through the analysis of salivary biomarkers. This is not only strengthening the diagnostic capabilities but also reducing the chances of human errors in the diagnostic process (Arya et al., 2023).

7. COMPARATIVE STUDIES ON ARTIFICIAL INTELLIGENCE–DRIVEN EPIDEMIOLOGY OF ENDODONTIC AND RESTORATIVE DISEASES: LINKING ORAL INFECTIONS TO SYSTEMIC HEALTH OUTCOMES.

Table 1.

Study Design & Setting	AI Platform / System	Target Conditions	Key Diagnostic Outcomes	Relevance to AI-Driven Epidemiology & Oral–Systemic Link
12-month retrospective observational study (single center) (Bhavna 2025).	Deep learning–based radiographic interpretation + EHR pattern recognition	Restorative treatment	Caries sensitivity: 94% (vs 82%); Periodontal accuracy: 91% (vs 74%); Periapical lesion accuracy: 92% ($\kappa = 0.86$)	Revealed probability of integrating AI-detected oral inflammatory burden with systemic risk indicators (diabetes, hypertension, cardiovascular disease); model for AI-enhanced epidemiological surveillance
Preliminary retrospective diagnostic study (Kazimierczak et al., 2024).	Diagnocat Ltd. (cloud-based AI)	Endodontic treatment	Overall accuracy for filling detection: 90.72%; F1 score: 95.12%; Lower accuracy for qualitative parameters (55–63%); Very low F1 for short filling (8.33%) & voids (14.29%)	Reliable for identifying treated teeth in large datasets; requires refinement for qualitative epidemiologic outcome assessment
Retrospective comparative study (multi-trial dataset) (Allihaibi, Koller, & Mannocci, 2025).	Diagnocat Ltd.	Detection of endodontic lesions	Higher sensitivity than clinicians (Tooth: 67.3% vs 49.3%; Root: 54.3% vs 43.8%); Lower specificity (Tooth: 82.3% vs 92.5%); Comparable overall accuracy (Tooth: 76.3% vs 75.3%)	Useful adjunct for detecting lesions potentially missed clinically; supports large-scale epidemiological mapping of periapical pathology
Randomized controlled crossover trial (Pul et al., 2025).	AI-assisted diagnostic system	Periapical radiolucencies	Accuracy improved (91.6% → 93.3%, $p<0.001$); False positives reduced (4.3% → 2.0%); Sensitivity unchanged (~46%)	AI based technique enhances diagnostic consistency, decreases overtreatment, and benefits junior clinicians—essential for standardized epidemiologic data collection

7.1. AI versus conventional diagnostic methods in endodontic and restorative disease epidemiology: a comparative retrospective study linking oral infections to systemic health outcomes.

A 12-month retrospective observational study evaluated the role of AI in the epidemiological assessment of endodontic and restorative diseases as well as their potential systemic associations. The study included 100 adult patients (20–70 years) whose records contained both conventional clinical diagnoses and AI-assisted analyses derived from deep learning–based radiographic interpretation and electronic health record pattern-recognition systems. Diagnostic accuracy for dental caries, periodontal disease, periapical lesions, and possibly malignant oral lesions was compared between AI and conventional methods. AI consistently demonstrated superior accuracy in detecting and diagnosing the aforementioned conditions with example, AI had sensitivity of 94% in detecting dental caries (compared to 82%), 91% accuracy in detecting periodontal disease (compared to 74%), 92% accuracy in detecting periapical lesions and 83% accuracy for detecting potentially malignant oral lesions (compared to 67%). Additionally, algorithmic integration enabled the identification of association between chronic oral inflammatory burden and systemic risk indicators, including diabetes mellitus, hypertension, and cardiovascular diseases (Bhavna 2025).

7.2. Comparative assessment of Diagnocat AI and expert consensus in evaluating endodontic treatment outcomes on panoramic radiographs.

This preliminary study evaluated the performance of the AI-based system designed by Diagnocat Ltd., which was used for the evaluation of the outcome of endodontic treatments based on panoramic radiographs. It was found that the AI system was capable of evaluating different endodontic parameters, such as the possibility of root canal filling, the effect of the endodontic treatment, the occurrence of overfilling, short filling, and the existence of any voids in the endodontic filling materials. By comparing the outcomes obtained through the AI system and the consensus opinion of two experienced human observers, the AI system was found to have high diagnostic potential for the evaluation of endodontic filling, with an accuracy of 90.72% and an F1 score of 95.12%. However, the accuracy rates of the AI system for the qualitative treatment characteristics were found to be 55.81% for adequate obturation and 62.79% for density. Furthermore, the F1 scores for short filling and the presence of spaces in the filling material were found to be very low at 8.33% and 14.29%, respectively. This implies that, although the AI platform is very reliable for the recognition of endodontically treated teeth, further refinement of the AI tool is necessary for enhancing the precision of the assessment of qualitative aspects of root canal therapy, thereby strengthening the potential of the AI tool for AI-based epidemiological research (Kazimierczak et al., 2024).

7.3. Comparative diagnostic accuracy of Diagnocat AI and endodontists in detecting periapical lesions using periapical radiographs and CBCT reference standard.

This retrospective study assessed the diagnostic performance of the AI-driven platform Diagnocat Ltd. against two calibrated endodontists, using periapical radiographs from 376 teeth (860 roots) obtained across four prospective clinical trials, with CBCT serving as the reference standard. Sensitivity, specificity, overall accuracy, and the area under the ROC curve were computed at both the tooth and root levels. The AI platform exhibited superior sensitivity relative to the clinicians (tooth level: 67.3% vs 49.3%, $P < .001$; root level: 54.3% vs 43.8%, $P = .003$), yet it demonstrated lower specificity (tooth: 82.3% vs 92.5%, $P < .001$; root: 86.7% vs 94.5%, $P < .001$). The accuracy of the AI was similar to that of clinicians at the tooth level (76.3% vs 75.3%, $P = .716$) but was slightly lower in the AI than in clinicians at the root level (78.5% vs 81.6%, $P = .021$). The ROC curve results showed similar area under the curve values in the AI and clinicians for the tooth level (0.75 vs 0.71) and the root level (0.71 vs 0.69), indicating that the AI can potentially be used as an additional tool in the detection of endodontic lesions that might have been missed by clinicians, but the lower specificity of the AI points to the importance of clinical judgement to prevent over-diagnosis (Allihaibi, Koller, & Mannocci, 2025).

7.4. Effect of AI assistance on dentists' diagnostic accuracy and confidence in detecting periapical radiolucency: a randomized controlled trial.

This randomized controlled trial evaluated the effect of AI assistance on the diagnostic performance and confidence of dentists in the detection of periapical radiolucency (PRs) on panoramic radiographs. Fifty radiographs were interpreted by 30 dentists with varying levels of experience with and without AI assistance using a crossover design and cone beam computed tomography as the reference standard. Sensitivity, specificity, predictive values, overall accuracy, and areas under the ROC and AFROC curves were analyzed using mixed-effects regression models. The findings showed that overall diagnostic accuracy was slightly improved with the assistance of AI, from 91.6% without to 93.3% with AI support ($p < 0.001$), mainly through a reduction in false positives, from 4.3% to 2.0%, with sensitivity remaining virtually unchanged at 46.0% and 45.8% without and with AI support, respectively. The benefits of using the assistance of AI were found to be greater for junior dentists in terms of confidence levels. In addition, it was found that assistance from AI affects treatment decisions (Pul et al., 2025).

8. ETHICAL AND REGULATORY CONSIDERATIONS

8.1 Data Privacy and Security

The integration of AI in dentistry supports the protection of patient information, which may include clinical information, radiographs, and biometric data. This can be achieved through effective data encryption and storage to conform to the international standards on data protection.

8.2 Algorithmic Bias

There are possibilities that AI may exhibit biases depending on the information used to train the model, which may cause inequalities in the outcomes of different classes of patients. It is imperative to ensure that there is diversity in the data sets as well as monitoring the performance of the models to ensure that there are no differences in the treatment provided.

8.3 Regulatory Frameworks

AI-based dental tools must comply with existing regulations for medical devices as well as digital health policies that are issued by national and international governments. The approval process for AI-based tools must consider safety, efficacy, transparency, and accountability.

8.4 Clinical Validation and Standardization

Complete clinical trials and external validation are essential to ensure the validity and reproducibility of AI systems. Standardization is a key aspect to ensure consistency, comparability, and safe clinical application of AI systems in dental practice (Rahim et al., 2024).

9. FUTURE DIRECTIONS

9.1 Precision Dentistry

Future advancements in AI are also likely to enhance precision dentistry, which is characterized by individualized risk prediction, individualized preventive strategies, and individualized treatment planning. Such integration will also facilitate a better understanding of susceptibility to endodontic and restorative diseases, thereby providing a better personalized outcome for therapy.

9.2 Real-Time Epidemiological Surveillance

It is also envisioned that AI-driven analytics technology integrated with EHRs and GIS technology will facilitate real-time surveillance of oral disease patterns. Such a technology platform is envisioned to facilitate real-time surveillance for early detection of oral diseases, thereby strengthening surveillance for oral-systemic disease associations.

9.3 Integration with Systemic Disease Monitoring

The future of AI technology in dentistry is anticipated to be integrated with a broader healthcare platform for monitoring systemic diseases. Such integration is envisioned to facilitate a better understanding of oral-systemic correlations for early detection of systemic complications from chronic oral infections.

10. CONCLUSION

Artificial intelligence-based epidemiology is an important step forward in the complex relationship between endodontic diseases, restorative diseases, and systemic health outcomes. This approach would bring about a paradigm shift in the current approach, where the focus would shift from the current 'reactive' approach towards 'proactive,' 'preventive,' and 'precision-based' oral healthcare delivery systems. Moreover, the current evidence regarding the relationship between chronic oral infections and systemic inflammatory and metabolic diseases emphasizes the importance of an integrated approach to different branches of sciences, including artificial intelligence-based epidemiology in the near future, in relation to precision dentistry, public health surveillance, and the role of oral health in relation to systemic health in general. Consequently, it can be noticed that there is remarkable potential in the convergence of artificial intelligence, epidemiology, and dental sciences in advancing precision dentistry, public health surveillance, and reinforcing oral health as a whole in relation to overall systemic health.

FUNDING STATEMENT

This work was supported by the Deanship of Scientific Research, Vice Presidency for Graduate Studies and Scientific Research, King Faisal University, Saudi Arabia [Grant No. KFU264121].

REFERENCES

Abdalla-Aslan, R., Yeshua, T., Kabla, D., Leichter, I., & Nadler, C. (2020). An artificial intelligence system using machine learning for automatic detection and classification of dental restorations in panoramic radiography. *Oral Surgery, Oral Medicine, Oral Pathology and Oral Radiology*, *130*(5), 593–602. DOI: 10.1016/j.oooo.2020.05.012 PMID: 32646672

Adeoye, J., & Su, Y. X. (2024). Artificial intelligence in salivary biomarker discovery and validation for oral diseases. *Oral Diseases*, *30*(1), 23–37. DOI: 10.1111/odi.14641 PMID: 37335832

Ahmed, Z. H., Almuharib, A. M., Abdulkarim, A. A., Alhassoon, A. H., Alanazi, A. F., Alhaqbani, M. A., Alshalawi, M. S., Almuqayrin, A. K., & Almahmoud, M. I. (2023). Artificial Intelligence and Its Application in Endodontics: A Review. *The Journal of Contemporary Dental Practice*, *24*(11), 912–917. DOI: 10.5005/jp-journals-10024-3593 PMID: 38238281

Albano, D., Galiano, V., Basile, M., Di Luca, F., Gitto, S., Messina, C., Cagetti, M. G., Del Fabbro, M., Tartaglia, G. M., & Sconfienza, L. M. (2024). Artificial intelligence for radiographic imaging detection of caries lesions: A systematic review. *BMC Oral Health*, *24*(1), 274. DOI: 10.1186/s12903-024-04046-7 PMID: 38402191

Allihaibi, M., Koller, G., & Mannocci, F. (2025). Diagnostic Accuracy of a Commercial AI-based Platform in Evaluating Endodontic Treatment Outcomes on Periapical Radiographs Using CBCT as the Reference Standard. *Journal of Endodontics*, *51*(7), 898–908.e8. DOI: 10.1016/j.joen.2025.03.007 PMID: 40180318

Aloyouny, A. Y., Almufarji, F., Almutairi, G. G., Alkait, S., Al-Mohaya, M. A., & Alserwi, R. (2022). Impact of Rheumatic Diseases on Oral Health-Related Quality of Life. *Cureus*, *14*(12), e32268. DOI: 10.7759/cureus.32268 PMID: 36483518

Aminoshariae, A., Kulild, J. C., Mickel, A., & Fouad, A. F. (2017). Association between Systemic Diseases and Endodontic Outcome: A Systematic Review. *Journal of Endodontics*, *43*(4), 514–519. DOI: 10.1016/j.joen.2016.11.008 PMID: 28190585

Aminoshariae, A., Nosrat, A., Nagendrababu, V., Dianat, O., Mohammad-Rahimi, H., O'Keefe, A. W., & Setzer, F. C. (2021). Artificial intelligence in endodontic education. *Journal of Endodontics*, *50*(5), 562–578. DOI: 10.1016/j.joen.2024.02.011 PMID: 38387793

Arya, S. S., Dias, S. B., Jelinek, H. F., Hadjileontiadis, L. J., & Pappa, A. M. (2023). The convergence of traditional and digital biomarkers through AI-assisted biosensing: A new era in translational diagnostics? *Biosensors & Bioelectronics*, *235*, 115387. DOI: 10.1016/j.bios.2023.115387 PMID: 37229842

Asiri, A. F., & Altuwalah, A. S. (2022). The role of neural artificial intelligence for diagnosis and treatment planning in endodontics: A qualitative review. *The Saudi Dental Journal*, *34*(4), 270–281. DOI: 10.1016/j.sdentj.2022.04.004 PMID: 35692236

Bender, I. B., Seltzer, S., & Yermish, M. (2003). The incidence of bacteremia in endodontic manipulation: Preliminary report. 1960. *Journal of Endodontics*, *29*(11), 697–696. DOI: 10.1097/00004770-200311000-00003 PMID: 14651273

Bhavna. (2025). Role of artificial intelligence in diagnosing oral and systemic diseases: A retrospective study. *International Journal of Current Pharmaceutical Review and Research, 17*(9), 1301–1305. https://www.ijcpr.com/

Boreak, N. (2020). Effectiveness of artificial intelligence applications designed for endodontic diagnosis, decision-making, and prediction of prognosis: A systematic review. *The Journal of Contemporary Dental Practice*, *21*(8), 926–934. DOI: 10.5005/jp-journals-10024-2894 PMID: 33568617

Carrillo-Rodriguez, P., Selheim, F., & Hernandez-Valladares, M. (2023). Mass Spectrometry-Based Proteomics Workflows in Cancer Research: The Relevance of Choosing the Right Steps. *Cancers (Basel)*, *15*(2), 555. DOI: 10.3390/cancers15020555 PMID: 36672506

Chan, A. K. Y., Tsang, Y. C., Jiang, C. M., Leung, K. C. M., Lo, E. C. M., & Chu, C. H. (2023). Integration of Oral Health into General Health Services for Older Adults. *Geriatrics (Basel, Switzerland)*, *8*(1), 20. DOI: 10.3390/geriatrics8010020 PMID: 36826362

Choi, R. Y., Coyner, A. S., Kalpathy-Cramer, J., Chiang, M. F., & Campbell, J. P. (2020). Introduction to machine learning, neural networks, and deep learning. *Translational Vision Science & Technology*, *9*(2), 14. DOI: 10.1167/tvst.9.2.14 PMID: 32704420

Collin, M., Christidis, N., Hagelberg, S., Arvidsson, L. Z., Larheim, T. A., Ernberg, M., & Hedenberg-Magnusson, B. (2024). Temporomandibular involvement in children and adolescents with juvenile idiopathic arthritis: A 2-year prospective cohort study. *Scientific Reports*, *14*(1), 5512. DOI: 10.1038/s41598-024-56174-3 PMID: 38448491

Das, S. (2022). Artificial intelligence in endodontics: A peek into the future. *RGUHS Journal of Dental Sciences*, *14*(3), 35–37. DOI: 10.26715/rjds.14_3_7

Deo, P. N., & Deshmukh, R. (2019). Oral microbiome: Unveiling the fundamentals. *Journal of Oral and Maxillofacial Pathology : JOMFP*, *23*(1), 122–128. DOI: 10.4103/jomfp.JOMFP_304_18 PMID: 31110428

Ding, H., Wu, J., Zhao, W., Matinlinna, J. P., Burrow, M. F., & Tsoi, J. K. H. (2021). Artificial intelligence in dentistry—A review. *Frontiers in Dental Medicine*, *4*, 1085251. DOI: 10.3389/fdmed.2023.1085251 PMID: 39935549

Ekert, T., Krois, J., Meinhold, L., Elhennawy, K., Emara, R., Golla, T., & Schwendicke, F. (2019). Deep learning for the radiographic detection of apical lesions. *Journal of Endodontics*, *45*(7), 917–922. DOI: 10.1016/j.joen.2019.03.016 PMID: 31160078

Elzayat, H., Mesto, G., & Al-Marzooq, F. (2023). Unraveling the Impact of Gut and Oral Microbiome on Gut Health in Inflammatory Bowel Diseases. *Nutrients*, *15*(15), 3377. DOI: 10.3390/nu15153377 PMID: 37571313

Esfanjani, M. T., Gilani, N., Esfanjani, A. T., Nourizadeh, A. M., Faramarzi, E., & Hekmatfar, S. (2023). Are oral health behaviors associated with metabolic syndrome in the Azar cohort population? *BMC Oral Health*, *23*(1), 370. DOI: 10.1186/s12903-023-03003-0 PMID: 37291532

Faiyazuddin, M., Rahman, S. J. Q., Anand, G., Siddiqui, R. K., Mehta, R., Khatib, M. N., Gaidhane, S., Zahiruddin, Q. S., Hussain, A., & Sah, R. (2025). The Impact of Artificial Intelligence on Healthcare: A Comprehensive Review of Advancements in Diagnostics, Treatment, and Operational Efficiency. *Health Science Reports*, *8*(1), e70312. DOI: 10.1002/hsr2.70312 PMID: 39763580

Fisher, S. (2021). Priorities for successful use of artificial intelligence by public health organizations: A literature review. *BMC Public Health*, *21*, 10422. DOI: 10.1186/s12889-021-10422-2 PMID: 36419010

Fontenele, R. C., & Jacobs, R. (2025). Unveiling the power of artificial intelligence for image-based diagnosis and treatment in endodontics: An ally or adversary? *International Endodontic Journal*, *58*(2), 155–170. DOI: 10.1111/iej.14163 PMID: 39526945

Garcia-Junior, M. A., Andrade, B. S., Lima, A. P., Soares, I. P., Notário, A. F. O., Bernardino, S. S., Guevara-Vega, M. F., Honório-Silva, G., Munoz, R. A. A., Jardim, A. C. G., Martins, M. M., Goulart, L. R., Cunha, T. M., Carneiro, M. G., & Sabino-Silva, R. (2025). Artificial-Intelligence Bio-Inspired Peptide for Salivary Detection of SARS-CoV-2 in Electrochemical Biosensor Integrated with Machine Learning Algorithms. *Biosensors (Basel)*, *15*(2), 75. DOI: 10.3390/bios15020075 PMID: 39996977

Guevara-Vega, M., Rosa, R. B., Caixeta, D. C., Costa, M. A., de Souza, R. C., Ferreira, G. M., Mundim Filho, A. C., Carneiro, M. G., Jardim, A. C. G., & Sabino-Silva, R. (2024). Salivary detection of Chikungunya virus infection using a portable and sustainable biophotonic platform coupled with artificial intelligence algorithms. *Scientific Reports*, *14*(1), 21546. DOI: 10.1038/s41598-024-71889-z PMID: 39278957

Guido, R., Ferrisi, S., Lofaro, D., & Conforti, D. (2024). An Overview on the Advancements of Support Vector Machine Models in Healthcare Applications: A Review. *Information (Basel)*, *15*(4), 235. DOI: 10.3390/info15040235

Ibraheem, W. I., Jain, S., Ayoub, M. N., Namazi, M. A., Alfaqih, A. I., Aggarwal, A., Meshni, A. A., Almarghlani, A., & Alhumaidan, A. A. (2025). Assessment of the Diagnostic Accuracy of Artificial Intelligence Software in Identifying Common Periodontal and Restorative Dental Conditions (Marginal Bone Loss, Periapical Lesion, Crown, Restoration, Dental Caries) in Intraoral Periapical Radiographs. *Diagnostics (Basel)*, *15*(11), 1432. DOI: 10.3390/diagnostics15111432 PMID: 40507004

Jing, Y., Bian, Y., Hu, Z., Wang, L., & Xie, X. Q. (2018). Deep Learning for Drug Design: An Artificial Intelligence Paradigm for Drug Discovery in the Big Data Era. *The AAPS Journal*, *20*(3), 58. DOI: 10.1208/s12248-018-0210-0 PMID: 29603063

Kang, S., Shon, B., Park, E. Y., Jeong, S., & Kim, E. K. (2024). Diagnostic accuracy of dental caries detection using ensemble techniques in deep learning with intraoral camera images. *PLoS One*, *19*(9), e0310004. DOI: 10.1371/journal.pone.0310004 PMID: 39241044

Karamüftüoğlu, N., Üçpunar, B. Y., Birben, İ., Altundağ, A. E., Mullaoğlu, K. Ö., & Bal, C. (2026). Artificial Intelligence in Pediatric Dentistry: A Systematic Review and Meta-Analysis. *Children (Basel, Switzerland)*, *13*(1), 152. DOI: 10.3390/children13010152 PMID: 41597160

Karobari, M. I., Adil, A. H., Basheer, S. N., Murugesan, S., Savadamoorthi, K. S., Mustafa, M., Abdulwahed, A., & Almokhatieb, A. A. (2023). Evaluation of the diagnostic and prognostic accuracy of artificial intelligence in endodontic dentistry: A comprehensive review of literature. *Computational and Mathematical Methods in Medicine, 7049360*(1), 7049360. Advance online publication. DOI: 10.1155/2023/7049360 PMID: 36761829

Kaushik, R., & Rapaka, R. (2025). AI-driven evolution in teledentistry: A comprehensive overview of technology and clinical applications. *Dentistry Review, 5*(2), 100154. DOI: 10.1016/j.dentre.2025.100154

Kazimierczak, W., Wajer, R., Wajer, A., Kalka, K., Kazimierczak, N., & Serafin, Z. (2024). Evaluating the diagnostic accuracy of an AI-driven platform for assessing endodontic treatment outcomes using panoramic radiographs: A preliminary study. *Journal of Clinical Medicine, 13*(12), 3401. DOI: 10.3390/jcm13123401 PMID: 38929931

Khanagar, S. B., Alfadley, A., Alfouzan, K., Awawdeh, M., Alaqla, A., & Jamleh, A. (2023). Developments and performance of artificial intelligence models designed for application in endodontics: A systematic review. *Diagnostics (Basel), 13*(3), 414. DOI: 10.3390/diagnostics13030414 PMID: 36766519

Khanagar, S. B., Alfadley, A., Alfouzan, K., Awawdeh, M., Alaqla, A., & Jamleh, A. (2023). Developments and Performance of Artificial Intelligence Models Designed for Application in Endodontics: A Systematic Review. *Diagnostics (Basel), 13*(3), 414. DOI: 10.3390/diagnostics13030414 PMID: 36766519

Li, H., Chen, S., Chang, B., Wang, X., He, Y., Xu, B., Sun, G., Yang, C., Li, G., Li, S., & Li, G. (2026). Application of artificial intelligence in oral health management: Challenges and opportunities. *Frontiers in Medicine, 13*, 1700529. DOI: 10.3389/fmed.2026.1700529 PMID: 41709905

Li, X., Kolltveit, K. M., Tronstad, L., & Olsen, I. (2000). Systemic diseases caused by oral infection. *Clinical Microbiology Reviews, 13*(4), 547–558. DOI: 10.1128/CMR.13.4.547 PMID: 11023956

Majeed, Z. N., Jassim, S. D., & Kamil, Z. H. (2023). Assessment of salivary and gingival crevicular fluids IL6, IL-8, IL-12, and IL-17 levels in healthy subjects and patients with periodontal disease. *Journal of Oral and Maxillofacial Pathology : JOMFP, 27*(3), 494–498. DOI: 10.4103/jomfp.jomfp_170_23 PMID: 38033941

McCarthy, J., Minsky, M. L., Rochester, N., & Shannon, C. E. (2006). A proposal for the Dartmouth summer research project on artificial intelligence, August 31, 1955. *AI Magazine*, *27*(4), 12. https://ojs.aaai.org/aimagazine/index.php/aimagazine/article/view/1904

Mei, F., Xie, M., Huang, X., Long, Y., Lu, X., Wang, X., & Chen, L. (2020). *Porphyromonas gingivalis* and Its Systemic Impact: Current Status. *Pathogens (Basel, Switzerland)*, *9*(11), 944. DOI: 10.3390/pathogens9110944 PMID: 33202751

Nair, P. N. (2004). Pathogenesis of apical periodontitis and the causes of endodontic failures. *Critical reviews in oral biology and medicine: an official publication of the American Association of Oral Biologists, 15*(6), 348–381. https://doi.org/.DOI: 10.1177/154411130401500604

Nguyen, T. T., Larrivée, N., Lee, A., Bilaniuk, O., & Durand, R. (2021). Use of Artificial Intelligence in Dentistry: Current Clinical Trends and Research Advances. *Journal - Canadian Dental Association*, *87*(2), l7. DOI: 10.12816/0059360 PMID: 34343070

Orhan, K., Bayrakdar, I. S., Ezhov, M., Kravtsov, A., & Özyürek, T. (2020). Evaluation of artificial intelligence for detecting periapical pathosis on cone-beam computed tomography scans. *International Endodontic Journal*, *53*(5), 680–689. DOI: 10.1111/iej.13265 PMID: 31922612

Ourang, S. A., Sohrabniya, F., Mohammad-Rahimi, H., Dianat, O., Aminoshariae, A., Nagendrababu, V., Dummer, P. M. H., Duncan, H. F., & Nosrat, A. (2024). Artificial intelligence in endodontics: Fundamental principles, workflow, and tasks. *International Endodontic Journal*, *57*(11), 1546–1565. DOI: 10.1111/iej.14127 PMID: 39056554

Panahi, O. (2024). AI: A New Frontier in Oral and Maxillofacial Surgery. *Acta Scientific Dental Sciences*, *8*(6), 40–42.

Parker, J. M., Mol, A., Rivera, E. M., & Tawil, P. Z. (2017). Cone-beam computed tomography uses in clinical endodontics: Observer variability in detecting periapical lesions. *Journal of Endodontics*, *43*(2), 184–187. DOI: 10.1016/j.joen.2016.10.007 PMID: 28024758

Patel, A., Shah, D., Patel, Z., Makwana, H. S., & Rajput, A. (2023). A comprehensive review on AI in endodontics. *International Journal for Research in Applied Science and Engineering Technology*, *11*(7), 165–170. DOI: 10.22214/ijraset.2023.54565

Pauwels, R., Brasil, D. M., Yamasaki, M. C., Jacobs, R., Bosmans, H., Freitas, D. Q., & Haiter-Neto, F. (2021). Artificial intelligence for detection of periapical lesions on intraoral radiographs: Comparison between convolutional neural networks and human observers. *Oral Surgery, Oral Medicine, Oral Pathology and Oral Radiology*, *131*(5), 610–616. DOI: 10.1016/j.oooo.2021.01.018 PMID: 33653645

Prasad, M., Manjunath, C., Murthy, A. K., Sampath, A., Jaiswal, S., & Mohapatra, A. (2019). Integration of oral health into primary health care: A systematic review. *Journal of Family Medicine and Primary Care*, *8*(6), 1838–1845. DOI: 10.4103/jfmpc.jfmpc_286_19 PMID: 31334142

Pul, U., Tichy, A., Pitchika, V., & Schwendicke, F. (2025). Impact of artificial intelligence assistance on diagnosing periapical radiolucencies: A randomized controlled trial. *Journal of Dentistry*, *160*, 105868. DOI: 10.1016/j.jdent.2025.105868 PMID: 40466762

Rahim, A., Khatoon, R., Khan, T. A., Syed, K., Khan, I., Khalid, T., & Khalid, B. (2024). Artificial intelligence-powered dentistry: Probing the potential, challenges, and ethicality of artificial intelligence in dentistry. *Digital Health*, *10*, 20552076241291345. DOI: 10.1177/20552076241291345 PMID: 39539720

Reyes, L. T., Knorst, J. K., Ortiz, F. R., & Ardenghi, T. M. (2022). Machine Learning in the Diagnosis and Prognostic Prediction of Dental Caries: A Systematic Review. *Caries Research*, *56*(3), 161–170. DOI: 10.1159/000524167 PMID: 35636386

Rokaya, D., Jaghsi, A. A., Jagtap, R., & Srimaneepong, V. (2024). Artificial intelligence in dentistry and dental biomaterials. *Frontiers in Dental Medicine*, *5*, 1525505. DOI: 10.3389/fdmed.2024.1525505 PMID: 39917699

Rosen, J., Sancheti, P., Fierlinger, A., Niazi, F., Johal, H., & Bedi, A. (2017). Response to: Important Considerations When Determining the Cost-effectiveness of Viscosupplements in the Treatment of Knee Osteoarthritis. *Advances in Therapy*, *33*(12), 2273–2276. DOI: 10.1007/s12325-016-0422-6 PMID: 27778299

Rydén, L., Buhlin, K., Ekstrand, E., de Faire, U., Gustafsson, A., Holmer, J., Kjellström, B., Lindahl, B., Norhammar, A., Nygren, Å., Näsman, P., Rathnayake, N., Svenungsson, E., & Klinge, B. (2016). Periodontitis Increases the Risk of a First Myocardial Infarction: A Report From the PAROKRANK Study. *Circulation*, *133*(6), 576–583. DOI: 10.1161/CIRCULATIONAHA.115.020324 PMID: 26762521

Sarvamangala, D. R., & Kulkarni, R. V. (2022). Convolutional neural networks in medical image understanding: A survey. *Evolutionary Intelligence*, *15*(1), 1–22. DOI: 10.1007/s12065-020-00540-3 PMID: 33425040

Setzer, F. C., Shi, K. J., Zhang, Z., Yan, H., Yoon, H., Mupparapu, M., & Li, J. (2020). Artificial Intelligence for the Computer-aided Detection of Periapical Lesions in Cone-beam Computed Tomographic Images. *Journal of Endodontics*, *46*(7), 987–993. DOI: 10.1016/j.joen.2020.03.025 PMID: 32402466

Tabatabaian, F., Vora, S. R., & Mirabbasi, S. (2023). Applications, functions, and accuracy of artificial intelligence in restorative dentistry: A literature review. *Journal of Esthetic and Restorative Dentistry : Official Publication of the American Academy of Esthetic Dentistry ... [et al.]*, *35*(6), 842–859. DOI: 10.1111/jerd.13079 PMID: 37522291

Taylor, G. W. (2001). Bidirectional interrelationships between diabetes and periodontal diseases: An epidemiologic perspective. *Annals of Periodontology*, *6*(1), 99–112. DOI: 10.1902/annals.2001.6.1.99 PMID: 11887478

Tyagi, M., Jain, S., Ranjan, M., Hassan, S., Prakash, N., Kumar, D., Kumar, A., & Singh, S. (2025). Artificial Intelligence Tools in Dentistry: A Systematic Review on Their Application and Outcomes. *Cureus*, *17*(5), e85062. DOI: 10.7759/cureus.85062 PMID: 40585609

U.S. Food and Drug Administration. (2023). *Artificial intelligence and machine learning (AI/ML)-enabled medical devices.* https://www.fda.gov/medical-devices/software-medical-device-samd/artificial-intelligence-and-machine-learning-aiml-enabled-medical-devices

Vashisht, R., Sharma, A., Kiran, T., Jolly, S. S., Brar, P. K., & Puri, J. V. (2024). Artificial intelligence in dentistry—A scoping review. *Journal of Oral and Maxillofacial Surgery, Medicine, and Pathology*, *36*(4), 579–592. DOI: 10.1016/j.ajoms.2024.04.009

Wang, C. H., Chueh, L. H., Chen, S. C., Feng, Y. C., Hsiao, C. K., & Chiang, C. P. (2011). Impact of diabetes mellitus, hypertension, and coronary artery disease on tooth extraction after nonsurgical endodontic treatment. *Journal of Endodontics*, *37*(1), 1–5. DOI: 10.1016/j.joen.2010.08.054 PMID: 21146066

Wang, Q., Nguyen, T.-T., Huang, J. Z., & Nguyen, T. T. (2018). An efficient random forests algorithm for high dimensional data classification. *Advances in Data Analysis and Classification*, *12*(4), 953–972. DOI: 10.1007/s11634-018-0318-1

Wang, X., Wang, X., Lou, Y., Liu, J., Huo, S., Pang, X., Wang, W., Wu, C., Chen, Y., Chen, Y., Chen, A., Bi, F., Xing, W., Deng, Q., Jia, L., & Chen, J. (2022). Constructing tongue coating recognition model using deep transfer learning to assist syndrome diagnosis and its potential in noninvasive ethnopharmacological evaluation. *Journal of Ethnopharmacology*, *285*, 114905. DOI: 10.1016/j.jep.2021.114905 PMID: 34896205

World Health Organization. (2023). *Global oral health status report: Towards universal health coverage for oral health by 2030*. World Health Organization.

Yeslam, H. E., Freifrau von Maltzahn, N., & Nassar, H. M. (2024). Revolutionizing CAD/CAM-based restorative dental processes and materials with artificial intelligence: A concise narrative review. *PeerJ*, *12*, e17793. DOI: 10.7717/peerj.17793 PMID: 39040936

Zhang, Q., Zhang, R., Xiong, Y., Sui, Y., Tong, C., & Lin, F. H. (2025). Generative AI Mental Health Chatbots as Therapeutic Tools: Systematic Review and Meta-Analysis of Their Role in Reducing Mental Health Issues. *Journal of Medical Internet Research*, *27*, e78238. DOI: 10.2196/78238 PMID: 41401240

Zhou, B., Yang, G., Shi, Z., & Ma, S. (2024). Natural Language Processing for Smart Healthcare. *IEEE Reviews in Biomedical Engineering*, *17*, 4–18. DOI: 10.1109/RBME.2022.3210270 PMID: 36170385

Zhu, J. (2021). Artificial intelligence in the diagnosis of dental diseases on panoramic radiographs: A preliminary study. *BMC Oral Health*, *21*, 158. DOI: 10.1186/s12903-021-01592-6 PMID: 37270488

Zhu, S., Gilbert, M., Chetty, I., & Siddiqui, F. (2022). The 2021 landscape of FDA-approved artificial intelligence/machine learning-enabled medical devices: An analysis of the characteristics and intended use. *International Journal of Medical Informatics*, *165*, 104828. DOI: 10.1016/j.ijmedinf.2022.104828 PMID: 35780651

Compilation of References

Aalizadeh, Y., Khamisi, N., Asghari, P., Safari, A., Mottaghi, M., Taherkhani, M. H., Alemi, A., Ghaderi, M., & Rahmanian, M. (2024). The Mediterranean diet and periodontitis: A systematic review and meta-analysis. *Heliyon*, *10*(15), e35633. DOI: 10.1016/j.heliyon.2024.e35633 PMID: 39170303

Abdalla-Aslan, R., Yeshua, T., Kabla, D., Leichter, I., & Nadler, C. (2020). An artificial intelligence system using machine learning for automatic detection and classification of dental restorations in panoramic radiography. *Oral Surgery, Oral Medicine, Oral Pathology and Oral Radiology*, *130*(5), 593–602. DOI: 10.1016/j.oooo.2020.05.012 PMID: 32646672

Abdelouahed, M., Yateem, D., Amzil, C., Aribi, I., Abdelwahed, E. H., & Fredericks, S. (2025). Integrating artificial intelligence into public health education and healthcare: Insights from the COVID-19 and monkeypox crises for future pandemic readiness. *Frontiers in Education*, *10*, 1518909. DOI: 10.3389/feduc.2025.1518909

AbdulRaheem, Y.AbdulRaheem Y. (2023). Unveiling the Significance and Challenges of Integrating Prevention Levels in Healthcare Practice. *Journal of Primary Care & Community Health*, *14*, 21501319231186500. DOI: 10.1177/21501319231186500 PMID: 37449436

Abe, M.. (2024). Detection of periodontal pathogens in wastewater: A pilot study. *Water Research*, *230*, 119532.

Abidin, C. (2018). *Internet celebrity: Understanding fame online*. Emerald., DOI: 10.1108/9781787560765

Abimbola, O. Y. (2023). Evaluating the impact of community-based oral health education programs on preventive dental behaviors among adults in the United States. *International Journal of Medical and Health Research*, *1*(1), 68–99. DOI: 10.61424/ijmhr.v1i1.605

Abodunrin, O. R., Olagunju, M. T., Alade, O. T., & Foláyan, M. O. (2023). Relationships between oral health and the sustainable development goals: A scoping review. *BioMed*, *3*(4), 460–470. DOI: 10.3390/biomed3040037

Abusleme, L., Dupuy, A. K., Dutzan, N., Silva, N., Burleson, J. A., Strausbaugh, L. D., Gamonal, J., & Diaz, P. I. (2013). The subgingival microbiome in health and periodontitis and its relationship with community biomass and inflammation. *The ISME Journal*, *7*(5), 1016–1025. DOI: 10.1038/ismej.2012.174 PMID: 23303375

Acipinar, S., & Yalcin, M. (2025). Correlation between aging, periodontal diagnoses and systemic diseases: A retrospective analysis of 3,000 patients. *BMC Oral Health*, *25*(1), 1832. DOI: 10.1186/s12903-025-07228-z PMID: 41291667

Adeoye, J., & Su, Y. X. (2024). Artificial intelligence in salivary biomarker discovery and validation for oral diseases. *Oral Diseases*, *30*(1), 23–37. DOI: 10.1111/odi.14641 PMID: 37335832

Ahlbom, A. (2021). Modern Epidemiology, 4th edition. TL Lash, TJ VanderWeele, S Haneuse, KJ Rothman. Wolters Kluwer, 2021. *European Journal of Epidemiology*, *36*(8), 767–768. DOI: 10.1007/s10654-021-00778-w

Ahmed, N., Abbasi, M. S., Zuberi, F., Qamar, W., Halim, M. S., Maqsood, A., & Khan, A. (2021). Artificial intelligence in dentistry: Unlocking new possibilities. *International Journal of Environmental Research and Public Health*, *18*(6), 2711.

Ahmed, Z. H., Almuharib, A. M., Abdulkarim, A. A., Alhassoon, A. H., Alanazi, A. F., Alhaqbani, M. A., Alshalawi, M. S., Almuqayrin, A. K., & Almahmoud, M. I. (2023). Artificial Intelligence and Its Application in Endodontics: A Review. *The Journal of Contemporary Dental Practice*, *24*(11), 912–917. DOI: 10.5005/jp-journals-10024-3593 PMID: 38238281

Alabdullah, J. H., & Daniel, S. J. (2018). Evidence for teledentistry in orthodontics: A systematic review. *The Angle Orthodontist*, *88*(6), 802–810. DOI: 10.2319/012218-52.1

Albani, V., Nishio, K., Ito, T., Kotronia, E., Moynihan, P., Robinson, L., Hanratty, B., Kingston, A., Abe, Y., Takayama, M., Iinuma, T., Arai, Y., & Ramsay, S. E. (2021). Associations of poor oral health with frailty and physical functioning in the oldest old: Results from two studies in England and Japan. *BMC Geriatrics*, *21*(1), 187. DOI: 10.1186/s12877-021-02081-5 PMID: 33736595

Albano, D., Galiano, V., Basile, M., Di Luca, F., Gitto, S., Messina, C., Cagetti, M. G., Del Fabbro, M., Tartaglia, G. M., & Sconfienza, L. M. (2024). Artificial intelligence for radiographic imaging detection of caries lesions: A systematic review. *BMC Oral Health, 24*(1), 274. DOI: 10.1186/s12903-024-04046-7 PMID: 38402191

Alderwick, H., Hutchings, A., Briggs, A., & Mays, N. (2021). The impacts of collaboration between local health care and non-health care organizations and factors shaping how they work: A systematic review of reviews. *BMC Public Health, 21*(1), 753. DOI: 10.1186/s12889-021-10630-1 PMID: 33874927

Alemán, J. O., Bokulich, N. A., Swann, J. R., Walker, J. M., De Rosa, J. C., Battaglia, T., Costabile, A., Pahlavans, A., Liang, Y., & Breslow, J. L. (2018). Fecal microbiota and bile acid interactions with systemic and adipose tissue metabolism in diet-induced weight loss of obese postmenopausal women. *Journal of Translational Medicine, 16*(1), 244. DOI: 10.1186/s12967-018-1619-z PMID: 30176893

AlHumaid, J.. (2020). Ethical considerations of artificial intelligence in healthcare: A focus on dentistry. *BMC Medical Ethics, 21*, 1–9.

Al-Hwsali, A., Alsaadi, B., Abdi, N., Khatab, S., Alzubaidi, M., Solaiman, B., & Househ, M. (2023). Scoping Review: Legal and Ethical Principles of Artificial Intelligence in Public Health. *Studies in Health Technology and Informatics, 305*, 640–643. DOI: 10.3233/SHTI230579 PMID: 37387113

Alkan, A., Cakmak, O., Yilmaz, S., Cebi, T., & Gurgan, C. (2015). Relationship between psychological factors and oral health status and behaviours. *Oral Health & Preventive Dentistry, 13*(4), 331–339. PMID: 25197739

All of Us Research Program Investigators. (2019). The "All of Us" Research Program. *The New England Journal of Medicine, 381*(7), 668–676. DOI: 10.1056/NEJMsr1809937 PMID: 31412182

Allihaibi, M., Koller, G., & Mannocci, F. (2025). Diagnostic Accuracy of a Commercial AI-based Platform in Evaluating Endodontic Treatment Outcomes on Periapical Radiographs Using CBCT as the Reference Standard. *Journal of Endodontics, 51*(7), 898–908.e8. DOI: 10.1016/j.joen.2025.03.007 PMID: 40180318

Alotiby, A. (2024). Immunology of Stress: A Review Article. *Journal of Clinical Medicine, 13*(21), 6394. DOI: 10.3390/jcm13216394 PMID: 39518533

Aloyouny, A. Y., Almufarji, F., Almutairi, G. G., Alkait, S., Al-Mohaya, M. A., & Alserwi, R. (2022). Impact of Rheumatic Diseases on Oral Health-Related Quality of Life. *Cureus, 14*(12), e32268. DOI: 10.7759/cureus.32268 PMID: 36483518

Álvarez-Gálvez, J., Ortega-Martín, E., Carretero-Bravo, J., Pérez-Muñoz, C., Suárez-Lledó, V., & Ramos-Fiol, B. (2023). Social determinants of multimorbidity patterns: A systematic review. *Frontiers in Public Health, 11*, 1081518. DOI: 10.3389/fpubh.2023.1081518 PMID: 37050950

Amaya, A., Medina, I., Mazzilli, S., D'Arcy, J., Cocco, N., Van Hout, M. C., Stöver, H., & Moazen, B. (2024). Oral health services in prison settings: A global scoping review of availability, accessibility, and model of delivery. *Journal of Community Psychology, 52*(8), 1108–1137. DOI: 10.1002/jcop.23081 PMID: 37566403

Aminoshariae, A., Kulild, J. C., Mickel, A., & Fouad, A. F. (2017). Association between Systemic Diseases and Endodontic Outcome: A Systematic Review. *Journal of Endodontics, 43*(4), 514–519. DOI: 10.1016/j.joen.2016.11.008 PMID: 28190585

Aminoshariae, A., Nosrat, A., Nagendrababu, V., Dianat, O., Mohammad-Rahimi, H., O'Keefe, A. W., & Setzer, F. C. (2021). Artificial intelligence in endodontic education. *Journal of Endodontics, 50*(5), 562–578. DOI: 10.1016/j.joen.2024.02.011 PMID: 38387793

Anil, S., Vellappally, S., Hashem, M., Preethanath, R. S., Patil, S., & Samaranayake, L. P. (2016). Xerostomia in geriatric patients: A burgeoning global concern. *Journal of Investigative and Clinical Dentistry, 7*(1), 5–12. DOI: 10.1111/jicd.12120 PMID: 25175324

Antoniadou, M., Manta, G., Kanellopoulou, A., Kalogerakou, T., Satta, A., & Mangoulia, P. (2024, December). Managing stress and somatization symptoms among students in demanding academic healthcare environments. [). MDPI.]. *Health Care, 12*(24), 2522. PMID: 39765949

Anyikwa, C. L., & Ogwo, C. E. (2025). Enhancing oral health outcomes through public health policy reform. *Frontiers in Oral Health, 6*, 1604465. DOI: 10.3389/froh.2025.1604465 PMID: 40551851

Arora, V., Mishra, S. S., Sahoo, J., Gupta, M., Joshi, A., Bajaj, K., Joshi, V., & Joshi, N. K. (2024). Effectiveness of M-Health in Improving Physical Activity: An Indian Perspective. *National Journal of Community Medicine, 1*(15), 1. DOI: 10.55489/njcm.150120243345

Arshed, M., Kazi, A. K., Ashraf, W., Kiran, M., Arshed, M., Kazi, A. K., Ashraf, W., & Kiran, M. (2025). *Universal Health Coverage: Progress Toward Achieving Universal Health Coverage and Lessons Learned* [Chapter]. Innovation and Transformation of Public Health. IGI Global Scientific Publishing. (universal-health-coverage). Https://Services.Igi-Global.Com/Resolvedoi/Resolve.Aspx?Doi=10.4018/979-8-3373-1992-6.Ch002. DOI: 10.4018/979-8-3373-1992-6.ch002

Arshed, M., Kazi, A. K., Kiran, M., Ali, S. M. F., Arshed, M., Kazi, A. K., Kiran, M., & Ali, S. M. F. (2025). *Challenges in Health Equity: Balancing Innovation With Fairness and Addressing Algorithmic Biases* [Chapter]. Innovation and Transformation of Public Health. IGI Global Scientific Publishing. (challenges-in-health-equity). Https://Services.Igi-Global.Com/Resolvedoi/Resolve.Aspx?Doi=10.4018/979-8-3373-1992-6.Ch004. DOI: 10.4018/979-8-3373-1992-6.ch004

Arshed, M., Kiran, M., Umer, M. F., Samkari, J. A., Hassan, S. M., Qamer, S., Gillani, A. H., Hameed, S., Ashraf, W., Mujtaba, H., & Khan, M. N. (2025). Prevalence and associated factors of adherence to antihypertensive medication: A nationwide cross-sectional study. *BMC Public Health*, *25*(1), 2364. Advance online publication. DOI: 10.1186/s12889-025-21456-6 PMID: 40610935

Arshed, M., Mahmud, A. B., Umer, M. F., Mashhadi, F., & Kawish, A. B. (2025). Study protocol for a randomized control trial investigating the effectiveness of a multifaceted mHealth approach on adherence to antihypertensive treatment among patients in Pakistan. *Pakistan Journal of Medical Sciences*, *41*(1), 1. Advance online publication. DOI: 10.12669/pjms.41.1.9272 PMID: 39867791

Arya, S. S., Dias, S. B., Jelinek, H. F., Hadjileontiadis, L. J., & Pappa, A. M. (2023). The convergence of traditional and digital biomarkers through AI-assisted biosensing: A new era in translational diagnostics? *Biosensors & Bioelectronics*, *235*, 115387. DOI: 10.1016/j.bios.2023.115387 PMID: 37229842

Ashley, E. A. (2016). Towards precision medicine. *Nature Reviews. Genetics*, *17*(9), 507–522. DOI: 10.1038/nrg.2016.86 PMID: 27528417

Asiri, A. F., & Altuwalah, A. S. (2022). The role of neural artificial intelligence for diagnosis and treatment planning in endodontics: A qualitative review. *The Saudi Dental Journal*, *34*(4), 270–281. DOI: 10.1016/j.sdentj.2022.04.004 PMID: 35692236

Atchison, K. A., Rozier, R. G., & Weintraub, J. A. (2019). Integration of oral health and primary care: Communication, coordination and referral. NAM Perspectives. Discussion Paper. National Academy of Medicine. https://doi.org/DOI: 10.31478/201905a

Avramova, N. T. (2022). Dental fear, anxiety, and phobia; causes, diagnostic criteria and the medical and social impact. *Journal of Mind and Medical Sciences*, *9*(2), 23. DOI: 10.22543/2392-7674.1348

Aydin, S., Karabacak, M., Vlachos, V., & Margetis, K. (2024). Large language models in patient education: A scoping review of applications in medicine. *Frontiers in Medicine*, *11*, 1477898. DOI: 10.3389/fmed.2024.1477898 PMID: 39534227

Baelum, V., & López, R. (2013). Periodontal disease epidemiology—Learn it, teach it, and use it. *Periodontology 2000, 62*(1), 7–15. DOI: 10.1111/j.1600-0757.2012.00449.x PMID: 23574461

Baima, G., Arce, M., Romandini, M., & Van Dyke, T. (2025). Inflammatory and immunological basis of periodontal diseases. *Journal of Periodontal Research*, jre.70040. Advance online publication. DOI: 10.1111/jre.70040 PMID: 41065279

Baima, G., Shin, H. S., Arrica, M., Laforí, A., Cordaro, M., & Romandini, M. (2023). The co-occurrence of the two main oral diseases: Periodontitis and dental caries. *Clinical Oral Investigations, 27*(11), 6483–6492. DOI: 10.1007/s00784-023-05253-2 PMID: 37714978

Bala, R., Sargaiyan, V., Rathi, S. A., Mankar, S. S., Jaiswal, A. K., & Mankar, S. A. (2023). Mobile dental clinic for oral health services to underserved rural Indian communities. *Bioinformation, 19*(13), 1383–1387. DOI: 10.6026/973206300191383 PMID: 38415028

Barranca-Enríquez, A., & Romo-Gonzâlez, T. (2022). Your health is in your mouth: A comprehensive view to promote general wellness. *Frontiers in Oral Health, 3*, 971223. DOI: 10.3389/froh.2022.971223 PMID: 36186536

Bashirian, S., Khoshravesh, S., Ayubi, E., Karimi-Shahanjarini, A., Shirahmadi, S., & Solaymani, P. F. (2023). The impact of health education interventions on oral health promotion among older people: A systematic review. *BMC Geriatrics, 23*(1), 548. DOI: 10.1186/s12877-023-04259-5 PMID: 37697260

Bates, D. W., Saria, S., Ohno-Machado, L., Shah, A., & Escobar, G. (2014). Big data in health care: Using analytics to identify and manage high-risk and high-cost patients. *Health Affairs (Project Hope), 33*(7), 1123–1131. DOI: 10.1377/hlthaff.2014.0041 PMID: 25006137

Beaglehole, R., Bonita, R., Horton, R., Adams, C., Alleyne, G., Asaria, P., Baugh, V., Bekedam, H., Billo, N., Casswell, S., Cecchini, M., Colagiuri, R., Colagiuri, S., Collins, T., Ebrahim, S., Engelgau, M., Galea, G., Gaziano, T., Geneau, R., & Watt, J. (2011). Priority actions for the non-communicable disease crisis. *Lancet, 377*(9775), 1438–1447. DOI: 10.1016/S0140-6736(11)60393-0 PMID: 21474174

Beam, A. L., & Kohane, I. S. (2018). Big Data and Machine Learning in Health Care. *Journal of the American Medical Association, 319*(13), 1317–1318. DOI: 10.1001/jama.2017.18391 PMID: 29532063

Beltrán, V., López, L., Acuña-Mardones, P., Silva, R., Acevedo, C., Bustos, J., Alarcón, C., von Marttens, R., Espinoza, I., & Mariño, R. (2025). A teledentistry care model for older populations in remote settings in Chile using satellite communication technology. *Frontiers in Oral Health*, *6*, 1699401. DOI: 10.3389/froh.2025.1699401 PMID: 41424661

Bender, I. B., Seltzer, S., & Yermish, M. (2003). The incidence of bacteremia in endodontic manipulation: Preliminary report. 1960. *Journal of Endodontics*, *29*(11), 697–696. DOI: 10.1097/00004770-200311000-00003 PMID: 14651273

Bernabe, E., & Marcenes, W. (2011). Income inequality and tooth loss in the United States. *Journal of Dental Research*, *90*(6), 724–729. DOI: 10.1177/0022034511400081 PMID: 21508433

Bernabe, E., Marcenes, W., Hernandez, C. R., Bailey, J., Abreu, L. G., Alipour, V., Amini, S., Arabloo, J., Arefi, Z., Arora, A., Ayanore, M. A., Bärnighausen, T. W., Bijani, A., Cho, D. Y., Chu, D.-T., Fischer, F., Folayan, M. O., Futran, N. D., Haagsma, J. A., & Kassebaum, N. J. (2020). Global, regional, and national levels and trends in the burden of oral conditions, 1990–2017. *Journal of Dental Research*, *99*(4), 362–373. PMID: 32122215

Berwick, D. M., Nolan, T. W., & Whittington, J. (2008). The triple aim: Care, health, and cost. *Health Affairs (Project Hope)*, *27*(3), 759–769. DOI: 10.1377/hlthaff.27.3.759 PMID: 18474969

Betts, K. J., & Moravec, L. (2023). Integration of oral health screening, intervention, and referral into the pediatric well-child visit. *Journal of Pediatric Health Care : Official Publication of National Association of Pediatric Nurse Associates & Practitioners*, *37*(6), 609–615. DOI: 10.1016/j.pedhc.2023.05.007 PMID: 37330729

Bhati, D., Deogade, M. S., & Kanyal, D. (2023). Improving Patient Outcomes through Effective Hospital Administration: A Comprehensive Review. *Cureus*, *15*(10), e47731. DOI: 10.7759/cureus.47731 PMID: 38021686

Bhavna. (2025). Role of artificial intelligence in diagnosing oral and systemic diseases: A retrospective study. *International Journal of Current Pharmaceutical Review and Research, 17*(9), 1301–1305. https://www.ijcpr.com/

Bibault, J.-E., Giraud, P., & Burgun, A. (2016). Big data and machine learning in radiation oncology: State of the art and future prospects. *Cancer Letters*, *382*(1), 110–117. DOI: 10.1016/j.canlet.2016.05.033 PMID: 27241666

Bida, S. M., Cre u, O. C., Bida, C., Tudorici, T., & Chirita, R. (2025). ORAL HEALTH CHALLENGES IN PATIENTS WITH PSYCHIATRIC DISORDERS: RISKS, BARRIERS, AND CLINICAL IMPLICATIONS. *Romanian Journal of Medical and Dental Education, 14*(2).

Bierman, A. S., Wang, J., O'Malley, P. G., & Moss, D. K. (2021). Transforming care for people with multiple chronic conditions: Agency for Healthcare Research and Quality's research agenda. *Health Services Research, 56*(S1, Suppl 1), 973–979. DOI: 10.1111/1475-6773.13863 PMID: 34378192

Bird, A. (2007). Perceptions of epigenetics. *Nature, 447*(7143), 396–398. DOI: 10.1038/nature05913 PMID: 17522671

Bisht, V., Das, B., Hussain, A., Kumar, V., & Navani, N. K. (2024). Understanding of probiotic origin antimicrobial peptides: a sustainable approach ensuring food safety. *npj Science of Food, 8*(1), 67.

Bitencourt, F. V., Nascimento, G. G., Costa, S. A., Andersen, A., Sandbæk, A., & Leite, F. R. M. (2023). Co-occurrence of Periodontitis and Diabetes-Related Complications. *Journal of Dental Research, 102*(10), 1088–1097. DOI: 10.1177/00220345231179897 PMID: 37448314

Bolton, D., & Gillett, G. (2019). *The biopsychosocial model of health and disease: New philosophical and scientific developments*. Springer. DOI: 10.1007/978-3-030-11899-0

Boreak, N. (2020). Effectiveness of artificial intelligence applications designed for endodontic diagnosis, decision-making, and prediction of prognosis: A systematic review. *The Journal of Contemporary Dental Practice, 21*(8), 926–934. DOI: 10.5005/jp-journals-10024-2894 PMID: 33568617

Borg-Bartolo, R., Roccuzzo, A., Tennert, C., Prasinou, M., Jäggi, M., Molinero-Mourelle, P., Bornstein, M. M., & Campus, G. (2025). Oral health-related quality of life of community-dwellers in the canton of Bern, Switzerland. *Acta Odontologica Scandinavica, 84*, 42707. DOI: 10.2340/aos.v84.42707

Borges do Nascimento, I. J., Marcolino, M. S., Abdulazeem, H. M., Weerasekara, I., Azzopardi-Muscat, N., Gonçalves, M. A., & Novillo-Ortiz, D. (2021). Impact of big data analytics on people's health: Overview of systematic reviews and recommendations for future studies. *Journal of Medical Internet Research, 23*(4), e27275. DOI: 10.2196/27275 PMID: 33847586

Borsa, L., Dubois, M., Sacco, G., & Lupi, L. (2021). Analysis the link between periodontal diseases and Alzheimer's disease: A systematic review. *International Journal of Environmental Research and Public Health*, *18*(17), 9312. DOI: 10.3390/ijerph18179312 PMID: 34501899

Botelho, J., Mascarenhas, P., Viana, J., Proença, L., Orlandi, M., Leira, Y., Chambrone, L., Mendes, J. J., & Machado, V. (2022). An umbrella review of the evidence linking oral health and systemic noncommunicable diseases. *Nature Communications*, *13*(1), 7614. DOI: 10.1038/s41467-022-35337-8 PMID: 36494387

Brabham, D. C., Ribisl, K. M., Kirchner, T. R., & Bernhardt, J. M. (2014). Crowdsourcing Applications for Public Health. *American Journal of Preventive Medicine*, *46*(2), 179–187. DOI: 10.1016/j.amepre.2013.10.016 PMID: 24439353

Brall, C., Berlin, C., & Schwappach, D. (2019). Ethics of artificial intelligence in public health: A conceptual framework. *BMC Medical Ethics*, *20*, 1–14.

Brower, T. (2025). Systemic diseases linked to oral health: A review of the epidemiology of periodontal disease, poor oral hygiene, and tooth caries. *Dental Science and Innovative Research*, *4*(1). Advance online publication. DOI: 10.61148/3065-7008/DSIR/051

Brownstein, J. S., Freifeld, C. C., & Madoff, L. C. (2009). Digital disease detection: Harnessing the Web for public health surveillance. *The New England Journal of Medicine*, *360*(21), 2153–2157. DOI: 10.1056/NEJMp0900702 PMID: 19423867

Brownstein, J. S., Freifeld, C. C., Reis, B. Y., & Mandl, K. D. (2008). Surveillance sans frontieres: Internet-based emerging infectious disease intelligence and the HealthMap project. *PLoS Medicine*, *5*(7), e151. DOI: 10.1371/journal.pmed.0050151 PMID: 18613747

Bruce, L. C., Frassl, M. A., Arhonditsis, G. B., Gal, G., Hamilton, D. P., Hanson, P. C., Hetherington, A. L., Melack, J. M., Read, J. S., Rinke, K., Rigosi, A., Trolle, D., Winslow, L., Adrian, R., Ayala, A. I., Bocaniov, S. A., Boehrer, B., Boon, C., Brookes, J. D., & Hipsey, M. R. (2018). A multi-lake comparative analysis of the General Lake Model (GLM): Stress-testing across a global observatory network. *Environmental Modelling & Software*, *102*, 274–291. DOI: 10.1016/j.envsoft.2017.11.016

Buehler, J. W., Hopkins, R. S., Overhage, J. M., Sosin, D. M., & Tong, V. (2003). Framework for evaluating public health surveillance systems for early detection of outbreaks. *MMWR. Recommendations and Reports*, *53*(RR-5), 1–11. PMID: 15129191

Buhlin, K., Hultin, M., Norderyd, O., Persson, L., Pockley, A. G., Rabe, P., Klinge, B., & Gustafsson, A. (2009). Risk factors for atherosclerosis in cases with severe periodontitis. *Journal of Clinical Periodontology*, *36*(7), 541–549. DOI: 10.1111/j.1600-051X.2009.01430.x PMID: 19538326

Bycroft, C., Freeman, C., Petkova, D., Band, G., Elliott, L. T., Sharp, K., Motyer, A., Vukcevic, D., Delaneau, O., O'Connell, J., Cortes, A., Welsh, S., Young, A., Effingham, M., McVean, G., Leslie, S., Allen, N., Donnelly, P., & Marchini, J. (2018). The UK Biobank resource with deep phenotyping and genomic data. *Nature*, *562*(7726), 203–209. DOI: 10.1038/s41586-018-0579-z PMID: 30305743

Cademartori, M. G., Gastal, M. T., Nascimento, G. G., Demarco, F. F., & Correa, M. B. (2018). Is depression associated with oral health outcomes in adults and elders? A systematic review and meta-analysis. *Clinical Oral Investigations*, *22*(8), 2685–2702. DOI: 10.1007/s00784-018-2611-y PMID: 30191327

Cao, L., van Nistelrooij, N., Chaves, E., Bergé, S., Cenci, M., Xi, T., Loomans, B., & Vinayahalingam, S. (2025). Automated chart filing on bitewings using deep learning: Enhancing clinical diagnosis in a multi-center study. *Journal of Dentistry*, *161*, 105919. DOI: 10.1016/j.jdent.2025.105919 PMID: 40550354

Cao, R., Lai, J., Fu, X., Qiu, P., Chen, J., & Liu, W. (2023). Association between psychological stress, anxiety and oral health status among college students during the Omicron wave: A cross-sectional study. *BMC Oral Health*, *23*(1), 470. DOI: 10.1186/s12903-023-03151-3 PMID: 37424009

Caron, R. M., Noel, K., Reed, R. N., Sibel, J., & Smith, H. J. (2023). Health Promotion, Health Protection, and Disease Prevention: Challenges and Opportunities in a Dynamic Landscape. *AJPM Focus*, *3*(1), 100167. DOI: 10.1016/j.focus.2023.100167 PMID: 38149078

Carrillo-Rodriguez, P., Selheim, F., & Hernandez-Valladares, M. (2023). Mass Spectrometry-Based Proteomics Workflows in Cancer Research: The Relevance of Choosing the Right Steps. *Cancers (Basel)*, *15*(2), 555. DOI: 10.3390/cancers15020555 PMID: 36672506

Carvalho, L. F. D. C. E. S., & Zanatta, R. F. (2024). Editorial: Technological innovations for improved prevention and diagnosis of oral disease. *Frontiers in Oral Health*, *5*, 1481890. DOI: 10.3389/froh.2024.1481890 PMID: 39355782

Cascini, F., Santaroni, F., Lanzetti, R., Failla, G., Gentili, A., & Ricciardi, W. (2021). Developing a data-driven approach in order to improve the safety and quality of patient care. *Frontiers in Public Health*, *9*, 667819. DOI: 10.3389/fpubh.2021.667819 PMID: 34095071

Castillo, E. G., Ijadi-Maghsoodi, R., Shadravan, S., Moore, E., Mensah, M. O.III, Docherty, M., Aguilera Nunez, M. G., Barcelo, N., Goodsmith, N., Halpin, L. E., Morton, I., Mango, J., Montero, A. E., Rahmanian Koushkaki, S., Bromley, E., Chung, B., Jones, F., Gabrielian, S., Gelberg, L., & Wells, K. B. (2019). Community Interventions to Promote Mental Health and Social Equity. *Current Psychiatry Reports*, *21*(5), 35. DOI: 10.1007/s11920-019-1017-0 PMID: 30927093

Celeste, R. K., Fernandes, I. B., & Nadanovsky, P. (2011). The contextual effect of neighborhood income on dental caries in adults: A multilevel analysis. *Community Dentistry and Oral Epidemiology*, *39*(3), 193–201. PMID: 21070318

Centers for Disease Control and Prevention. (2023). *National diabetes statistics report*. U.S. Department of Health and Human Services. https://www.cdc.gov/diabetes/php/data-research/index.html

Centers for Disease Control and Prevention. (2024). *Health disparities*. https://www.cdc.gov/healthy-youth/health-disparities/index.html

Chan, A. K. Y., Chu, C. H., Ogawa, H., & Lai, E. H. H. (2023). Improving oral health of older adults for healthy ageing. *Journal of Dental Sciences*, *19*(1), 1–7. DOI: 10.1016/j.jds.2023.10.018 PMID: 38303786

Chan, A. K. Y., Hui, J. C. Y., Hu, L. L., & Chu, C. H. (2026). The Mouth–Mind Connection: Interplay of Oral and Mental Health in Older Adults. *Geriatrics (Basel, Switzerland)*, *11*(1), 8. DOI: 10.3390/geriatrics11010008 PMID: 41562791

Chan, A. K. Y., Tsang, Y. C., Jiang, C. M., Leung, K. C. M., Lo, E. C. M., & Chu, C. H. (2023). Integration of Oral Health into General Health Services for Older Adults. *Geriatrics (Basel, Switzerland)*, *8*(1), 20. DOI: 10.3390/geriatrics8010020 PMID: 36826362

Chang, Y., Lee, J. S., Lee, K.-J., Woo, H. G., & Song, T.-J. (2020). Improved oral hygiene is associated with decreased risk of new-onset diabetes: A nationwide population-based cohort study. *Diabetologia*, *63*(5), 924–933. DOI: 10.1007/s00125-020-05112-9 PMID: 32128623

Chapple, I. L. C., & Genco, R. (2013). Diabetes and periodontal diseases: Consensus report. *Journal of Periodontology*, *84*(4S, 4-s), S106–S112. DOI: 10.1902/jop.2013.1340011 PMID: 23631572

Chapple, I. L. C., & Genco, R. J. (2022). Diabetes and periodontal diseases: Consensus report of the Joint EFP/AAP Workshop on Periodontitis and Systemic Diseases. *Journal of Clinical Periodontology*, *40*(s14, S14), S106–S112. DOI: 10.1111/jcpe.12077 PMID: 23627322

Chen, J., Ge, X., Yuan, C., Chen, Y., Li, X., Zhang, X., Chen, S., Zheng, W. Y., & Miao, C. (2025). Comparing orthodontic pretreatment information provided by large language models. *BMC Oral Health*, *25*(1), 838. DOI: 10.1186/s12903-025-06246-1 PMID: 40437500

Chen, S., Yu, J., Chamouni, S., Wang, Y., & Li, Y. (2024). Integrating machine learning and artificial intelligence in life-course epidemiology: Pathways to innovative public health solutions. *BMC Medicine*, *22*(1), 354. Advance online publication. DOI: 10.1186/s12916-024-03566-x PMID: 39218895

Chen, W. A., Dou, Y., Fletcher, H. M., & Boskovic, D. S. (2023). Local and systemic effects of *Porphyromonas gingivalis* infection. *Microorganisms*, *11*(2), 470. DOI: 10.3390/microorganisms11020470 PMID: 36838435

Chen, W., Li, C., Jin, D., Shi, Y., Zhang, M., Bo, M., Qian, D., Wang, M., & Li, G. (2022). Metabolomics combined with a network pharmacology-based strategy to reveal the underlying mechanism of Zhenhua submicron emulsion in treating oropharyngeal mucositis complications of radiation therapy for head and neck cancer. *Drug Design, Development and Therapy*, *16*, 3169–3182. DOI: 10.2147/DDDT.S376984 PMID: 36158237

Chen, W., Lin, G., Chen, Y., Cheng, F., Li, X., Ding, J., Zhong, Y., Kong, C., Chen, M., Xia, S., Lu, C., & Ji, J. (2024). Prediction of the Ki-67 expression level in head and neck squamous cell carcinoma with machine learning-based multiparametric MRI radiomics: A multicenter study. *BMC Cancer*, *24*(1), 418. DOI: 10.1186/s12885-024-12026-x PMID: 38580939

Chen, X., Orom, H., Hay, J. L., Waters, E. A., Schofield, E., Li, Y., & Kiviniemi, M. T. (2019). Differences in Rural and Urban Health Information Access and Use. *The Journal of Rural Health : Official Journal of the American Rural Health Association and the National Rural Health Care Association*, *35*(3), 405–417. DOI: 10.1111/jrh.12335 PMID: 30444935

Cheung, M. K., Chan, J. Y. K., Wong, M. C. S., Wong, P. Y., Lei, P., Cai, L., Lan, L., Ho, W. C. S., Yeung, A. C. M., Chan, P. K. S., & Chen, Z. (2022). Determinants and interactions of oral bacterial and fungal microbiota in healthy Chinese adults. *Microbiology Spectrum*, *10*(1), e0241021. DOI: 10.1128/spectrum.02410-21 PMID: 35107355

Choi, R. Y., Coyner, A. S., Kalpathy-Cramer, J., Chiang, M. F., & Campbell, J. P. (2020). Introduction to machine learning, neural networks, and deep learning. *Translational Vision Science & Technology*, *9*(2), 14. DOI: 10.1167/tvst.9.2.14 PMID: 32704420

Christen, P. (2012). A survey of indexing techniques for scalable record linkage and deduplication. *IEEE Transactions on Knowledge and Data Engineering*, *24*(9), 1537–1555. DOI: 10.1109/TKDE.2011.127

Chung, E., Yang, B., Kang, S., Kim, Y., Na, J., Park, S., On, S., & Byun, S. (2024). Validation of 2D lateral cephalometric analysis using artificial intelligence-processed low-dose cone beam computed tomography. *Heliyon*, *10*(21), e39445. DOI: 10.1016/j.heliyon.2024.e39445 PMID: 39583802

Chung, E., Yang, B., Park, I., Yi, S., On, S., Kim, Y., Kang, S., & Byun, S. (2022). Effectiveness of cone-beam computed tomography-generated cephalograms using artificial intelligence cephalometric analysis. *Scientific Reports*, *12*(1), 20585. Advance online publication. DOI: 10.1038/s41598-022-25215-0 PMID: 36446924

Clemente-Suárez, V. J., Redondo-Flórez, L., Beltrán-Velasco, A. I., Martín-Rodríguez, A., Martínez-Guardado, I., Navarro-Jiménez, E., Laborde-Cárdenas, C. C., & Tornero-Aguilera, J. F. (2023). The Role of Adipokines in Health and Disease. *Biomedicines*, *11*(5), 1290. DOI: 10.3390/biomedicines11051290 PMID: 37238961

Clish, C. B. (2015). Metabolomics: An emerging but powerful tool for precision medicine. *Cold Spring Harbor Molecular Case Studies*, *1*(1), a000588. DOI: 10.1101/mcs.a000588 PMID: 27148576

Cogburn, C. D. (2019). Culture, Race, and Health: Implications for Racial Inequities and Population Health. *The Milbank Quarterly*, *97*(3), 736–761. DOI: 10.1111/1468-0009.12411 PMID: 31512293

Cohen, D., Huynh, T., Sebold, A., Harvey, J., Neudorf, C., & Brown, A. (2014). The population health approach: A qualitative study of conceptual and operational definitions for leaders in Canadian healthcare. *SAGE Open Medicine*, *2*, 2050312114522618. DOI: 10.1177/2050312114522618 PMID: 26770704

Collin, M., Christidis, N., Hagelberg, S., Arvidsson, L. Z., Larheim, T. A., Ernberg, M., & Hedenberg-Magnusson, B. (2024). Temporomandibular involvement in children and adolescents with juvenile idiopathic arthritis: A 2-year prospective cohort study. *Scientific Reports*, *14*(1), 5512. DOI: 10.1038/s41598-024-56174-3 PMID: 38448491

Collins, F. S., & Varmus, H. (2015). A new initiative on precision medicine. *The New England Journal of Medicine*, *372*(9), 793–795. DOI: 10.1056/NEJMp1500523 PMID: 25635347

Cowie, M. R., Blomster, J. I., Curtis, L. H., Duclaux, S., Ford, I., Fritz, F., & Zalewski, A. (2017). Electronic health records to facilitate clinical research. *Clinical Research in Cardiology : Official Journal of the German Cardiac Society*, *106*(1), 1–9. DOI: 10.1007/s00392-016-1025-6 PMID: 27557678

Curran, G. M., Bauer, M., Mittman, B., Pyne, J. M., & Stetler, C. (2012). Effectiveness-implementation hybrid designs: Combining elements of clinical effectiveness and implementation research to enhance public health impact. *Medical Care*, *50*(3), 217–226. DOI: 10.1097/MLR.0b013e3182408812 PMID: 22310560

Da Silva, R. G. L. (2024). The advancement of artificial intelligence in biomedical research and health innovation: Challenges and opportunities in emerging economies. *Globalization and Health*, *20*(1), 44. DOI: 10.1186/s12992-024-01049-5 PMID: 38773458

Dai, X., Dai, M., Liang, Y., Li, X., & Zhao, W. (2025). Global burden and trends of oral disorders among adolescent and young adults (10–24 years old) from 1990 to 2021. *BMC Oral Health*, *25*(1), 486. DOI: 10.1186/s12903-025-05864-z PMID: 40186217

Danforth, K., Ahmad, A. M., Blanchet, K., Khalid, M., Means, A. R., Memirie, S. T., Alwan, A., & Watkins, D. (2023). Monitoring and evaluating the implementation of essential packages of health services. *BMJ Global Health*, *8*(Suppl 1), e010726. DOI: 10.1136/bmjgh-2022-010726 PMID: 36977532

Dankwa-Mullan, I. (2024). Health Equity and Ethical Considerations in Using Artificial Intelligence in Public Health and Medicine. *Preventing Chronic Disease*, *21*, 240245. Advance online publication. DOI: 10.5888/pcd21.240245 PMID: 39173183

Dao, A. T., Do, L. G., Stormon, N., Dhanapriyanka, M., & Ha, D. H. (2025). Causal analyses in longitudinal observational studies in oral health: A scoping review. *Community Dentistry and Oral Epidemiology*, *53*(1), 7–16. DOI: 10.1111/cdoe.13002 PMID: 39248439

Dash, S., Shakyawar, S. K., Sharma, M., & Kaushik, S. (2019). Big data in healthcare: Management, analysis and future prospects. *Journal of Big Data*, *6*(1), 1–25. DOI: 10.1186/s40537-019-0217-0

Dashti, M., Londono, J., Ghasemi, S., Zare, N., Samman, M., Ashi, H., Amirzade-Iranaq, M., Khosraviani, F., Sabeti, M., & Khurshid, Z. (2024). Comparative analysis of deep learning algorithms for dental caries detection and prediction from radiographic images: A comprehensive umbrella review. *PeerJ. Computer Science*, *10*, e2371. DOI: 10.7717/peerj-cs.2371 PMID: 39650341

Das, S. (2022). Artificial intelligence in endodontics: A peek into the future. *RGUHS Journal of Dental Sciences*, *14*(3), 35–37. DOI: 10.26715/rjds.14_3_7

de Abreu, M. H. N. G., Cruz, A. J. S., Borges-Oliveira, A. C., Martins, R. C., & Mattos, F. F. (2021). Perspectives on Social and Environmental Determinants of Oral Health. *International Journal of Environmental Research and Public Health*, *18*(24), 13429. DOI: 10.3390/ijerph182413429 PMID: 34949037

de Carvalho, R. D. P., Casarin, R. C. V., de Lima, P. O., & Cogo-Müller, K. (2021). Statins with potential to control periodontitis: From biological mechanisms to clinical studies. *Journal of Oral Biosciences*, *63*(3), 232–244. DOI: 10.1016/j.job.2021.06.002 PMID: 34146687

Delgado-Rodríguez, M., & Llorca, J. (2004). Bias. *Journal of Epidemiology and Community Health*, *58*(8), 635–641. DOI: 10.1136/jech.2003.008466 PMID: 15252064

Deng, K., Zonta, F., Yang, H., Pelekos, G., & Tonetti, M. S. (2024). Development of a machine learning multiclass screening tool for periodontal health status based on non-clinical parameters and salivary biomarkers. *Journal of Clinical Periodontology*, *51*(12), 1547–1560. DOI: 10.1111/jcpe.13856 PMID: 37697491

Deo, P. N., & Deshmukh, R. (2019). Oral microbiome: Unveiling the fundamentals. *Journal of Oral and Maxillofacial Pathology : JOMFP*, *23*(1), 122–128. DOI: 10.4103/jomfp.JOMFP_304_18 PMID: 31110428

Dewhirst, F. E., Chen, T., Izard, J., Paster, B. J., Tanner, A. C. R., Yu, W.-H., Lakshmanan, A., & Wade, W. G. (2010). The human oral microbiome. *Journal of Bacteriology*, *192*(19), 5002–5017. DOI: 10.1128/JB.00542-10 PMID: 20656903

Di Stefano, M., Polizzi, A., Santonocito, S., Romano, A., Lombardi, T., & Isola, G. (2022). Impact of oral microbiome in periodontal health and periodontitis: A critical review on prevention and treatment. *International Journal of Molecular Sciences*, *23*(9), 5142. DOI: 10.3390/ijms23095142 PMID: 35563531

Diez Roux, A. V. (2012). Conceptual approaches to the study of health disparities. *Annual Review of Public Health*, *33*(1), 41–58. DOI: 10.1146/annurev-publhealth-031811-124534 PMID: 22224879

Ding, H., Wu, J., Zhao, W., Matinlinna, J. P., Burrow, M. F., & Tsoi, J. K. H. (2021). Artificial intelligence in dentistry—A review. *Frontiers in Dental Medicine*, *4*, 1085251. DOI: 10.3389/fdmed.2023.1085251 PMID: 39935549

Divaris, K. (2016). Precision dentistry: Moving toward personalized oral health care. *Journal of Dental Research*, *95*(9), 965–970.

Divaris, K. (2019). Predicting dental caries outcomes in children: A "risky" concept. *Journal of Dental Research, 98*(13), 1405–1406. PMID: 31746686

Divaris, K., Lee, J. Y., Baker, A. D., & Vann, W. F.Jr. (2017). Precision oral health in the era of omics and systems biology. *Journal of Dental Research, 96*(5), 487–493. PMID: 28425840

Dix, A., Hünniger, K., Weber, M., Guthke, R., Kurzai, O., & Linde, J. (2015). Biomarker-based classification of bacterial and fungal whole-blood infections in a genome-wide expression study. *Frontiers in Microbiology, 6*, 171. DOI: 10.3389/fmicb.2015.00171 PMID: 25814982

Djekic, D., Shi, L., Brolin, H., Carlsson, F., Särnqvist, C., Savolainen, O., Cao, Y., Bäckhed, F., Tremaroli, V., Landberg, R., & Frøbert, O. (2020). Effects of a vegetarian diet on cardiometabolic risk factors, gut microbiota, and plasma metabolome in subjects with ischemic heart disease: A randomized crossover study. *Journal of the American Heart Association, 9*(18), e016518. DOI: 10.1161/JAHA.120.016518 PMID: 32893710

Dong, J., Li, Y., Xiao, H., Zhang, S., Wang, B., Wang, H., Li, Y., Fan, S., & Cui, M. (2021). Oral microbiota affects the efficacy and prognosis of radiotherapy for colorectal cancer in mouse models. *Cell Reports, 37*(4), 109886. DOI: 10.1016/j.celrep.2021.109886 PMID: 34706245

Donia, M. S., Cimermancic, P., Schulze, C. J., Wieland Brown, L. C., Martin, J., Mitreva, M., Clardy, J., Linington, R. G., & Fischbach, M. A. (2014). A systematic analysis of biosynthetic gene clusters in the human microbiome reveals a common family of antibiotics. *Cell, 158*(6), 1402–1414. DOI: 10.1016/j.cell.2014.08.032 PMID: 25215495

Dopelt, K., Avni, N., Haimov-Sadikov, Y., Golan, I., & Davidovitch, N. (2021). Telemedicine and eHealth Literacy in the Era of COVID-19: A Cross-Sectional Study in a Peripheral Clinic in Israel. *International Journal of Environmental Research and Public Health, 18*(18), 9556. DOI: 10.3390/ijerph18189556 PMID: 34574480

Doshi-Velez, F., & Kim, B. (2017). Towards a rigorous science of interpretable machine learning. arXiv preprint arXiv:1702.08608.

Dove, E. S., Knoppers, B. M., & Zawati, M. H. (2015). An ethics safe harbor for international genomics research? *Genome Medicine, 7*(1), 1–4. DOI: 10.1186/s13073-015-0204-4 PMID: 25606059

Dühring, S., Germerodt, S., Skerka, C., Zipfel, P. F., Dandekar, T., & Schuster, S. (2015). Host–pathogen interactions between the human innate immune system and *Candida albicans*: Understanding and modeling defense and evasion strategies. *Frontiers in Microbiology*, *6*, 625. DOI: 10.3389/fmicb.2015.00625 PMID: 26175718

Duley, S. I., Fitzpatrick, P. G., Zornosa, X., & Barnes, W. G. (2012). A center for oral health promotion: Establishing an inter-professional paradigm for dental hygiene, health care management and nursing education. *Journal of Dental Hygiene*, *86*(2), 63–70. PMID: 22584443

Durmuş, S., Çakır, T., Özgür, A., & Guthke, R. (2015). A review on computational systems biology of pathogen–host interactions. *Frontiers in Microbiology*, *6*, 235. PMID: 25914674

Dwork, C., & Roth, A. (2014). The algorithmic foundations of differential privacy. *Foundations and Trends in Theoretical Computer Science*, *9*(3-4), 211–407. DOI: 10.1561/0400000042

Edfeldt, K., Swedenborg, J., Hansson, G. K., & Yan, Z. (2002). Expression of Toll-like receptors in human atherosclerotic lesions: A possible pathway for plaque activation. *Circulation*, *105*(10), 1158–1161. DOI: 10.1161/circ.105.10.1158 PMID: 11889007

Edo-Osagie, O., De La Iglesia, B., Lake, I., & Edeghere, O. (2020). A scoping review of the use of Twitter for public health research. *Computers in Biology and Medicine*, *122*, 103770. DOI: 10.1016/j.compbiomed.2020.103770 PMID: 32502758

Eicher, T. P., & Mohajeri, M. H. (2022). Overlapping mechanisms of action of brain-active bacteria and bacterial metabolites in the pathogenesis of common brain diseases. *Nutrients*, *14*(13), 2661. DOI: 10.3390/nu14132661 PMID: 35807841

Eichner, M., & Dietz, K. (2003). Transmission potential of smallpox: Estimates based on detailed data from an outbreak. *American Journal of Epidemiology*, *158*(2), 110–117. DOI: 10.1093/aje/kwg103 PMID: 12851223

Ekert, T., Krois, J., Meinhold, L., Elhennawy, K., Emara, R., Golla, T., & Schwendicke, F. (2019). Deep learning for the radiographic detection of apical lesions. *Journal of Endodontics*, *45*(7), 917–922. DOI: 10.1016/j.joen.2019.03.016 PMID: 31160078

Elzayat, H., Mesto, G., & Al-Marzooq, F. (2023). Unraveling the Impact of Gut and Oral Microbiome on Gut Health in Inflammatory Bowel Diseases. *Nutrients*, *15*(15), 3377. DOI: 10.3390/nu15153377 PMID: 37571313

Emadi, M., Delavari, S., & Bayati, M. (2021). Global socioeconomic inequality in the burden of communicable and non-communicable diseases and injuries: An analysis on global burden of disease study 2019. *BMC Public Health*, *21*(1), 1771. DOI: 10.1186/s12889-021-11793-7 PMID: 34583668

Epelde, F. (2024). How AI Could Help Us in the Epidemiology and Diagnosis of Acute Respiratory Infections? *Pathogens (Basel, Switzerland)*, *13*(11), 940. DOI: 10.3390/pathogens13110940 PMID: 39599493

Esfanjani, M. T., Gilani, N., Esfanjani, A. T., Nourizadeh, A. M., Faramarzi, E., & Hekmatfar, S. (2023). Are oral health behaviors associated with metabolic syndrome in the Azar cohort population? *BMC Oral Health*, *23*(1), 370. DOI: 10.1186/s12903-023-03003-0 PMID: 37291532

Esteva, A., Robicquet, A., Ramsundar, B., Kuleshov, V., DePristo, M., Chou, K., Cui, C., Corrado, G., Thrun, S., & Dean, J. (2019). A guide to deep learning in healthcare. *Nature Medicine*, *25*(1), 24–29. DOI: 10.1038/s41591-018-0316-z PMID: 30617335

Etches, V., Frank, J., Di Ruggiero, E., & Manuel, D. (2006). Measuring population health: A review of indicators. *Annual Review of Public Health*, *27*(1), 29–55. DOI: 10.1146/annurev.publhealth.27.021405.102141 PMID: 16533108

European Commission. (2022). *European Health Data Space. Proposal for a Regulation of the European Parliament and of the Council (COM/2022/197 final)*. Publications Office of the European Union.

Eysenbach, G. (2009). Infodemiology and infoveillance: Framework for an emerging set of public health informatics methods to analyze search, communication and publication behavior on the internet. *Journal of Medical Internet Research*, *11*(1), e11. DOI: 10.2196/jmir.1157 PMID: 19329408

Ezzati, M., & Riboli, E. (2012). Can noncommunicable diseases be prevented? Lessons from studies of populations and individuals. *Science*, *337*(6101), 1482–1487. DOI: 10.1126/science.1227001 PMID: 22997325

Faggion, C. M.Jr. (2017). Methodological issues in periodontal research: Causal inference and evidence hierarchies. *Journal of Clinical Periodontology*, *44*(9), 868–875.

Fairchild, G., Tasseff, B., Khalsa, H., Generous, N., Daughton, A. R., Velappan, N., Priedhorsky, R., & Deshpande, A. (2018). Epidemiological Data Challenges: Planning for a More Robust Future Through Data Standards. *Frontiers in Public Health*, *6*, 336. DOI: 10.3389/fpubh.2018.00336 PMID: 30533407

Faiyazuddin, M., Rahman, S. J. Q., Anand, G., Siddiqui, R. K., Mehta, R., Khatib, M. N., Gaidhane, S., Zahiruddin, Q. S., Hussain, A., & Sah, R. (2025). The Impact of Artificial Intelligence on Healthcare: A Comprehensive Review of Advancements in Diagnostics, Treatment, and Operational Efficiency. *Health Science Reports*, *8*(1), e70312. DOI: 10.1002/hsr2.70312 PMID: 39763580

Falbe, J., Grummon, A. H., & Krieger, J. W. (2022). Sugar-sweetened beverage taxes and population health outcomes. *JAMA Pediatrics*, *176*(2), 129–131. DOI: 10.1001/jamapediatrics.2021.5051 PMID: 34902011

Fanelli, F., Saleh, M., Santamaria, P., Zhurakivska, K., Nibali, L., & Troiano, G. (2025). Development and comparative evaluation of a reinstructed GPT-4o model specialized in periodontology. *Journal of Clinical Periodontology*, *52*(5), 707–716. DOI: 10.1111/jcpe.14101 PMID: 39723544

Fan, Y., & Pedersen, O. (2021). Gut microbiota in human metabolic health and disease. *Nature Reviews. Microbiology*, *19*(1), 55–71. DOI: 10.1038/s41579-020-0433-9 PMID: 32887946

Farahani, B., Firouzi, F., Chang, V., Badaroglu, M., Constant, N., & Mankodiya, K. (2018). Towards fog-driven IoT eHealth: Promises and challenges of IoT in medicine and healthcare. *Future Generation Computer Systems*, *78*, 659–676. DOI: 10.1016/j.future.2017.04.036

Farid, A., Fatima, Z., Fareed, Z., Athar, Z., Manzoor, A., & Sheharyar, M. F. H. (2026). Emerging Infectious Control Technologies: A Global Perspective Surveillance and Response to Hospital Acquired Infections. In *Innovation and Transformation of Public Health* (pp. 459-496). IGI Global Scientific Publishing.

Farid, A., Han, W., Kwan, J. K., & Yeung, K. L. (2025). Enhancing bedding hygiene in long-term care facilities: Investigating the impact of multilevel antimicrobial polymers (MAP-1) on bacterial and MDRO reduction. *Antimicrobial Resistance and Infection Control*, *14*(1), 36. DOI: 10.1186/s13756-025-01555-0 PMID: 40270052

Farid, A., Han, W., Lai, C. K. C., Kwan, J. K. C., & Yeung, K. L. (2025). Clinical evaluation of MAP-1 antimicrobial coating on patient privacy curtains: Insights from a randomized trial in a Hong Kong hospital. *The Journal of Hospital Infection*, *162*, 223–231. DOI: 10.1016/j.jhin.2025.05.012 PMID: 40456490

Fathima, F., & Sakthi, D. S. (2023, March). Personality Traits and Its Effect On Oral Health of Outpatients Visiting a Private Dental Institution in Chennai. In *2023 International Conference on Business Analytics for Technology and Security (ICBATS)* (pp. 1-4). IEEE. https://doi.org/DOI: 10.1109/ICBATS57792.2023.10111302 fatima, G., Allami, R. H., & Yousif, M. G. (2023). *Integrative AI-Driven Strategies for Advancing Precision Medicine in Infectious Diseases and Beyond: A Novel Multidisciplinary Approach* (Version 1). arXiv. DOI: 10.48550/ARXIV.2307.15228

Featherstone, J. D. B. (2003). The caries balance: Contributing factors and early detection. *Journal of the California Dental Association*, *31*(2), 129–133. DOI: 10.1080/19424396.2003.12224144 PMID: 12636316

Fedele, D. A.. (2020). Mobile apps for oral health promotion. *Community Dentistry and Oral Epidemiology*, *48*(5), 432–440. DOI: 10.2196/11432

Fejerskov, O., & Kidd, E. (Eds.). (2008). *Dental caries: The disease and its clinical management* (2nd ed.). Blackwell Munksgaard.

Fisher-Owens, S. A., Gansky, S. A., Platt, L. J., Weintraub, J. A., Soobader, M.-J., Bramlett, M. D., & Newacheck, P. W. (2007). Influences on children's oral health: A conceptual model. *Pediatrics*, *120*(3), e510–e520. DOI: 10.1542/peds.2006-3084 PMID: 17766495

Fisher, S. (2021). Priorities for successful use of artificial intelligence by public health organizations: A literature review. *BMC Public Health*, *21*, 10422. DOI: 10.1186/s12889-021-10422-2 PMID: 36419010

Fitzgerald, K. A., & Kagan, J. C. (2020). Toll-like receptors and the control of immunity. *Cell*, *180*(6), 1044–1066. DOI: 10.1016/j.cell.2020.02.041 PMID: 32164908

Fitzpatrick, P. J. (2023). Improving health literacy using the power of digital communications to achieve better health outcomes for patients and practitioners. *Frontiers in Digital Health*, *5*, 1264780. DOI: 10.3389/fdgth.2023.1264780 PMID: 38046643

Fletcher-Lartey, S. M., & Caprarelli, G. (2016). Application of GIS technology in public health: Successes and challenges. *Parasitology*, *143*(4), 401–415. DOI: 10.1017/S0031182015001869 PMID: 26831619

Floridi, L., Cowls, J., Beltrametti, M., Chatila, R., Chazerand, P., Dignum, V., Luetge, C., Madelin, R., Pagallo, U., Rossi, F., Schafer, B., Valcke, P., & Vayena, E. (2018). An ethical framework for a good AI society: Opportunities, risks, principles, and recommendations. *Minds and Machines*, *28*(4), 689–707. DOI: 10.1007/s11023-018-9482-5 PMID: 30930541

Foláyan, M. O., Bernard, O. T., Titus, O. S., Alade, O., Aliyu, T. K., Bhayat, A., Ndembi, N., Fasiku, G., & El Tantawi, M. (2025). Cultural practices, oral health service utilisation and oral health policy and guidelines development in Africa: Insights from the yorùbá ethnic group. *Frontiers in Oral Health*, *6*, 1539827. DOI: 10.3389/froh.2025.1539827 PMID: 40045959

Foláyan, M. O., & Starr, J. R. (2024). Grand challenges and future oral epidemiology research. *Frontiers in Oral Health, 4,* 1349252. DOI: 10.3389/froh.2023.1349252 PMID: 38268765

Fontenele, R. C., & Jacobs, R. (2025). Unveiling the power of artificial intelligence for image-based diagnosis and treatment in endodontics: An ally or adversary? *International Endodontic Journal, 58*(2), 155–170. DOI: 10.1111/iej.14163 PMID: 39526945

Freeman, M. (Ed.). (2018). *The Ethics of Public Health* (1st ed.). Routledge., DOI: 10.4324/9781315239927

Frenk, J., Chen, L., Bhutta, Z., Cohen, J., Crisp, N., Evans, T., Fineberg, H., Garcia, P., Ke, Y., Kelley, P., Kistnasamy, B., Meleis, A., Naylor, D., Pablos-Mendez, A., Reddy, S., Scrimshaw, S., Sepulveda, J., Serwadda, D., & Zurayk, H. (2010). Health professionals for a new century: Transforming education to strengthen health systems in an interdependent world. *Lancet, 376*(9756), 1923–1958. DOI: 10.1016/S0140-6736(10)61854-5 PMID: 21112623

Frenk, J., & Moon, S. (2013). Governance challenges in global health. *The New England Journal of Medicine, 368*(10), 936–942. DOI: 10.1056/NEJMra1109339 PMID: 23465103

Frieden, T. R. (2010). A framework for public health action: The health impact pyramid. *American Journal of Public Health, 100*(4), 590–595. DOI: 10.2105/AJPH.2009.185652 PMID: 20167880

Friedman, C. P., Wong, A. K., & Blumenthal, D. (2010). Achieving a nationwide learning health system. *Science Translational Medicine, 2*(57), 57cm29. Advance online publication. DOI: 10.1126/scitranslmed.3001456 PMID: 21068440

Friis, R. H., & Sellers, T. A. (2021). *Epidemiology for public health practice* (6th ed.). Jones & Bartlett Learning.

Fu, D., Shu, X., Zhou, G., Ji, M., Liao, G., & Zou, L. (2025). Connection between oral health and chronic diseases. *MedComm, 6*(1), e70052. DOI: 10.1002/mco2.70052 PMID: 39811802

Fuster, V., García-Álvarez, A., Devesa, A., Mass, V., Owen, R., Quesada, A., Fuster, J. J., García-Lunar, I., Pocock, S., Sánchez-González, J., Sartori, S., Peyra, C., Andres, V., Muntendam, P., & Ibanez, B. (2024). Influence of Subclinical Atherosclerosis Burden and Progression on Mortality. *Journal of the American College of Cardiology, 84*(15), 1391–1403. DOI: 10.1016/j.jacc.2024.06.045 PMID: 39357937

Galié, S., García-Gavilán, J., Camacho-Barcía, L., Atzeni, A., Muralidharan, J., Papandreou, C., Arcelin, P., Palau-Galindo, A., Garcia, D., Basora, J., Arias-Vasquez, A., & Bulló, M. (2021). Effects of the Mediterranean diet or nut consumption on gut microbiota composition and fecal metabolites and their relationship with cardiometabolic risk factors. *Molecular Nutrition & Food Research*, *65*(19), e2000982. DOI: 10.1002/mnfr.202000982 PMID: 34331403

Ganesan, A., Kumar, G., Gauthaman, J., Lakshmi, K. C., & Kumbalaparambil, Y. A. (2024). Exploring the relationship between psychoneuroimmunology and oral diseases: A comprehensive review and analysis. *Journal of Lifestyle Medicine*, *14*(1), 13–19. DOI: 10.15280/jlm.2024.14.1.13 PMID: 38665319

García-Cruz, I.. (2024). Wastewater surveillance for sugar consumption and caries risk assessment. *Environmental Science & Technology Letters*, *11*(3), 215–221.

Garcia-Junior, M. A., Andrade, B. S., Lima, A. P., Soares, I. P., Notário, A. F. O., Bernardino, S. S., Guevara-Vega, M. F., Honório-Silva, G., Munoz, R. A. A., Jardim, A. C. G., Martins, M. M., Goulart, L. R., Cunha, T. M., Carneiro, M. G., & Sabino-Silva, R. (2025). Artificial-Intelligence Bio-Inspired Peptide for Salivary Detection of SARS-CoV-2 in Electrochemical Biosensor Integrated with Machine Learning Algorithms. *Biosensors (Basel)*, *15*(2), 75. DOI: 10.3390/bios15020075 PMID: 39996977

Garza, M., Del Fiol, G., Tenenbaum, J., Walden, A., & Zozus, M. N. (2016). Evaluating common data models for use with a longitudinal community registry. *Journal of Biomedical Informatics*, *64*, 333–341. DOI: 10.1016/j.jbi.2016.10.016 PMID: 27989817

Gatto, A., Liu, K., Milan, N., & Wong, S. (2025). The Effects of GLP-1 Agonists on Musculoskeletal Health and Orthopedic Care. *Current Reviews in Musculoskeletal Medicine*, *18*(10), 469–480. DOI: 10.1007/s12178-025-09978-3 PMID: 40372699

Gawande, M. S., Zade, N., Kumar, P., Gundewar, S., Weerarathna, I. N., & Verma, P. (2025). The role of artificial intelligence in pandemic responses: From epidemiological modeling to vaccine development. *Molecular Biomedicine*, *6*(1), 1. DOI: 10.1186/s43556-024-00238-3 PMID: 39747786

GBD 2017 Oral Disorders Collaborators, Bernabe, E., Marcenes, W., Hernandez, C. R., Bailey, J., Abreu, L. G., Alipour, V., Amini, S., Arabloo, J., Arefi, Z., Arora, A., Ayanore, M. A., Bärnighausen, T. W., Bijani, A., Cho, D. Y., Chu, D. T., Crowe, C. S., Demoz, G. T., Demsie, D. G., … Kassebaum, N. J. (2020). Global, Regional, and National Levels and Trends in Burden of Oral Conditions from 1990 to 2017: A Systematic Analysis for the Global Burden of Disease 2017 Study. *Journal of Dental Research, 99*(4), 362–373. DOI: 10.1177/0022034520908533

GBD 2019 Diseases and Injuries Collaborators (2020). Global burden of 369 diseases and injuries in 204 countries and territories, 1990-2019: a systematic analysis for the Global Burden of Disease Study 2019. *Lancet (London, England), 396*(10258), 1204–1222. https://doi.org/.DOI: 10.1016/S0140-6736(20)30925-9

GBD 2023 Disease and Injury and Risk Factor Collaborators (2025). Burden of 375 diseases and injuries, risk-attributable burden of 88 risk factors, and healthy life expectancy in 204 countries and territories, including 660 subnational locations, 1990-2023: a systematic analysis for the Global Burden of Disease Study 2023. *Lancet (London, England), 406*(10513), 1873–1922. https://doi.org/DOI: 10.1016/S0140-6736(25)01637-X

Geng, Q. S., Liu, R. J., Shen, Z. B., Wei, Q., Zheng, Y. Y., Jia, L. Q., Wang, L. H., Li, L. F., Li, J., & Xue, W. H. (2021). Transcriptome sequencing and metabolome analysis reveal the mechanism of Huanghua Baihe Tablet in the treatment of oral mucositis. *Chinese Journal of Natural Medicines*, *19*(12), 930–943. DOI: 10.1016/S1875-5364(22)60150-X PMID: 34961591

Ghoneim, A., Ebnahmady, A., D'Souza, V., Parbhakar, K. K., He, H., Gerbig, M., Singhal, S., & Quiñonez, C. (2022). The impact of dental care programs on healthcare system and societal outcomes: A scoping review. *BMC Health Services Research*, *22*(1), 1574. DOI: 10.1186/s12913-022-08951-x PMID: 36564768

Giannobile, W. V., & Lang, N. P. (2016). Are dental implants a panacea or should we better strive to save teeth? *Journal of Dental Research*, *95*(1), 5–6. DOI: 10.1177/0022034515618942 PMID: 26701917

Gil, A. J., Rodrigo-Moya, B., & Morcillo-Bellido, J. (2018). The effect of leadership in the development of innovation capacity: A learning organization perspective. *Leadership and Organization Development Journal*, *39*(6), 694–711. DOI: 10.1108/LODJ-12-2017-0399

Gillani, A. H., Arshad, H., Arshed, M., Jairoun, A., Shukar, S., Akbar, J., Hussain, A. K., Malik, H. M. A., Ibrahim, M. I. M., & Fang, Y. (2024). Cross-sectional assessment of perception and attitude of pharmacy students towards pharmaceutical promotion: A study from developing country, Pakistan. *Frontiers in Medicine*, *11*, 1424352. Advance online publication. DOI: 10.3389/fmed.2024.1424352 PMID: 39554505

Ginsburg, G. S., & Willard, H. F. (2009). Genomic and personalized medicine: Foundations and applications. *Translational Research : The Journal of Laboratory and Clinical Medicine*, *154*(6), 277–287. DOI: 10.1016/j.trsl.2009.09.005 PMID: 19931193

Glick, M., Urquhart, O., Bhosale, A. S., Carrasco-Labra, A., & Edelson, J. T. (2023). A unified voice to drive global improvements in oral health. *BMC Global and Public Health*, *1*(1), 19. DOI: 10.1186/s44263-023-00019-0 PMID: 39681896

Goodwin, S., McPherson, J. D., & McCombie, W. R. (2016). Coming of age: Ten years of next-generation sequencing technologies. *Nature Reviews. Genetics*, *17*(6), 333–351. DOI: 10.1038/nrg.2016.49 PMID: 27184599

Gosling, R., Davies, S. M., & Hussey, J. A. (2016). How integrating primary care and public health could improve population health outcomes: A view from Liverpool, UK. *Public Health Research & Practice*, *26*(1), e2611602. DOI: 10.17061/phrp2611602 PMID: 26863165

Gottlieb, S., & Silvis, L. (2023). Regulators face novel challenges as artificial intelligence tools enter medical practice. *JAMA Health Forum*, *4*(6), e232300. DOI: 10.1001/jamahealthforum.2023.2300 PMID: 37289461

Green, C. A., Duan, N., Gibbons, R. D., Hoagwood, K. E., Palinkas, L. A., & Wisdom, J. P. (2015). Approaches to Mixed Methods Dissemination and Implementation Research: Methods, Strengths, Caveats, and Opportunities. *Administration and Policy in Mental Health*, *42*(5), 508–523. DOI: 10.1007/s10488-014-0552-6 PMID: 24722814

Gualtero, D. F., Lafaurie, G. I., Buitrago, D. M., Castillo, Y., Vargas-Sanchez, P. K., & Castillo, D. M. (2023). Oral microbiome mediated inflammation, a potential inductor of vascular diseases: A comprehensive review. *Frontiers in Cardiovascular Medicine*, *10*, 1250263. DOI: 10.3389/fcvm.2023.1250263 PMID: 37711554

Guan, W., Li, J., Liang, Q., Huang, Y., Li, S., Xu, X., Zhang, Y., Wang, F., & Xu, X. (2024). Disease burden and health inequality of older adults with edentulism and the projected trend until 2040: Based on the Global Burden of Disease study 2021. *Clinical Oral Investigations*, *29*(1), 22. DOI: 10.1007/s00784-024-06111-5 PMID: 39699767

Guevara-Vega, M., Rosa, R. B., Caixeta, D. C., Costa, M. A., de Souza, R. C., Ferreira, G. M., Mundim Filho, A. C., Carneiro, M. G., Jardim, A. C. G., & Sabino-Silva, R. (2024). Salivary detection of Chikungunya virus infection using a portable and sustainable biophotonic platform coupled with artificial intelligence algorithms. *Scientific Reports*, *14*(1), 21546. DOI: 10.1038/s41598-024-71889-z PMID: 39278957

Guido, R., Ferrisi, S., Lofaro, D., & Conforti, D. (2024). An Overview on the Advancements of Support Vector Machine Models in Healthcare Applications: A Review. *Information (Basel)*, *15*(4), 235. DOI: 10.3390/info15040235

Gummin, D. D., Mowry, J. B., Beuhler, M. C., Spyker, D. A., Rivers, L. J., Feldman, R., Brown, K., Pham, N. P. T., Bronstein, A. C., & DesLauriers, C. (2023). 2022 Annual report of the national poison data system®(NPDS) from America's Poison Centers®: 40th annual report. *Clinical Toxicology : The Official Journal of the American Academy of Clinical Toxicology and European Association of Poisons Centres and Clinical Toxicologists*, *61*(10), 717–939. DOI: 10.1080/15563650.2023.2268981 PMID: 38084513

Gwathmey, T. M., Williams, K. L., Caban-Holt, A., Starks, T. D., Foy, C. G., Mathews, A., & Byrd, G. S. (2024). Building a Community Partnership for the Development of Health Ministries Within the African American Community: The Triad Pastors Network. *Journal of Community Health*, *49*(3), 559–567. DOI: 10.1007/s10900-023-01315-4 PMID: 38265538

Hajat, C. (2011). An introduction to epidemiology. *Methods in Molecular Biology (Clifton, N.J.)*, *713*, 27–39. DOI: 10.1007/978-1-60327-416-6_3 PMID: 21153609

Hajishengallis, G. (2015). Periodontitis: From microbial immune subversion to systemic inflammation. *Nature Reviews. Immunology*, *15*(1), 30–44. DOI: 10.1038/nri3785 PMID: 25534621

Hajishengallis, G. (2022). Interconnection of periodontal disease and comorbidities: Evidence, mechanisms, and implications. *Periodontology 2000*, *89*(1), 9–18. DOI: 10.1111/prd.12430 PMID: 35244969

Hajishengallis, G., & Chavakis, T. (2021). Local and systemic mechanisms linking periodontal disease and inflammatory comorbidities. *Nature Reviews. Immunology*, *21*(7), 426–440. DOI: 10.1038/s41577-020-00488-6 PMID: 33510490

Haldane, V., Ariyarajah, A., Berry, I., Loutet, M., Salamanca-Buentello, F., & Upshur, R. E. G. (2023). Global inequity creates local insufficiency: A qualitative study of COVID-19 vaccine implementation challenges in low-and-middle-income countries. *PLoS One*, *18*(2), e0281358. DOI: 10.1371/journal.pone.0281358 PMID: 36780502

Hasin, Y., Seldin, M., & Lusis, A. (2017). Multi-omics approaches to disease. *Genome Biology*, *18*(1), 83. DOI: 10.1186/s13059-017-1215-1 PMID: 28476144

Hendrickx, J., Gracea, R., Vanheers, M., Winderickx, N., Preda, F., Shujaat, S., & Jacobs, R. (2024). Can artificial intelligence-driven cephalometric analysis replace manual tracing? A systematic review and meta-analysis. *European Journal of Orthodontics*, *46*(5), cjae029. Advance online publication. DOI: 10.1093/ejo/cjae029 PMID: 38895901

Henning, K. J. (2004). Overview of syndromic surveillance: What is syndromic surveillance? MMWR Supplements, 53, 5-11.

Henning-Smith, C., Moscovice, I., & Kozhimannil, K. (2019). Differences in social isolation and its relationship to health by rurality: Rural–urban differences in social isolation. *The Journal of Rural Health : Official Journal of the American Rural Health Association and the National Rural Health Care Association*, *35*(4), 540–549. DOI: 10.1111/jrh.12344 PMID: 30609155

Hernán, M. A., & Robins, J. M. (2020). *Causal inference: What if?* Chapman & Hall/CRC.

Herrera, D., Sanz, M., Shapira, L., Brotons, C., Chapple, I., Frese, T., Graziani, F., Hobbs, F. D. R., Huck, O., Hummers, E., Jepsen, S., Kravtchenko, O., Madianos, P., Molina, A., Ungan, M., Vilaseca, J., Windak, A., & Vinker, S. (2024). Periodontal diseases and cardiovascular diseases, diabetes, and respiratory diseases: Summary of the consensus report by the European Federation of Periodontology and WONCA Europe. *The European Journal of General Practice*, *30*(1), 2320120. DOI: 10.1080/13814788.2024.2320120 PMID: 38511739

Hoagland, A., & Kipping, S. (2024). Challenges in promoting health equity and reducing disparities in access across new and established technologies. *The Canadian Journal of Cardiology*, *40*(6), 1154–1167. DOI: 10.1016/j.cjca.2024.02.014 PMID: 38417572

Hobson, G., Adamson, J., Adler, H., Firth, R., Gould, S., Houlihan, C., Johnson, C., Porter, D., Rampling, T., Ratcliffe, L., Russell, K., Shankar, A. G., & Wingfield, T. (2021). Family cluster of three cases of monkeypox imported from Nigeria to the United Kingdom, May 2021. *Eurosurveillance*, *26*(32), 2100745. DOI: 10.2807/1560-7917.ES.2021.26.32.2100745 PMID: 34387184

Howard, A. G., Attard, S. M., Herring, A. H., Wang, H., Du, S., & Gordon-Larsen, P. (2021). Socioeconomic gradients in the Westernization of diet in China over 20 years. *SSM - Population Health*, *16*, 100943. DOI: 10.1016/j.ssmph.2021.100943 PMID: 34703875

Huang, C., Wang, J., Wang, S., & Zhang, Y. (2023). A review of deep learning in dentistry. *Neurocomputing*, *554*, 126629. DOI: 10.1016/j.neucom.2023.126629

Hu, M., Shu, X., Yu, G., Wu, X., Välimäki, M., & Feng, H. (2021). A risk prediction model based on machine learning for cognitive impairment among Chinese community-dwelling elderly people with normal cognition: Development and validation study. *Journal of Medical Internet Research*, *23*(2), e20298. DOI: 10.2196/20298 PMID: 33625369

Hung, M., Voss, M., Rosales, M., Li, W., Su, W., Xu, J., Bounsanga, J., Ruiz-Negrón, B., Lauren, E., & Licari, F. W. (2019). Application of machine learning for diagnostic prediction of root caries. *Gerodontology*, *36*(4), 395–404. DOI: 10.1111/ger.12432 PMID: 31274221

Hünniger, K., Lehnert, T., Bieber, K., Martin, R., Figge, M. T., & Kurzai, O. (2014). A virtual infection model quantifies innate effector mechanisms and *Candida albicans* immune escape in human blood. *PLoS Computational Biology*, *10*(2), e1003479. DOI: 10.1371/journal.pcbi.1003479 PMID: 24586131

Hunsrisakhun, J., Naorungroj, S., Tangkuptanon, W., Wattanasit, P., Pupong, K., & Pithpornchaiyakul, S. (2025). Impact of oral health chatbot with and without toothbrushing training on childhood caries. *International Dental Journal*, *75*(2), 1348–1359. DOI: 10.1016/j.identj.2024.09.028 PMID: 39443262

Huynh, T. M., & Cohen, D. (2013). Innovators and early adopters of population health in healthcare: Real and present opportunities for healthcare-public health collaboration. *Healthcare Papers*, *13*(3), 53–89. DOI: 10.12927/hcpap.2014.23683 PMID: 24524572

Ibraheem, W. I., Jain, S., Ayoub, M. N., Namazi, M. A., Alfaqih, A. I., Aggarwal, A., Meshni, A. A., Almarghlani, A., & Alhumaidan, A. A. (2025). Assessment of the Diagnostic Accuracy of Artificial Intelligence Software in Identifying Common Periodontal and Restorative Dental Conditions (Marginal Bone Loss, Periapical Lesion, Crown, Restoration, Dental Caries) in Intraoral Periapical Radiographs. *Diagnostics (Basel)*, *15*(11), 1432. DOI: 10.3390/diagnostics15111432 PMID: 40507004

Ide, M., & Papapanou, P. N. (2013). Epidemiology of the association between maternal periodontal disease and adverse pregnancy outcomes—Systematic review. *Journal of Periodontology*, *84*(4S, 4-s), S181–S194. DOI: 10.1902/jop.2013.134009 PMID: 23631578

Ioannidis, J. P. A. (2005). Why most published research findings are false. *PLoS Medicine*, *2*(8), e124. DOI: 10.1371/journal.pmed.0020124 PMID: 16060722

Isiaka, A. B., Anakwenze, V. N., Ilodinso, C. R., Anaukwu, C. G., Ezeokoli, C. M.-V., Noi, S. M., Agboola, G. O., & Adonu, R. M.Amarachukwu Bernaldine IsiakaVivian Nonyelum AnakwenzeChiamaka Rosemary IlodinsoChikodili Gladys AnaukwuChukwuebuka Mary-Vin EzeokoliSamuel Mensah NoiGazali Oluwasegun AgboolaRichard Mensah Adonu. (2024). Harnessing Artificial Intelligence for Early Detection and Management of Infectious Disease Outbreaks. *International Journal of Innovative Research and Development*. Advance online publication. DOI: 10.24940/ijird/2024/v13/i2/FEB24016

Islam, S. (2025). Evaluating the impact of AI-generated educational content on patient understanding and anxiety in endodontics and restorative dentistry: A comparative study. *BMC Oral Health*, *25*(1), 689. DOI: 10.1186/s12903-025-06069-0 PMID: 40335999

Iwelunmor, J., Newsome, V., & Airhihenbuwa, C. O. (2014). Framing the impact of culture on health: A systematic review of the PEN-3 cultural model and its application in public health research and interventions. *Ethnicity & Health*, *19*(1), 20–46. DOI: 10.1080/13557858.2013.857768 PMID: 24266638

Jafari, P., & Azuaje, F. (2006). An assessment of recently published gene expression data analyses: Reporting experimental design and statistical factors. *BMC Medical Informatics and Decision Making*, *6*(1), 27. DOI: 10.1186/1472-6947-6-27 PMID: 16790051

Jain, N., Dutt, U., Radenkov, I., & Jain, S. (2024). WHO's global oral health status report 2022: Actions, discussion and implementation. *Oral Diseases*, *30*(2), 73–79. DOI: 10.1111/odi.14516 PMID: 36680388

Jamieson, L., Haag, D., Schuch, H., Kapellas, K., Arantes, R., & Thomson, W. M. (2020). Indigenous Oral Health Inequalities at an International Level: A Commentary. *International Journal of Environmental Research and Public Health*, *17*(11), 3958. DOI: 10.3390/ijerph17113958 PMID: 32503229

Janssens, B., Vanobbergen, J., Petrovic, M., Jacquet, W., Schols, J. M. G. A., & De Visschere, L. (2017). The oral health condition and treatment needs assessment of nursing home residents in Flanders (Belgium). *Community Dental Health, 34*(3), 143–151. DOI: 10.1922/CDH_4086Janssens09 PMID: 28872808

Javed, F., Rahman, I., & Romanos, G. E. (2019). Tobacco-product usage as a risk factor for dental implants. *Periodontology 2000, 81*(1), 48–56. DOI: 10.1111/prd.12282 PMID: 31407428

Jeong, J., Kim, K., Gu, Y., Yoon, D., Zhang, M., Wang, L., & Kim, J.-H. (2025). Deep learning for automated dental plaque index assessment: Validation against expert evaluations. *BMC Oral Health, 25*(1), 1000. DOI: 10.1186/s12903-025-06350-2 PMID: 40604649

Jepsen, S., Suvan, J., & Deschner, J. (2020). The association of periodontal diseases with metabolic syndrome and obesity. *Periodontology 2000, 83*(1), 125–153. DOI: 10.1111/prd.12326 PMID: 32385882

Jia, S., Li, X., & Du, Q. (2023). Host insulin resistance caused by *Porphyromonas gingivalis*—Review of recent progresses. *Frontiers in Cellular and Infection Microbiology, 13*, 1209381. DOI: 10.3389/fcimb.2023.1209381 PMID: 37520442

Jindal, M., Chaiyachati, K. H., Fung, V., Manson, S. M., & Mortensen, K. (2023). Eliminating health care inequities through strengthening access to care. *Health services research, 58 Suppl 3*(Suppl 3), 300–310. .DOI: 10.1111/1475-6773.14202

Jing, Y., Bian, Y., Hu, Z., Wang, L., & Xie, X. Q. (2018). Deep Learning for Drug Design: An Artificial Intelligence Paradigm for Drug Discovery in the Big Data Era. *The AAPS Journal, 20*(3), 58. DOI: 10.1208/s12248-018-0210-0 PMID: 29603063

Jin, L. J., Lamster, I. B., Greenspan, J. S., Pitts, N. B., Scully, C., & Warnakulasuriya, S. (2016). Global burden of oral diseases: Emerging concepts, management and interplay with systemic health. *Oral Diseases, 22*(7), 609–619. DOI: 10.1111/odi.12428 PMID: 26704694

Joda, T., & Spallek, H. (2023). Editorial: Precision dentistry and ehealth in oral healthcare. *Frontiers in Oral Health, 4*, 1155166. DOI: 10.3389/froh.2023.1155166 PMID: 36960387

Johansson, C., Beckman, L., Rystedt, I., Kramer, A. C. A., & Lindmark, U. (2025). Oral health and oral health needs among patients with serious mental illness: Reflections and experiences of psychiatric staff in Sweden. *BMC Psychology, 13*(1), 446. DOI: 10.1186/s40359-025-02780-3 PMID: 40296173

Johnson, P.. (2025). Metagenomic detection of oral pathogens in municipal wastewater: A feasibility study. *The Science of the Total Environment, 850*, 157962.

Joseph, B. K., Kullman, L., & Sharma, P. N. (2016). The oral-systemic disease connection: A retrospective study. *Clinical Oral Investigations, 20*(8), 2267–2273. DOI: 10.1007/s00784-016-1725-3 PMID: 26841905

Joshi, V., Matthews, C., Aspiras, M., de Jager, M., Ward, M., & Kumar, P. (2014). Smoking decreases structural and functional resilience in the subgingival ecosystem. *Journal of Clinical Periodontology, 41*(11), 1037–1047. DOI: 10.1111/jcpe.12300 PMID: 25139209

Junaid, S. B., Imam, A. A., Balogun, A. O., De Silva, L. C., Surakat, Y. A., Kumar, G., Abdulkarim, M., Shuaibu, A. N., Garba, A., Sahalu, Y., Mohammed, A., Mohammed, T. Y., Abdulkadir, B. A., Abba, A. A., Kakumi, N. A. I., & Mahamad, S. (2022). Recent Advancements in Emerging Technologies for Healthcare Management Systems: A Survey. *Healthcare (Basel), 10*(10), 1940. DOI: 10.3390/healthcare10101940 PMID: 36292387

Kahn, M. G., Callahan, T. J., Barnard, J., Bauck, A. E., Brown, J., Davidson, B. N., & Zozus, M. N. (2016). A harmonized data quality assessment terminology and framework for the secondary use of electronic health record data. *EGEMS (Washington, DC), 4*(1), 1244. DOI: 10.13063/2327-9214.1244 PMID: 27713905

Kalenderian, E.. (2013). BigMouth: A multi-institutional dental data repository. *The Journal of the American Dental Association, 144*(12), 144–153.

Kang, J. W., Tang, X., Walton, C. J., Brown, M. J., Brewer, R. A., Maddela, R. L., Zheng, J. J., Agus, J. K., & Zivkovic, A. M. (2022). Multi-omic analyses reveal bifidogenic effects and metabolomic shifts in a healthy human cohort supplemented with a prebiotic dietary fiber blend. *Frontiers in Nutrition, 9*, 908534. DOI: 10.3389/fnut.2022.908534 PMID: 35782954

Kang, S., Shon, B., Park, E. Y., Jeong, S., & Kim, E. K. (2024). Diagnostic accuracy of dental caries detection using ensemble techniques in deep learning with intraoral camera images. *PLoS One, 19*(9), e0310004. DOI: 10.1371/journal.pone.0310004 PMID: 39241044

Kapila, Y. L. (2021). Oral health's inextricable connection to systemic health: Special populations bring to bear multimodal relationships and factors connecting periodontal disease to systemic diseases and conditions. *Periodontology 2000, 87*(1), 11–16. DOI: 10.1111/prd.12398 PMID: 34463994

Kaptoge, S., Seshasai, S. R. K., Gao, P., Freitag, D. F., Butterworth, A. S., Borglykke, A., Di Angelantonio, E., Gudnason, V., Rumley, A., Lowe, G. D. O., Jorgensen, T., & Danesh, J. (2014). Inflammatory cytokines and risk of coronary heart disease: New prospective study and updated meta-analysis. *European Heart Journal*, *35*(9), 578–589. DOI: 10.1093/eurheartj/eht367 PMID: 24026779

Karamüftüoğlu, N., Üçpunar, B. Y., Birben, İ., Altundağ, A. E., Mullaoğlu, K. Ö., & Bal, C. (2026). Artificial Intelligence in Pediatric Dentistry: A Systematic Review and Meta-Analysis. *Children (Basel, Switzerland)*, *13*(1), 152. DOI: 10.3390/children13010152 PMID: 41597160

Karobari, M. I., Adil, A. H., Basheer, S. N., Murugesan, S., Savadamoorthi, K. S., Mustafa, M., Abdulwahed, A., & Almokhatieb, A. A. (2023). Evaluation of the diagnostic and prognostic accuracy of artificial intelligence in endodontic dentistry: A comprehensive review of literature. *Computational and Mathematical Methods in Medicine*, *7049360*(1), 7049360. Advance online publication. DOI: 10.1155/2023/7049360 PMID: 36761829

Kassebaum, N. J., Smith, A. G. C., Bernabé, E., Fleming, T. D., Reynolds, A. E., Vos, T., Murray, C. J. L., Marcenes, W., Abyu, G. Y., Alsharif, U., Asayesh, H., Benzian, H., Dandona, L., Dandona, R., Kasaeian, A., Khader, Y. S., Khang, Y. H., Kokubo, Y., Kotsakis, G. A., & Yonemoto, N. (2017). Global, Regional, and National Prevalence, Incidence, and Disability-Adjusted Life Years for Oral Conditions for 195 Countries, 1990-2015: A Systematic Analysis for the Global Burden of Diseases, Injuries, and Risk Factors. *Journal of Dental Research*, *96*(4), 380–387. DOI: 10.1177/0022034517693566 PMID: 28792274

Katsumata, A. (2023). Deep learning and artificial intelligence in dental diagnostic imaging. *Japanese Dental Science Review*, *59*, 329–333. DOI: 10.1016/j.jdsr.2023.09.004 PMID: 37811196

Kau, A. L., Ahern, P. P., Griffin, N. W., Goodman, A. L., & Gordon, J. I. (2011). Human nutrition, the gut microbiome and the immune system. *Nature*, *474*(7351), 327–336. DOI: 10.1038/nature10213 PMID: 21677749

Kaushik, R., & Rapaka, R. (2025). AI-driven evolution in teledentistry: A comprehensive overview of technology and clinical applications. *Dentistry Review*, *5*(2), 100154. DOI: 10.1016/j.dentre.2025.100154

Kaye, J., Whitley, E. A., Lund, D., Morrison, M., Teare, H., & Melham, K. (2015). Dynamic consent: A patient interface for twenty-first century research networks. *European Journal of Human Genetics : EJHG*, *23*(2), 141–146. DOI: 10.1038/ejhg.2014.71 PMID: 24801761

Kazimierczak, W., Wajer, R., Wajer, A., Kalka, K., Kazimierczak, N., & Serafin, Z. (2024). Evaluating the diagnostic accuracy of an AI-driven platform for assessing endodontic treatment outcomes using panoramic radiographs: A preliminary study. *Journal of Clinical Medicine*, *13*(12), 3401. DOI: 10.3390/jcm13123401 PMID: 38929931

Kearns, C., Peres, M. A., & Watt, R. G. (2021). The future of dental public health: Precision, prevention, and integration. *Community Dentistry and Oral Epidemiology*, *49*(5), 369–375.

Keesara, S., Jonas, A., & Schulman, K. (2020). Covid-19 and health care's digital revolution. *The New England Journal of Medicine*, *382*(23), e82. DOI: 10.1056/NEJMp2005835 PMID: 32240581

Khadka, S., Khan, S., King, A., Goldberg, L. R., Crocombe, L., & Bettiol, S. (2021). Poor oral hygiene, oral microorganisms and aspiration pneumonia risk in older people in residential aged care: A systematic review. *Age and Ageing*, *50*(1), 81–87. DOI: 10.1093/ageing/afaa102 PMID: 32677660

Khairunnisa, Z., Siluvai, S., Kanakavelan, K., Agnes, L., Indumathi, K. P., & Krishnaprakash, G. (2024). Mental and oral health: a dual frontier in healthcare integration and prevention. *Cureus, 16*(12). Afroz, T., Beyene, J., Zaheer, K., Alameddine, M., Nabi, M. H., Hawlader, M. D. H., & Hossain, A. (2025). Oral health care challenges in individuals with severe mental illness: a qualitative meta-synthesis. *Frontiers in Oral Health*, *6*, 1655450.

Khammissa, R. A. G., & Andriankaja, O. M. (2025). Deepening the relationship between diabetes, oral health and periodontal disease. *Frontiers in Oral Health*, *6*, 1752592. DOI: 10.3389/froh.2025.1752592 PMID: 41584962

Khan, A., Barapatre, A. R., Babar, N., Doshi, J., Ghaly, M., Patel, K. G., Nawaz, S. M., Hasana, U. M., Khatri, S. P. M., Pathange, S. M., Pesaru, A. R., Puvvada, C. S., Billoo, M., & Jamil, U. (2025). Genomic medicine and personalized treatment: A narrative review. *Annals of Medicine and Surgery (London)*, *87*(3), 1406–1414. DOI: 10.1097/MS9.0000000000002965 PMID: 40213198

Khanagar, S. B., Al-Ehaideb, A., Maganur, P. C., Vishwanathaiah, S., Patil, S., & Naik, S. (2021). Developments, applications, and performance of artificial intelligence in dentistry – A systematic review. *Journal of Dental Sciences*, *16*(1), 508–522. DOI: 10.1016/j.jds.2020.06.019 PMID: 33384840

Khanagar, S. B., Alfadley, A., Alfouzan, K., Awawdeh, M., Alaqla, A., & Jamleh, A. (2023). Developments and performance of artificial intelligence models designed for application in endodontics: A systematic review. *Diagnostics (Basel)*, *13*(3), 414. DOI: 10.3390/diagnostics13030414 PMID: 36766519

Khoury, M. J., Bowen, M. S., Clyne, M., Dotson, W. D., Gwinn, M. L., Green, R. F., Kolor, K., Rodriguez, J. L., Wulf, A., & Yu, W. (2018). From public health genomics to precision public health: A 20-year journey. *Genetics in Medicine : Official Journal of the American College of Medical Genetics*, *20*(6), 574–582. DOI: 10.1038/gim.2017.211 PMID: 29240076

Khoury, M. J., Iademarco, M. F., & Riley, W. T. (2016). Precision public health for the era of precision medicine. *American Journal of Preventive Medicine*, *50*(3), 398–401. DOI: 10.1016/j.amepre.2015.08.031 PMID: 26547538

Kilian, M., Chapple, I. L. C., Hannig, M., Marsh, P. D., Meuric, V., Pedersen, A. M. L., Tonetti, M. S., Wade, W. G., & Zaura, E. (2016). The oral microbiome—An update for oral healthcare professionals. *British Dental Journal*, *221*(10), 657–666. DOI: 10.1038/sj.bdj.2016.865 PMID: 27857087

Kim, H. S., Choi, E. H., Khan, J., Roilides, E., Francesconi, A., Kasai, M., Sein, T., Schaufele, R. L., Sakurai, K., Son, C. G., Greer, B. T., Chanock, S., Lyman, C. A., & Walsh, T. J. (2005). Expression of genes encoding innate host defense molecules in normal human monocytes in response to *Candida albicans*. *Infection and Immunity*, *73*(6), 3714–3724. DOI: 10.1128/IAI.73.6.3714-3724.2005 PMID: 15908401

Kinane, D. F., Stathopoulou, P. G., & Papapanou, P. N. (2017). Periodontal diseases. *Nature Reviews. Disease Primers*, *3*(1), 17038. DOI: 10.1038/nrdp.2017.38 PMID: 28805207

Kisely, S. (2016). No mental health without oral health. *Canadian Journal of Psychiatry. Revue Canadienne de Psychiatrie*, *61*(5), 277–282. DOI: 10.1177/0706743716632523 PMID: 27254802

Kisely, S. (2023). Periodontal health and psychiatric disorders. *Current Oral Health Reports*, *10*(3), 111–116. DOI: 10.1007/s40496-023-00339-y

Kisely, S., Sawyer, E., Siskind, D., & Lalloo, R. (2016). The oral health of people with anxiety and depressive disorders–a systematic review and meta-analysis. *Journal of Affective Disorders*, *200*, 119–132. DOI: 10.1016/j.jad.2016.04.040 PMID: 27130961

Knight, E. T., Liu, J., Seymour, G. J., Faggion, C. M.Jr, & Cullinan, M. P. (2016). Risk factors that may modify the innate and adaptive immune responses in periodontal diseases. *Periodontology 2000*, *71*(1), 22–51. DOI: 10.1111/prd.12110 PMID: 27045429

Kocher, T., Meisel, P., Baumeister, S., & Holtfreter, B. (2024). Impact of public health and patient-centered prevention strategies on periodontitis and caries as causes of tooth loss in high-income countries. *Periodontology 2000*, *98*(1), 65–99. DOI: 10.1111/prd.12592 PMID: 39323071

Kosan, E., Krois, J., Wingenfeld, K., Deuter, C. E., Gaudin, R., & Schwendicke, F. (2022). Patients' perspectives on artificial intelligence in dentistry: A controlled study. *Journal of Clinical Medicine*, *11*(8), 2143. DOI: 10.3390/jcm11082143 PMID: 35456236

Kraemer, M., Tsui, J. L.-H., Chang, S. Y., Lytras, S., Khurana, M. P., Vanderslott, S., Bajaj, S., Scheidwasser, N., Curran-Sebastian, J. L., Semenova, E., Zhang, M., Unwin, H. J. T., Watson, O. J., Mills, C., Dasgupta, A., Ferretti, L., Scarpino, S. V., Koua, E., Morgan, O., & Bhatt, S. (2025). Artificial intelligence for modelling infectious disease epidemics. *Nature*, *638*(8051), 623–635. DOI: 10.1038/s41586-024-08564-w PMID: 39972226

Kranz, A. M., Gahlon, G., Dick, A. W., & Stein, B. D. (2019). Characteristics of US adults who delay dental care due to cost. *Journal of Public Health Dentistry*, *79*(4), 331–339. PMID: 31407343

Krenz, A., & Strulik, H. (2023). Physiological aging in India: The role of the epidemiological transition. *PLoS One*, *18*(7), e0287259. DOI: 10.1371/journal.pone.0287259 PMID: 37467173

Kreuter, M. W., Thompson, T., McQueen, A., & Garg, R. (2021). Addressing Social Needs in Health Care Settings: Evidence, Challenges, and Opportunities for Public Health. *Annual Review of Public Health*, *42*(1), 329–344. DOI: 10.1146/annurev-publhealth-090419-102204 PMID: 33326298

Krüger, T., Luo, T., Schmidt, H., Shopova, I., & Kniemeyer, O. (2015). Challenges and strategies for proteome analysis of the interaction of human pathogenic fungi with host immune cells. *Proteomes*, *3*(4), 467–495. DOI: 10.3390/proteomes3040467 PMID: 28248281

Kruk, M. E., Gage, A. D., Arsenault, C., Jordan, K., Leslie, H. H., Roder-DeWan, S., Adeyi, O., Barker, P., Daelmans, B., Doubova, S. V., English, M., García-Elorrio, E., Guanais, F., Gureje, O., Hirschhorn, L. R., Jiang, L., Kelley, E., Lemango, E. T., Liljestrand, J., & Pate, M. (2018). High-quality health systems in the sustainable development goals era: Time for a revolution. *The Lancet. Global Health*, *6*(11), e1196–e1252. DOI: 10.1016/S2214-109X(18)30386-3 PMID: 30196093

Kruse, C. S., Goswamy, R., Raval, Y. J., & Basha, S. (2016). Challenges and opportunities of big data in health care: A systematic review. *JMIR Medical Informatics*, *4*(4), e5359. DOI: 10.2196/medinform.5359 PMID: 27872036

Labus, A., Radenković, B., Rodić, B., Barać, D., & Malešević, A. (2021). Enhancing smart healthcare in dentistry: An approach to managing patients' stress. *Informatics for Health & Social Care*, *46*(3), 306–319. DOI: 10.1080/17538157.2021.1893322 PMID: 33784958

Lampe, N. M., Barbee, H., Tran, N. M., Bastow, S., & McKay, T. (2024). Health Disparities among Lesbian, Gay, Bisexual, Transgender, and Queer Older Adults: A Structural Competency Approach. *International Journal of Aging & Human Development*, *98*(1), 39–55. DOI: 10.1177/00914150231171838 PMID: 37122150

Lamster, I. B. (2021). Oral health's inextricable connection to systemic health. *Periodontology 2000*, *87*(1), 11–16. PMID: 34463994

Lamster, I. B. (2021). The 2021 WHO Resolution on Oral Health. *International Dental Journal*, *71*(4), 279–280. DOI: 10.1016/j.identj.2021.06.003 PMID: 34256923

Lamster, I. B. (2022). The nexus of oral and general health: Review and future directions. *Periodontology 2000*, *89*(1), 9–15. PMID: 35244969

Lamster, I. B., & Meyerowitz, C. (2021). The 2021 WHO resolution on oral health: Implications for global oral health. *Journal of Public Health Dentistry*, *81*(3), 177–179.

Lan, R., Zhang, M.-J., Liu, K., Meng, F.-F., Xu, X.-H., & Wang, C.-C.. (2024). Cytochrome P450-derived epoxyeicosatrienoic acid, the regulation of cardiovascular-related diseases, and the implication for pulmonary hypertension. *Cardiovascular Drugs and Therapy*, •••, 1–17. DOI: 10.1007/s10557-024-07655-0 PMID: 39652233

Lappalainen, H. K., Baklanov, A., Bäck, J., Arvanitidis, C., Basart, S., Bernier, N., Berod, D., Bornman, T., Buttigieg, P. L., Carmichael, G., Dañobeitia, J., De Roeck, Y.-H., Dey, S., Gerasopoulos, E., Feig, G., Gani, S., Glaves, H., Häme, S., Juurola, E., & Kulmala, M. (2025). Towards a Global Ground-Based Earth Observatory (GG-BEO): Leveraging existing systems and networks. *Big Earth Data*, *9*(4), 615–650. DOI: 10.1080/20964471.2025.2574174

Lazaro-Mojica, J., & Fernandez, R. (2021). Review paper on the future of the food sector through education, capacity building, knowledge translation and open innovation. *Current Opinion in Food Science, 38*, 162–167. DOI: 10.1016/j.cofs.2020.11.009

Lazer, D., Kennedy, R., King, G., & Vespignani, A. (2014). The parable of Google Flu: Traps in big data analysis. *Science, 343*(6176), 1203–1205. DOI: 10.1126/science.1248506 PMID: 24626916

Ledger, D., & McCaffrey, D. (2014). Inside wearables: How the science of human behavior change offers the secret to long-term engagement. *Endeavour Partners, 200*(93), 1–17.

Lee, J. H., Kim, D. H., Jeong, S. N., & Choi, S. H. (2018). Detection and diagnosis of dental caries using a deep learning-based convolutional neural network algorithm. *Journal of Dentistry, 77*, 106–111. DOI: 10.1016/j.jdent.2018.07.015 PMID: 30056118

Lee, J. H., Kim, Y. T., & Lee, J. B. (2024). Identification of dental implant systems from low-quality and distorted dental radiographs using AI trained on a large multi-center dataset. *Scientific Reports, 14*(1), 12606. DOI: 10.1038/s41598-024-63422-z PMID: 38824187

Lehnert, T., Timme, S., Pollmächer, J., Hünniger, K., Kurzai, O., & Figge, M. T. (2015). Bottom-up modeling approach for the quantitative estimation of parameters in pathogen–host interactions. *Frontiers in Microbiology, 6*, 608. DOI: 10.3389/fmicb.2015.00608 PMID: 26150807

Lei, Y., Li, M., Zhang, H., Deng, Y., Dong, X., Chen, P., Li, Y., Zhang, S., Li, C., Wang, S., & Tao, R. (2025). Comparative analysis of the human microbiome from four different regions of China and machine learning-based geographical inference. *MSphere, 10*(1), e00672–e24. DOI: 10.1128/msphere.00672-24 PMID: 39699186

Libbrecht, M. W., & Noble, W. S. (2015). Machine learning applications in genetics and genomics. *Nature Reviews. Genetics, 16*(6), 321–332. DOI: 10.1038/nrg3920 PMID: 25948244

Li, H., Chen, S., Chang, B., Wang, X., He, Y., Xu, B., Sun, G., Yang, C., Li, G., Li, S., & Li, G. (2026). Application of artificial intelligence in oral health management: Challenges and opportunities. *Frontiers in Medicine, 13*, 1700529. DOI: 10.3389/fmed.2026.1700529 PMID: 41709905

Li, L., Novillo-Ortiz, D., Azzopardi-Muscat, N., & Kostkova, P. (2021). Digital data sources and their impact on people's health: A systematic review of systematic reviews. *Frontiers in Public Health*, *9*, 645260. DOI: 10.3389/fpubh.2021.645260 PMID: 34026711

Lim, C. S., Rosli, R., Seow, H. F., & Chong, P. P. (2011). Transcriptome profiling of endothelial cells during infections with high and low densities of *Candida albicans* cells. *International Journal of Medical Microbiology : IJMM*, *301*(6), 536–546. DOI: 10.1016/j.ijmm.2010.12.002 PMID: 21371935

Linden, G. J., & Herzberg, M. C., & Working Group 4 of the Joint EFP/AAP Workshop. (2013). Periodontitis and systemic diseases: Clinical evidence. *Journal of Clinical Periodontology*, *40*(s14), S20–S29. PMID: 23627330

Lipsky, M. S., Singh, T., Zakeri, G., & Hung, M. (2024). Oral health and older adults: A narrative review. *Dentistry Journal*, *12*(2), 30. DOI: 10.3390/dj12020030 PMID: 38392234

Listl, S.. (2019). Value-based oral healthcare: Concepts and application. *Community Dentistry and Oral Epidemiology*, *47*(6), 515–523.

Listl, S., & Filho, A. (2020). *Big Data and Machine Learning*. Textbooks in Contemporary Dentistry., DOI: 10.1007/978-3-030-50123-5_23

Listl, S., Galloway, J., Mossey, P. A., & Marcenes, W. (2015). Global economic impact of dental diseases. *Journal of Dental Research*, *94*(10), 1355–1361. DOI: 10.1177/0022034515602879 PMID: 26318590

Liu, J., Zhang, M., Zhu, M., Tan, S., Luo, X., Liu, J., & Zeng, H. (2025). Comparative analysis of diagnostic techniques and treatment modalities for early-stage esophageal carcinoma: A comprehensive review. *Frontiers in Oncology*, *15*, 1650965. DOI: 10.3389/fonc.2025.1650965 PMID: 40963869

Liu, T., Lee, K., Mukundan, A., Karmakar, R., Dhiman, H., & Wang, H.-C. (2025). AI in dentistry: Innovations, ethical considerations, and integration barriers. *Bioengineering (Basel, Switzerland)*, *12*(9), 928. DOI: 10.3390/bioengineering12090928 PMID: 41007172

Li, X., Kolltveit, K. M., Tronstad, L., & Olsen, I. (2000). Systemic diseases caused by oral infection. *Clinical Microbiology Reviews*, *13*(4), 547–558. DOI: 10.1128/CMR.13.4.547 PMID: 11023956

Li, Y., Wu, X., Liu, M., Deng, K., Tullini, A., Zhang, X., Shi, J., Lai, H., & Tonetti, M. S. (2024). Enhanced control of periodontitis by an artificial intelligence-enabled multimodal-sensing toothbrush and targeted mHealth micromessages: A randomized trial. *Journal of Clinical Periodontology*, *51*(12), 1632–1643. DOI: 10.1111/jcpe.13987 PMID: 38631679

Li, Y., Ye, H., Wu, W., Li, J., Zhao, X., Liu, Y., & Zhou, Y. (2025). Effectiveness and methodologies of virtual reality dental simulators for veneer tooth preparation training: Randomized controlled trial. *Journal of Medical Internet Research*, *27*, e63961. DOI: 10.2196/63961 PMID: 40402564

Li, Y., Zou, Y., & Xu, H. (2024). *From Data to Decisions: The Integration of AI in Epidemiological Research*. Frontiers in Computing and Intelligent Systems., DOI: 10.54097/7jktck77

Love-Koh, J., Griffin, S., Kataika, E., Revill, P., Sibandze, S., & Walker, S. (2020). Methods to promote equity in health resource allocation in low- and middle-income countries: An overview. *Globalization and Health*, *16*(1), 6. DOI: 10.1186/s12992-019-0537-z PMID: 31931823

Lowenstein, A., Singh, M. L., & Papas, A. S. (2025). Addressing disparities in oral health access and outcomes for aging adults in the United States. *Frontiers in Dental Medicine*, *6*, 1522892. DOI: 10.3389/fdmed.2025.1522892 PMID: 40236738

Lv, X., Zhang, X., Li, Y., Ding, X., Lai, H., & Shi, J. (2024). Leveraging large language models for improved patient access and self-management: Assessor-blinded comparison between expert- and AI-generated content. *Journal of Medical Internet Research*, *26*, e55847. DOI: 10.2196/55847 PMID: 38663010

MacCallum, D. M. (2009). Massive induction of innate immune response to *Candida albicans* in the kidney in a murine intravenous challenge model. *FEMS Yeast Research*, *9*(7), 1111–1122. DOI: 10.1111/j.1567-1364.2009.00576.x PMID: 19845042

Mainas, G., Ide, M., Rizzo, M., Magan-Fernandez, A., Mesa, F., & Nibali, L. (2022). Managing the systemic impact of periodontitis. *Medicina (Kaunas, Lithuania)*, *58*(5), 621. DOI: 10.3390/medicina58050621 PMID: 35630038

Maiti, N., Chawla, R., Toure, B., Agrawal, P., & Abba, S. H. (2025, November). Federated Learning for Collaborative Dental Diagnosis Across Hospitals Without Compromising Privacy. In *2025 Tenth International Conference on Science Technology Engineering and Mathematics (ICONSTEM)* (pp. 1-8). IEEE. DOI: 10.1109/ICONSTEM65670.2025.11374623

Majeed, Z. N., Jassim, S. D., & Kamil, Z. H. (2023). Assessment of salivary and gingival crevicular fluids IL6, IL-8, IL-12, and IL-17 levels in healthy subjects and patients with periodontal disease. *Journal of Oral and Maxillofacial Pathology : JOMFP, 27*(3), 494–498. DOI: 10.4103/jomfp.jomfp_170_23 PMID: 38033941

Majmundar, A., Le, N., Moran, M. B., Unger, J. B., & Reuter, K. (2020). Public response to a social media tobacco prevention campaign: Content analysis. *JMIR Public Health and Surveillance, 6*(4), e20649. DOI: 10.2196/20649 PMID: 33284120

Malicka, B., Skośkiewicz-Malinowska, K., & Kaczmarek, U. (2022). The impact of socioeconomic status, general health and oral health on health-related quality of life, oral health-related quality of life and mental health among Polish older adults. *BMC Geriatrics, 22*(1), 2. DOI: 10.1186/s12877-021-02716-7 PMID: 34979959

Mallineni, S., Sethi, M., Punugoti, D., Kotha, S., Alkhayal, Z., Mubaraki, S., Almotawah, F. N., Kotha, S. L., Sajja, R., Nettam, V., Thakare, A. A., & Sakhamuri, S. (2024). Artificial intelligence in dentistry: A descriptive review. *Bioengineering (Basel, Switzerland), 11*(12), 1267. DOI: 10.3390/bioengineering11121267 PMID: 39768085

Mandl, K. D., Gottlieb, D., & Ellis, A. (2020). SMART on FHIR: A standards-based, interoperable apps platform for electronic health records. *Journal of the American Medical Informatics Association : JAMIA, 23*(5), 899–908. DOI: 10.1093/jamia/ocv189 PMID: 26911829

Manolio, T. A., Abramowicz, M., Al-Mulla, F., Anderson, W., Balling, R., Berger, A. C., Bleyl, S., Chakravarti, A., Chantratita, W., Chisholm, R. L., Dissanayake, V. H. W., Dunn, M., Dzau, V. J., Han, B.-G., Hubbard, T., Kolbe, A., Korf, B., Kubo, M., Lasko, P., & Ginsburg, G. S. (2015). Global implementation of genomic medicine: We are not alone. *Science Translational Medicine, 7*(290), 290ps13. DOI: 10.1126/scitranslmed.aab0194 PMID: 26041702

Maranville, J. C., & Di Rienzo, A. (2014). Combining genetic and nongenetic biomarkers to realize the promise of pharmacogenomics for inflammatory diseases. *Pharmacogenomics, 15*(15), 1931–1940. DOI: 10.2217/pgs.14.129 PMID: 25495413

Marashi, S., Hidarnia, A., Kazemi, S., & Shakerinejad, G. (2024). The effect of educational intervention based on self-efficacy theory on promoting adolescent oral health behaviors through mobile application: A randomized controlled trial study. *BMC Oral Health, 24*(1), 1283. DOI: 10.1186/s12903-024-04970-8 PMID: 39448943

Marmot, M. (2017). Social justice, epidemiology, and health inequalities. *European Journal of Epidemiology, 32*(7), 537–546. DOI: 10.1007/s10654-017-0286-3 PMID: 28776115

Martínez, M., Postolache, T. T., García-Bueno, B., Leza, J. C., Figuero, E., Lowry, C. A., & Malan-Müller, S. (2022). The role of the oral microbiota related to periodontal diseases in anxiety, mood and trauma-and stress-related disorders. *Frontiers in Psychiatry*, *12*, 814177. DOI: 10.3389/fpsyt.2021.814177 PMID: 35153869

Martínez-Peláez, R., Ochoa-Brust, A., Rivera, S., Félix, V. G., Ostos, R., Brito, H., Félix, R. A., & Mena, L. J. (2023). Role of Digital Transformation for Achieving Sustainability: Mediated Role of Stakeholders, Key Capabilities, and Technology. *Sustainability (Basel)*, *15*(14), 11221. DOI: 10.3390/su151411221

Martinez, R., Soliz, P., Caixeta, R., & Ordunez, P. (2019). Reflection on modern methods: Years of life lost due to premature mortality-a versatile and comprehensive measure for monitoring non-communicable disease mortality. *International Journal of Epidemiology*, *48*(4), 1367–1376. DOI: 10.1093/ije/dyy254 PMID: 30629192

Martin, N., & Mulligan, S. (2022). Environmental sustainability through good-quality oral healthcare. *International Dental Journal*, *72*(1), 26–30. DOI: 10.1016/j.identj.2021.06.005 PMID: 34412896

Martin, S. S., Aday, A. W., Allen, N. B., Almarzooq, Z. I., Anderson, C. A. M., Arora, P., Avery, C. L., Baker-Smith, C. M., Bansal, N., Beaton, A. Z., Commodore-Mensah, Y., Currie, M. E., Elkind, M. S. V., Fan, W., Generoso, G., Barone Gibbs, B., Heard, D. G., Hiremath, S., Johansen, M. C., & Palaniappan, L. P. (2025). 2025 heart disease and stroke statistics: A report of US and global data from the American Heart Association. *Circulation*, *151*(8), e41–e660. DOI: 10.1161/CIR.0000000000001303 PMID: 39866113

Martins, J., Onofre, M., & Hallal, P. C. (2023). Launch of the Global Observatory for Physical Education (GoPE!). *Journal of Physical Activity & Health*, *20*(7), 573–574. DOI: 10.1123/jpah.2023-0099 PMID: 37130590

Marwaha, K., Cain, R., Asmis, K., Czaplinski, K., Holland, N., Mayer, D. C. G., & Chacon, J. (2025). Exploring the complex relationship between psychosocial stress and the gut microbiome: Implications for inflammation and immune modulation. *Journal of Applied Physiology (Bethesda, Md.)*, *138*(2), 518–535. DOI: 10.1152/japplphysiol.00652.2024 PMID: 39813028

Mathur, M. R., Bhosale, A. S., Abel, S. N., Fisher, J., Listl, S., Carrasco-Labra, A., Urquhart, O., & Glick, M. (2025). Envisioning sustainable oral health through effective advocacy. *BMC Global and Public Health*, *3*(1), 15. DOI: 10.1186/s44263-025-00133-1 PMID: 39972337

Matsuo, H.. (2021). Spatial distribution of dental caries and socioeconomic status in an urban setting: A GIS-based study. *Community Dental Health*, *38*(2), 101–107.

McCarthy, J., Minsky, M. L., Rochester, N., & Shannon, C. E. (2006). A proposal for the Dartmouth summer research project on artificial intelligence, August 31, 1955. *AI Magazine*, *27*(4), 12. https://ojs.aaai.org/aimagazine/index.php/aimagazine/article/view/1904

McDowell, I. (2023). Theoretical models of health behavior. *Understanding health determinants: Explanatory theories for social epidemiology*, 253-306.

McGuire, A. L., Caulfield, T., & Cho, M. K. (2008). Research ethics and the challenge of whole-genome sequencing. *Nature Reviews. Genetics*, *9*(2), 152–156. DOI: 10.1038/nrg2302 PMID: 18087293

McRae, M. P., Kerr, A. R., Janal, M. N., Thornhill, M. H., Redding, S. W., Vigneswaran, N., Kang, S. K., Niederman, R., Christodoulides, N. J., Trochesset, D. A., Murdoch, C., Dapkins, I., Bouquot, J., Modak, S. S., Simmons, G. W., & McDevitt, J. T. (2021). Nuclear F-actin cytology in oral epithelial dysplasia and oral squamous cell carcinoma. *Journal of Dental Research*, *100*(5), 479–486. DOI: 10.1177/0022034520973162 PMID: 33179547

Mei, F., Xie, M., Huang, X., Long, Y., Lu, X., Wang, X., & Chen, L. (2020). *Porphyromonas gingivalis* and Its Systemic Impact: Current Status. *Pathogens (Basel, Switzerland)*, *9*(11), 944. DOI: 10.3390/pathogens9110944 PMID: 33202751

Menon, S., & Koura, K. G. (2025). Artificial intelligence for tuberculosis control: A scoping review of applications in public health. *Journal of Global Health*, *15*, 04192. DOI: 10.7189/jogh.15.04192 PMID: 40709592

Menon, T., Gopalakrishnan, S. N., Balasubramanian, R., & Justin, S. R. (2017). Characterisation of the human oral microbiome in patients with coronary artery disease using next-generation sequencing of 16S rRNA amplicons. *Indian Journal of Medical Microbiology*, *35*(1), 101–104. DOI: 10.4103/ijmm.IJMM_16_370 PMID: 28303827

Mertz, E. A.. (2017). Data systems and oral health surveillance: Opportunities and challenges. *Journal of Public Health Dentistry*, *77*(S1), S59–S69.

Meskó, B., Drobni, Z., Benyei, E., Gergely, B., & Gyorffy, Z. (2017). Digital health is a cultural transformation of traditional healthcare. *mHealth*, *3*, 38. DOI: 10.21037/mhealth.2017.08.07 PMID: 29184890

Meurman, J. H., & Bascones-Martínez, A. (2021). Oral infections and systemic health—More than just links to cardiovascular diseases. *Oral Health & Preventive Dentistry*, *19*(1), 441–448. DOI: 10.3290/j.ohpd.b1993965 PMID: 34505498

Michie, S., Van Stralen, M. M., & West, R. (2011). The behaviour change wheel. *Implementation Science : IS, 6*(1), 42. DOI: 10.1186/1748-5908-6-42 PMID: 21513547

Mittelstadt, B. D., & Floridi, L. (2016). The ethics of big data: Current and foreseeable issues in biomedical contexts. *Science and Engineering Ethics, 22*(2), 303–341. DOI: 10.1007/s11948-015-9652-2 PMID: 26002496

Miura, F., van Ewijk, C. E., Backer, J. A., Xiridou, M., Franz, E., de Coul, E. O., Banwart, D., van Cleef, B., van Rijckevorsel, G., & Swan, C. (2022). Estimated incubation period for monkeypox cases confirmed in the Netherlands, May 2022. *Eurosurveillance, 27*(24), 2200448. DOI: 10.2807/1560-7917.ES.2022.27.24.2200448 PMID: 35713026

Mohammed, S., Mohammed, N., Balammagary, S., Kolla, S., Ganta, S., & Khader, S. (2025). Harnessing artificial intelligence for public health and epidemiology: Opportunities, barriers, and pathways to equitable global impact. *International Journal of Computer Science and Information Technologies, 17*(5), 37–52. DOI: 10.5121/ijcsit.2025.17504

Molete, M. M., Malele-Kolisa, Y., Thekiso, M., Lang, A. Y., Kong, A., & George, A. (2024). The role of community health workers in promoting oral health at school settings: A scoping review. *Journal of Public Health Dentistry, 84*(2), 175–186. DOI: 10.1111/jphd.12612 PMID: 38558304

Montero, E., Bujaldón, R., Montanya, E., Calle-Pascual, A. L., Rojo-Martínez, G., Castaño, L., Franch-Nadal, J., Delgado, E., Chaves, F., Alonso, B., Sanz, M., & Herrera, D. (2024). Cross-sectional association between severe periodontitis and diabetes mellitus: A nation-wide cohort study. *Journal of Clinical Periodontology, 51*(4), 368–379. DOI: 10.1111/jcpe.13937 PMID: 38140803

Moran, A. P., Prendergast, M. M., & Appelmelk, B. J. (1996). Molecular mimicry of host structures by bacterial lipopolysaccharides and its contribution to disease. *FEMS Immunology and Medical Microbiology, 16*(2), 105–115. DOI: 10.1111/j.1574-695X.1996.tb00127.x PMID: 8988391

Morze, J., Wittenbecher, C., Schwingshackl, L., Danielewicz, A., Rynkiewicz, A., Hu, F. B., & Guasch-Ferré, M. (2022). Metabolomics and type 2 diabetes risk: An updated systematic review and meta-analysis of prospective cohort studies. *Diabetes Care, 45*(4), 1013–1024. DOI: 10.2337/dc21-1705 PMID: 35349649

Moynihan, P. J., & Kelly, S. M. (2014). Effect on caries of restricting sugars intake: Systematic review to inform WHO guidelines. *Journal of Dental Research, 93*(1), 8–18. DOI: 10.1177/0022034513508954 PMID: 24323509

Müller, V., Viemann, D., Schmidt, M., Endres, N., Ludwig, S., Leverkus, M., Roth, J., & Goebeler, M. (2007). *Candida albicans* triggers activation of distinct signaling pathways to establish a proinflammatory gene expression program in primary human endothelial cells. *The Journal of Immunology : Official Journal of the American Association of Immunologists*, *179*(12), 8435–8445. DOI: 10.4049/jimmunol.179.12.8435 PMID: 18056390

Murray, P. E., Coffman, J. A., & Garcia-Godoy, F. (2024). Oral pathogens' substantial burden on cancer, cardiovascular diseases, Alzheimer's, diabetes, and other systemic diseases: A public health crisis—A comprehensive review. *Pathogens (Basel, Switzerland)*, *13*(12), 1084. DOI: 10.3390/pathogens13121084 PMID: 39770344

Murugesan, S., Al Ahmad, S. F., Singh, P., Saadaoui, M., Kumar, M., & Al Khodor, S. (2020). Profiling the salivary microbiome of the Qatari population. *Journal of Translational Medicine*, *18*(1), 127. DOI: 10.1186/s12967-020-02291-2 PMID: 32169076

Naicker, S., Plange-Rhule, J., Tutt, R. C., & Eastwood, J. B. (2009). Shortage of healthcare workers in developing countries: Africa. Ethnicity & Disease, 19(1 Suppl 1), S1-60-4.

Nair, P. N. (2004). Pathogenesis of apical periodontitis and the causes of endodontic failures. *Critical reviews in oral biology and medicine: an official publication of the American Association of Oral Biologists, 15*(6), 348–381. https://doi.org/.DOI: 10.1177/154411130401500604

Nair, L., & Adetayo, O. A. (2019). Cultural competence and ethnic diversity in healthcare. *Plastic and Reconstructive Surgery. Global Open*, *7*(5), e2219. DOI: 10.1097/GOX.0000000000002219 PMID: 31333951

Narayanan, A., & Shmatikoff, V. (2008). Robust de-anonymization of large sparse datasets. *2008 IEEE Symposium on Security and Privacy*, 111-125. https://doi.org/ DOI: 10.1109/SP.2008.33

Nassar, H. M.. (2024). A panorama of machine learning in dentistry. *Journal of Clinical and Translational Research*, *10*(4), 1–22.

National Cancer Institute. (2026). *SEER cancer stat facts: Oral cavity and pharynx cancer*. Surveillance, Epidemiology, and End Results (SEER) Program. https://seer.cancer.gov/statfacts/html/oralcav.html

National Institute of Dental and Craniofacial Research (US). (2021). *Oral health in America: Advances and challenges*. Bethesda, MD: Author. https://www.ncbi.nlm.nih.gov/books/NBK576535/

Nazir, M. A. (2017). Prevalence of periodontal disease, its association with systemic diseases, and prevention. *International Journal of Health Sciences (Qassim)*, *11*(2), 72–80. PMID: 28539867

Nelson, S., Kim, E. G. R., & Kaelber, D. C. (2023). Integrating oral health into primary care: Perspectives for older adults. *Journal of Dental Research*, *102*(8), 849–853. DOI: 10.1177/00220345231165011 PMID: 37085982

Newman, M. G., Takei, H. H., Klokkevold, P. R., & Carranza, F. A. (Eds.). (2019). *Newman and Carranza's clinical periodontology* (13th ed.). Elsevier.

Nghayo, H. A., Palanyandi, C. E., Ramphoma, K. J., & Maart, R. (2024). Oral health community engagement programs for rural communities: A scoping review. *PLoS One*, *19*(2), e0297546. DOI: 10.1371/journal.pone.0297546 PMID: 38319914

Ng, S. K., & Leung, W. K. (2008). A community study on the relationship of dental anxiety with oral health status and oral health-related quality of life. *Community Dentistry and Oral Epidemiology*, *36*(4), 347–356. DOI: 10.1111/j.1600-0528.2007.00412.x PMID: 19145721

Nguyen, T. T., Larrivée, N., Lee, A., Bilaniuk, O., & Durand, R. (2021). Use of Artificial Intelligence in Dentistry: Current Clinical Trends and Research Advances. *Journal - Canadian Dental Association*, *87*(2), l7. DOI: 10.12816/0059360 PMID: 34343070

Nicholson, J. K., & Lindon, J. C. (2008). Systems biology: Metabonomics. *Nature*, *455*(7216), 1054–1056. DOI: 10.1038/4551054a PMID: 18948945

Niknam, F., Sharifian, R., Bashiri, A., Mardani, M., Akbari, R., Tuffaha, H., Do, L., & Bastani, P. (2023). Tele-dentistry, its trends, scope, and future framework in oral medicine; a scoping review during January 1999 to December 2021. *Archives of public health = Archives belges de sante publique*, *81*(1), 104. https://doi.org/ .DOI: 10.1186/s13690-023-01128-w

Ni, Y., Alwell, K., & Kravitz, N. D. (2022). Deep learning for cephalometric landmark detection in orthodontics: A systematic review. *The Angle Orthodontist*, *92*(5), 659–667.

Nunez, S. G., Rabelo, S. P., Subotic, N., Caruso, J. W., & Knezevic, N. N. (2025). Chronic stress and autoimmunity: The role of HPA axis and cortisol dysregulation. *International Journal of Molecular Sciences*, *26*(20), 9994. DOI: 10.3390/ijms26209994 PMID: 41155288

Nuzzo, R. (2020). How participatory approaches can make epidemiology more equitable and ethical. *Nature Medicine*, *26*(11), 1669–1672. DOI: 10.1038/s41591-020-1145-1

Nykiforuk, C. I. J., & Flaman, L. M. (2011). Geographic Information Systems (GIS) for Health Promotion and Public Health: A Review. *Health Promotion Practice*, *12*(1), 63–73. DOI: 10.1177/1524839909334624 PMID: 19546198

Obermeyer, Z., Powers, B., Vogeli, C., & Mullainathan, S. (2019). Dissecting racial bias in an algorithm used to manage the health of populations. *Science*, *366*(6464), 447–453. DOI: 10.1126/science.aax2342 PMID: 31649194

Obi, C. O., Jiakor, I. E., Etiaba, E., & Onwujekwe, O. (2024). Collaborations and networks within communities for improved utilization of primary healthcare centers: On the road to universal health coverage. *International Journal of Public Health*, *69*, 1606810. DOI: 10.3389/ijph.2024.1606810 PMID: 38887723

Öçbe, M., Çelebi, E., & Öçbe, Ç. B. (2025). An overlooked connection: Oral health status in patients with chronic diseases. *BMC Oral Health*, *25*(1), 314. DOI: 10.1186/s12903-025-05673-4 PMID: 40016657

Odone, A., Buttigieg, S., Ricciardi, W., Azzopardi-Muscat, N., & Staines, A. (2019). Public health digitalization in Europe. *European Journal of Public Health*, *29*(Supplement_3), 28–35. DOI: 10.1093/eurpub/ckz161 PMID: 31738441

Offenbacher, S., Katz, V., Fertik, G., Collins, J., Boyd, D., Maynor, G., McKaig, R., & Beck, J. (1996). Periodontal infection as a possible risk factor for preterm low birth weight. *Journal of Periodontology*, *67*(10, Suppl), 1103–1113. DOI: 10.1902/jop.1996.67.10.1103

Omran, A. R. (2005). The epidemiologic transition: A theory of the epidemiology of population change. 1971. *The Milbank Quarterly*, *83*(4), 731–757. DOI: 10.1111/j.1468-0009.2005.00398.x PMID: 16279965

Oni, T., & Unwin, N. (2015). Why the communicable/non-communicable disease dichotomy is problematic for public health control strategies: Implications of multimorbidity for health systems in an era of health transition. *International Health*, *7*(6), 390–399. DOI: 10.1093/inthealth/ihv040 PMID: 26103981

Orhan, K., Bayrakdar, I., Ezhov, M., Kravtsov, A., & Özyürek, T. (2020). Evaluation of artificial intelligence for detecting periapical pathosis on cone-beam computed tomography scans. *International Endodontic Journal*, *53*(5), 680–689. Advance online publication. DOI: 10.1111/iej.13265 PMID: 31922612

Ourang, S. A., Sohrabniya, F., Mohammad-Rahimi, H., Dianat, O., Aminoshariae, A., Nagendrababu, V., Dummer, P. M. H., Duncan, H. F., & Nosrat, A. (2024). Artificial intelligence in endodontics: Fundamental principles, workflow, and tasks. *International Endodontic Journal*, *57*(11), 1546–1565. DOI: 10.1111/iej.14127 PMID: 39056554

Oyekunle, D. O. T., Okwudili Matthew, U., Preston, D., & Boohene, D. (2024). Trust beyond technology algorithms: A theoretical exploration of consumer trust and behaviour in technological consumption and AI projects. *Journal of Computer and Communications*, *12*(06), 10–4236. DOI: 10.4236/jcc.2024.126006

Oyeyemi, A. L., Ramirez Varela, A., Lambert, E. V., Kohn, E. R., Hallal, P. C., & Pratt, M. (2024). An Overview of Physical Activity Research Evolution in Africa: The Global Observatory for Physical Activity—GoPA! *Journal of Physical Activity & Health*, *21*(5), 434–444. DOI: 10.1123/jpah.2023-0455 PMID: 38412851

Panahi, O. (2024). AI: A New Frontier in Oral and Maxillofacial Surgery. *Acta Scientific Dental Sciences*, *8*(6), 40–42.

Parker, J. M., Mol, A., Rivera, E. M., & Tawil, P. Z. (2017). Cone-beam computed tomography uses in clinical endodontics: Observer variability in detecting periapical lesions. *Journal of Endodontics*, *43*(2), 184–187. DOI: 10.1016/j.joen.2016.10.007 PMID: 28024758

Patel, A., Shah, D., Patel, Z., Makwana, H. S., & Rajput, A. (2023). A comprehensive review on AI in endodontics. *International Journal for Research in Applied Science and Engineering Technology*, *11*(7), 165–170. DOI: 10.22214/ijraset.2023.54565

Patel, V. A., Bhattacharya, P., Tanwar, S., Gupta, R., Sharma, G., Bokoro, P. N., & Sharma, R. (2022). Adoption of federated learning for healthcare informatics: Emerging applications and future directions. *IEEE Access : Practical Innovations, Open Solutions*, *10*, 90792–90826. DOI: 10.1109/ACCESS.2022.3201876

Patra, D., Banerjee, D., Ramprasad, P., Roy, S., Pal, D., & Dasgupta, S. (2023). Recent insights of obesity-induced gut and adipose tissue dysbiosis in type 2 diabetes. *Frontiers in Molecular Biosciences*, *10*, 1224982. DOI: 10.3389/fmolb.2023.1224982 PMID: 37842639

Patrick, D. L., Lee, R. S. Y., Nucci, M., Grembowski, D., Jolles, C. Z., & Milgrom, P. (2006). Reducing oral health disparities: A focus on social and cultural determinants. *BMC Oral Health*, *6*(S1, Suppl 1), S4. DOI: 10.1186/1472-6831-6-S1-S4 PMID: 16934121

Paul, M. J., & Dredze, M. (2011). You are what you tweet: Analyzing Twitter for public health. *Proceedings of the Fifth International AAAI Conference on Weblogs and Social Media*, 265-272.

Paul, S. M., Mytelka, D. S., Dunwiddie, C. T., Persinger, C. C., Munos, B. H., Lindborg, S. R., & Schacht, A. L. (2010). How to improve R&D productivity: The pharmaceutical industry's grand challenge. *Nature Reviews. Drug Discovery*, *9*(3), 203–214. DOI: 10.1038/nrd3078 PMID: 20168317

Pauwels, R., Brasil, D. M., Yamasaki, M. C., Jacobs, R., Bosmans, H., Freitas, D. Q., & Haiter-Neto, F. (2021). Artificial intelligence for detection of periapical lesions on intraoral radiographs: Comparison between convolutional neural networks and human observers. *Oral Surgery, Oral Medicine, Oral Pathology and Oral Radiology*, *131*(5), 610–616. DOI: 10.1016/j.oooo.2021.01.018 PMID: 33653645

Pavlou, I. A., Spandidos, D. A., Zoumpourlis, V., & Papakosta, V. K. (2024). Neurobiology of bruxism: The impact of stress. *Biomedical Reports*, *20*(4), 1–10. DOI: 10.3892/br.2024.1747 PMID: 38414628

Pearl, J., Glymour, M., & Jewell, N. P. (2016). *Causal inference in statistics: A primer*. Wiley.

Peres, M. A., Macpherson, L. M. D., Weyant, R. J., Daly, B., Venturelli, R., Mathur, M. R., Listl, S., Celeste, R. K., Guarnizo-Herreño, C. C., Kearns, C., Benzian, H., Allison, P., & Watt, R. G. (2019). Oral diseases: A global public health challenge. *Lancet*, *394*(10194), 249–260. DOI: 10.1016/S0140-6736(19)31146-8 PMID: 31327369

Petersen, P. E. (2003). The World Oral Health Report 2003: Continuous improvement of oral health in the 21st century—The approach of the WHO Global Oral Health Programme. *Community Dentistry and Oral Epidemiology*, *31*(s1, Suppl. 1), 3–23. DOI: 10.1046/j..2003.com122.x PMID: 15015736

Petersen, P. E. (2014). Strengthening of oral health systems: Oral health through primary health care. *Medical Principles and Practice : International Journal of the Kuwait University, Health Science Centre*, *23*(S1), 3–9. DOI: 10.1159/000356937 PMID: 24525450

Petersen, P. E., & Baez, R. J. (2013). *Oral health surveys: Basic methods* (5th ed.). World Health Organization.

Petersen, P. E., Bourgeois, D., Ogawa, H., Estupinan-Day, S., & Ndiaye, C. (2005). The global burden of oral diseases and risks to oral health. *Bulletin of the World Health Organization*, *83*(9), 661–669. PMID: 16211157

Pietiäinen, M., Liljestrand, J. M., Kopra, E., & Pussinen, P. J. (2018). Mediators between oral dysbiosis and cardiovascular diseases. *European Journal of Oral Sciences*, *126*(S1), 26–36. DOI: 10.1111/eos.12423 PMID: 30178551

Polizzi, A., & Leonardi, R. (2024). Automatic cephalometric landmark identification with artificial intelligence: An umbrella review of systematic reviews. *Journal of Dentistry*, *146*, 105056. DOI: 10.1016/j.jdent.2024.105056 PMID: 38729291

Prabhu, S. R., Warnakulasuriya, S., & Bhardwaj, S. (Eds.). (2026). *Lifestyle in Oral Health and Disease: A Comprehensive Guide for Oral Healthcare Providers*. Springer Nature.

Prainsack, B., & Buyx, A. (2017). *Solidarity in biomedicine and beyond*. Cambridge University Press. DOI: 10.1017/9781139696593

Prasad, M., Manjunath, C., Murthy, A. K., Sampath, A., Jaiswal, S., & Mohapatra, A. (2019). Integration of oral health into primary health care: A systematic review. *Journal of Family Medicine and Primary Care*, *8*(6), 1838–1845. DOI: 10.4103/jfmpc.jfmpc_286_19 PMID: 31334142

Pratt, M., Ramírez Varela, A., & Hallal, P. C. (2024). Celebrating 10 Years of the Global Observatory for Physical Activity—GoPA! *Journal of Physical Activity & Health*, *21*(5), 423–424. DOI: 10.1123/jpah.2024-0233 PMID: 38621673

Preshaw, P. M., Alba, A. L., Herrera, D., Jepsen, S., Konstantinidis, A., Makrilakis, K., & Taylor, R. (2012). Periodontitis and diabetes: A two-way relationship. *Diabetologia*, *55*(1), 21–31. DOI: 10.1007/s00125-011-2342-y PMID: 22057194

Proctor, E., Silmere, H., Raghavan, R., Hovmand, P., Aarons, G., Bunger, A., Griffey, R., & Hensley, M. (2011). Outcomes for implementation research: Conceptual distinctions, measurement challenges, and research agenda. *Administration and Policy in Mental Health*, *38*(2), 65–76. DOI: 10.1007/s10488-010-0319-7 PMID: 20957426

Pul, U., Tichy, A., Pitchika, V., & Schwendicke, F. (2025). Impact of artificial intelligence assistance on diagnosing periapical radiolucencies: A randomized controlled trial. *Journal of Dentistry*, *160*, 105868. DOI: 10.1016/j.jdent.2025.105868 PMID: 40466762

Pushalkar, S., Paul, B., Li, Q., Yang, J., Vasconcelos, R., Makwana, S., González, J. M., Shah, S., Xie, C., Janal, M. N., Queiroz, E., Bederoff, M., Leinwand, J., Solarewicz, J., Xu, F., Aboseria, E., Guo, Y., Aguallo, D., Gomez, C., & Saxena, D. (2020). Electronic cigarette aerosol modulates the oral microbiome and increases the risk of infection. *iScience*, *23*(3), 100884. DOI: 10.1016/j.isci.2020.100884 PMID: 32105635

Rädsch, T., Seidlitz, S., Moosbauer, J., Rasche, L., & Tolios, I. (2022). Federated learning in dentistry: Chances and challenges. *Journal of Dental Research, 101*(12), 1524–1532. DOI: 10.1177/00220345221108186 PMID: 35912725

Raghupathi, W., & Raghupathi, V. (2014). Big data analytics in healthcare: Promise and potential. *Health Information Science and Systems, 2*(1), 1–10. DOI: 10.1186/2047-2501-2-3 PMID: 25825667

Rahim, A., Khatoon, R., Khan, T. A., Syed, K., Khan, I., Khalid, T., & Khalid, B. (2024). Artificial intelligence-powered dentistry: Probing the potential, challenges, and ethicality of artificial intelligence in dentistry. *Digital Health, 10*, 20552076241291345. DOI: 10.1177/20552076241291345 PMID: 39539720

Rajkomar, A., Hardt, M., Howell, M. D., Corrado, G., & Chin, M. H. (2018). Ensuring fairness in machine learning to advance health equity. *Annals of Internal Medicine, 169*(12), 866–872. DOI: 10.7326/M18-1990 PMID: 30508424

Ramírez Varela, A., Hallal, P. C., Mejía Grueso, J., Pedišić, Ž., Salvo, D., Nguyen, A., Klepac, B., Bauman, A., Siefken, K., Hinckson, E., Oyeyemi, A. L., Richards, J., Salih Khidir, E. D., Inoue, S., Amagasa, S., Jauregui, A., Da Silva, M. C., Lee, I.-M., Ding, M., & Pratt, M. (2023). Status and Trends of Physical Activity Surveillance, Policy, and Research in 164 Countries: Findings From the Global Observatory for Physical Activity—GoPA! 2015 and 2020 Surveys. *Journal of Physical Activity & Health, 20*(2), 112–128. DOI: 10.1123/jpah.2022-0464 PMID: 36535269

Ramirez Varela, A., Salvo, D., Pratt, M., Milton, K., Siefken, K., Bauman, A., Kohl, H. W.III, Lee, I.-M., Heath, G., Foster, C., Powell, K., & Hallal, P. C. (2018). Worldwide use of the first set of physical activity Country Cards: The Global Observatory for Physical Activity - GoPA! *The International Journal of Behavioral Nutrition and Physical Activity, 15*(1), 29. DOI: 10.1186/s12966-018-0663-7 PMID: 29587783

Ramirez-Montoya, M. S. (2020). Challenges for Open Education with Educational Innovation: A Systematic Literature Review. *Sustainability (Basel), 12*(17), 7053. DOI: 10.3390/su12177053

Rani, H., Azizan, A. A., Walad, N. I. A., Hassan, S. A. A., Dom, T. N. M., Yeoh, D. S. H., Tay, J. W. C., Rosli, M. S. A., Aun, N. S. M., Aziz, A. F. A., Thwin, K. M., & Tew, I. M. (2025). Challenges and recommendations for oral healthcare of older adults in a long-term care facility. *Health Care, 13*(20), 2642. DOI: 10.3390/healthcare13202642 PMID: 41154320

Ray, R. R. (2023). Periodontitis: An oral disease with severe consequences. *Applied Biochemistry and Biotechnology, 195*(1), 17–32. DOI: 10.1007/s12010-022-04127-9 PMID: 36098930

Redd, T. K., Campbell, J. P., Brown, J. M., Kim, S. J., Ostmo, S., Chan, R. V. P., & Kalpathy-Cramer, J. (2021). Prediction of referral-warranted retinopathy of prematurity using a deep learning model trained on wide-field retinal images. *Nature Communications*, *12*(1), 1–11. PMID: 33397941

Remmele, C. W., Luther, C. H., Balkenhol, J., Dandekar, T., Müller, T., & Dittrich, M. T. (2015). Integrated inference and evaluation of host–fungi interaction networks. *Frontiers in Microbiology*, *6*, 764. DOI: 10.3389/fmicb.2015.00764 PMID: 26300851

Reyes, L. T., Knorst, J. K., Ortiz, F. R., & Ardenghi, T. M. (2022). Machine Learning in the Diagnosis and Prognostic Prediction of Dental Caries: A Systematic Review. *Caries Research*, *56*(3), 161–170. DOI: 10.1159/000524167 PMID: 35636386

Reynolds, M. G., Yorita, K. L., Kuehnert, M. J., Davidson, W. B., Huhn, G. D., Holman, R. C., & Damon, I. K. (2006). Clinical manifestations of human monkeypox influenced by route of infection. *The Journal of Infectious Diseases*, *194*(6), 773–780. DOI: 10.1086/505880 PMID: 16941343

Riccomini, F. E., Cirani, C. B. S., Carvalho, C. C. D., & Storopoli, J. E. (2021). Educational innovation: Trends for higher education in Brazil. *International Journal of Educational Management*, *35*(3), 564–578. DOI: 10.1108/IJEM-07-2019-0245

Rieke, N., Hancox, J., Li, W., Milletari, F., Roth, H. R., Albarqouni, S., Bakas, S., Galtier, M. N., Landman, B. A., Maier-Hein, K., Ourselin, S., Sheller, M., Summers, R. M., Trask, A., Xu, D., Baust, M., & Cardoso, M. J. (2020). The future of digital health with federated learning. npj. *Digital Medicine*, *3*(1), 1–7. DOI: 10.1038/s41746-020-00323-1 PMID: 33015372

Riley, P., Lamont, T., Worthington, H., Clarkson, J. E., & Beirne, P. (2017). Recall intervals for oral health in primary care patients. *Cochrane Database of Systematic Reviews*, *2017*(12), CD004346. PMID: 24353242

Rockett, I. R. (1999). Population and health: An introduction to epidemiology (2nd ed.). *Population Bulletin*, *54*(4), 1–44.

Rogers, A. A., Willumsen, T., Strømme, H., & Johnsen, J. A. K. (2022). Top-down self-regulation processes as determinants of oral hygiene self-care behaviour: A systematic scoping review. *Clinical and Experimental Dental Research*, *8*(4), 807–826. DOI: 10.1002/cre2.548 PMID: 35396799

Rokaya, D., Jaghsi, A. A., Jagtap, R., & Srimaneepong, V. (2024). Artificial intelligence in dentistry and dental biomaterials. *Frontiers in Dental Medicine*, *5*, 1525505. DOI: 10.3389/fdmed.2024.1525505 PMID: 39917699

Romero-Laorden, J. I., Lorenzo, F., Solis, J. H., & Lopez-Berges, M. (2022). Integration of dental and medical electronic health records: A systematic review of the evidence and challenges. *The Journal of the American Dental Association, 153*(8), 741–753.

Rosen, J., Sancheti, P., Fierlinger, A., Niazi, F., Johal, H., & Bedi, A. (2017). Response to: Important Considerations When Determining the Cost-effectiveness of Viscosupplements in the Treatment of Knee Osteoarthritis. *Advances in Therapy, 33*(12), 2273–2276. DOI: 10.1007/s12325-016-0422-6 PMID: 27778299

Rothman, K. J., Greenland, S., & Lash, T. L. (2008). *Modern epidemiology* (3rd ed.). Lippincott Williams & Wilkins.

Rutter, H., Savona, N., Glonti, K., Bibby, J., Cummins, S., Finegood, D. T., Greaves, F., Harper, L., Hawe, P., Moore, L., Petticrew, M., Rehfuess, E., Shiell, A., Thomas, J., & White, M. (2017). The need for a complex systems model of evidence for public health. *Lancet, 390*(10112), 2602–2604. DOI: 10.1016/S0140-6736(17)31267-9 PMID: 28622953

Rydén, L., Buhlin, K., Ekstrand, E., de Faire, U., Gustafsson, A., Holmer, J., Kjellström, B., Lindahl, B., Norhammar, A., Nygren, Å., Näsman, P., Rathnayake, N., Svenungsson, E., & Klinge, B. (2016). Periodontitis increases the risk of a first myocardial infarction: A report from the PAROKRANK study. *Circulation, 133*(6), 576–583. DOI: 10.1161/CIRCULATIONAHA.115.020324 PMID: 26762521

Sabharwal, A., Stellrecht, E., & Scannapieco, F. A. (2021). Associations between dental caries and systemic diseases: A scoping review. *BMC Oral Health, 21*(1), 472. DOI: 10.1186/s12903-021-01803-w PMID: 34563194

Sahoo, R. K., Sahoo, K. C., Dash, G. C., Kumar, G., Baliarsingh, S. K., Panda, B., & Pati, S. (2024). Diagnostic performance of artificial intelligence in detecting oral potentially malignant disorders and oral cancer using medical diagnostic imaging: A systematic review and meta-analysis. *Frontiers in Oral Health, 5*, 1494867. DOI: 10.3389/froh.2024.1494867 PMID: 39568787

Sahyoun, N. R., Krall, E., & Russell, R. M. (2003). Poor dentition in community-dwelling elderly was associated with malnutrition but not with a specific nutritional deficiency. *The American Journal of Clinical Nutrition, 77*(2), 411–416. PMID: 12540402

Salathé, M. (2018). Digital epidemiology: What is it, and where is it going? *Life Sciences, Society and Policy, 14*(1), 1–5. DOI: 10.1186/s40504-017-0065-7 PMID: 29302758

Salathé, M., Bengtsson, L., Bodnar, T. J., Brewer, D. D., Brownstein, J. S., Buckee, C., Campbell, E. M., Cattuto, C., Khandelwal, S., Mabry, P. L., & Vespignani, A. (2012). Digital epidemiology. *PLoS Computational Biology*, *8*(7), e1002616. DOI: 10.1371/journal.pcbi.1002616 PMID: 22844241

Salvador, S. M., & Toassi, R. F. C. (2021). Oral health self-perception: Physical, social and cultural expressions of a body in interaction with the world. *Physis (Rio de Janeiro, Brazil)*, *31*(1), e310122. DOI: 10.1590/s0103-73312021310122

Sandlund, M., Huss, L., & Theorell-Haglow, J. (2021). Nordic register-based research in dentistry: A systematic review of study designs and applications. *Acta Odontologica Scandinavica*, *79*(1), 1–10. PMID: 32401086

Santosa, A., Wall, S., Fottrell, E., Högberg, U., & Byass, P. (2014). The development and experience of epidemiological transition theory over four decades: A systematic review. *Global Health Action*, *7*(1), 23574. DOI: 10.3402/gha.v7.23574 PMID: 24848657

Sanz, M., Marco del Castillo, A., Jepsen, S., Gonzalez-Juanatey, J. R., D'Aiuto, F., Bouchard, P., Chapple, I., Dietrich, T., Gotsman, I., Graziani, F., Herrera, D., Loos, B., Madianos, P., Michel, J.-B., Perel, P., Pieske, B., Shapira, L., Shechter, M., Tonetti, M., & Wimmer, G. (2020). Periodontitis and cardiovascular diseases: Consensus report. *Journal of Clinical Periodontology*, *47*(3), 268–288. DOI: 10.1111/jcpe.13189 PMID: 32011025

Sarvamangala, D. R., & Kulkarni, R. V. (2022). Convolutional neural networks in medical image understanding: A survey. *Evolutionary Intelligence*, *15*(1), 1–22. DOI: 10.1007/s12065-020-00540-3 PMID: 33425040

Sato, Y., Saijo, Y., & Yoshioka, E. (2021). Work stress and oral conditions: A systematic review of observational studies. *BMJ Open*, *11*(5), e046532. DOI: 10.1136/bmjopen-2020-046532 PMID: 34049917

Scales, B. S., Erb-Downward, J. R., Huffnagle, I. M., LiPuma, J. J., & Huffnagle, G. B. (2015). Comparative genomics of Pseudomonas fluorescens subclade III strains from human lungs. *BMC Genomics*, *16*(1), 1032. DOI: 10.1186/s12864-015-2261-2 PMID: 26644001

Schack, L. M. H., Naderi, E., Fachal, L., Dorling, L., Luccarini, C., Dunning, A. M., Barnett, G., Barrera, M. E. A., Burnet, N. G., Calvo, L. M., Diergaarde, B., Dudding, T., Dunning, A., Duprez, F., Kerns, S. L., Kiang, M. C. L., Langendijk, H., Mehanna, H., Ness, A., & Alsner, J.The Head and Neck Group of the Radiogenomics Consortium. (2022). A genome-wide association study of radiotherapy-induced toxicity in head and neck cancer patients identifies a susceptibility locus associated with mucositis. *British Journal of Cancer, 126*(7), 1082–1090. DOI: 10.1038/s41416-021-01670-w PMID: 35039627

Schatz, M. C. (2015). Biological data sciences in genome research. *Genome Research, 25*(10), 1417–1422. DOI: 10.1101/gr.191684.115 PMID: 26430150

Scheerman, J. F. M., Meijel, B. V., Empelen, P. V., Verrips, G. H. W., Loveren, C. V., Twisk, J. W. R., Pakpour, J. H., Braak, V. N., & Kramer, G. J. C. (2018). Digital interventions for oral health behaviour. *Caries Research, 52*(6), 507–517. DOI: 10.1111/idh.12415 PMID: 31291683

Scheerman, J. F. M., van Loveren, C., van Meijel, B., Dusseldorp, E., Wartewig, E., Verrips, G. H. W., & van Empelen, P. (2018). Psychosocial correlates of oral hygiene behaviour in people aged 9-19: A systematic review with meta-analysis. *Community Dentistry and Oral Epidemiology, 46*(1), 43–55. DOI: 10.1111/cdoe.12325

Schirle, M., Bantscheff, M., & Kuster, B. (2012). Mass spectrometry-based proteomics in preclinical drug discovery. *Chemistry & Biology, 19*(1), 72–84. DOI: 10.1016/j.chembiol.2012.01.002 PMID: 22284356

Schmidt, A.. (2023). Community-level periodontal disease monitoring using wastewater-based epidemiology. *Environmental Research, 220*, 115164.

Schmidt, T. S. B., Hayward, M. R., Coelho, L. P., Li, S. S., Costea, P. I., Voigt, A. Y., Wirbel, J., Maistrenko, O. M., Alves, R. J., Bergsten, E., de Beaufort, C., Sobhani, I., Heintz-Buschart, A., Sunagawa, S., Zeller, G., Wilmes, P., & Bork, P. (2019). Extensive transmission of microbes along the gastrointestinal tract. *eLife, 8*, e42693. DOI: 10.7554/eLife.42693 PMID: 30747106

Schwarz, C., Hajdu, A. I., Dumitrescu, R., Sava-Rosianu, R., Bolchis, V., Anusca, D., Hanghicel, A., Fratila, A. D., Oancea, R., Jumanca, D., Galuscan, A., & Leretter, M. (2023). Link between Oral Health, Periodontal Disease, Smoking, and Systemic Diseases in Romanian Patients. *Healthcare (Basel), 11*(16), 2354. DOI: 10.3390/healthcare11162354 PMID: 37628551

Schwendicke, F., Giannakakis, A., Parthasarathy, S., Krois, J., & Samek, W. (2021). Explainable artificial intelligence in dentistry. *Journal of Dental Research, 100*(10), 1074–1081.

Schwendicke, F., Golla, T., Dreher, M., & Krois, J. (2019). Convolutional neural networks for dental image diagnostics: A scoping review. *Journal of Dentistry*, *91*, 103226. DOI: 10.1016/j.jdent.2019.103226 PMID: 31704386

Schwendicke, F., Samek, W., & Krois, J. (2020). Artificial intelligence in dentistry: Chances and challenges. *Journal of Dental Research*, *99*(7), 769–774. DOI: 10.1177/0022034520915714 PMID: 32315260

Segata, N., Haake, S. K., Mannon, P., Lemon, K. P., Waldron, L., Gevers, D., Huttenhower, C., & Izard, J. (2012). Composition of the adult digestive tract bacterial microbiome based on seven mouth surfaces, tonsils, throat, and stool samples. *Genome Biology*, *13*(6), R42. DOI: 10.1186/gb-2012-13-6-r42 PMID: 22698087

Segers, K., Declerck, S., Mangelings, D., Van den Heyden, Y., & Van Eeckhaut, A. (2019). Analytical techniques for metabolomic studies: A review. *Bioanalysis*, *11*(24), 2297–2318. DOI: 10.4155/bio-2019-0014 PMID: 31845604

Sekhar, P., & Prabakar, J. (2023). Knowledge and Practice of Preventive Measures for Oral Health Care among 14-16 Year Old School Children in Chennai - An Observational Study. *2nd International Conference on Business Analytics for Technology and Security, ICBATS 2023*. DOI: 10.1109/ICBATS57792.2023.10111394

Selwitz, R. H., Ismail, A. I., & Pitts, N. B. (2007). Dental caries. *Lancet*, *369*(9555), 51–59. DOI: 10.1016/S0140-6736(07)60031-2 PMID: 17208642

Setzer, F. C., Shi, K. J., Zhang, Z., Yan, H., Yoon, H., Mupparapu, M., & Li, J. (2020). Artificial Intelligence for the Computer-aided Detection of Periapical Lesions in Cone-beam Computed Tomographic Images. *Journal of Endodontics*, *46*(7), 987–993. DOI: 10.1016/j.joen.2020.03.025 PMID: 32402466

Shadmi, E., Chen, Y., Dourado, I., Faran-Perach, I., Furler, J., Hangoma, P., Hanvoravongchai, P., Obando, C., Petrosyan, V., Rao, K. D., Ruano, A. L., Shi, L., de Souza, L. E., Spitzer-Shohat, S., Sturgiss, E., Suphanchaimat, R., Uribe, M. V., & Willems, S. (2020). Health equity and COVID-19: Global perspectives. *International Journal for Equity in Health*, *19*(1), 104. DOI: 10.1186/s12939-020-01218-z PMID: 32586388

Shaffer, J. R., Wang, X., Feingold, E., Lee, M., Begum, F., Weeks, D. E., Cuenco, K. T., Barmada, M. M., Wendell, S. K., Crosslin, D. R., Laurie, C. C., Doheny, K. F., Pugh, E. W., Zhang, Q., Feenstra, B., Geller, F., Boyd, H. A., Zhang, H., Melbye, M., & Marazita, M. L. (2011). Genome-wide association scan for childhood caries implicates novel genes. *Journal of Dental Research*, *90*(12), 1457–1462. DOI: 10.1177/0022034511422910 PMID: 21940522

Shahzad, M., Upshur, R., Donnelly, P., Bharmal, A., Wei, X., Feng, P., & Brown, A. D. (2019). A population-based approach to integrated healthcare delivery: A scoping review of clinical care and public health collaboration. *BMC Public Health, 19*(1), 708. DOI: 10.1186/s12889-019-7002-z PMID: 31174501

Sheiham, A., & Watt, R. G. (2000). The common risk factor approach. *Community Dentistry and Oral Epidemiology, 28*(6), 399–406. DOI: 10.1034/j.1600-0528.2000.028006399.x PMID: 11106011

Shrestha, R. M.. (2022). Environmental and occupational determinants of periodontal disease: A systematic review. *International Journal of Environmental Research and Public Health, 19*(4), 1938. PMID: 35206125

Silness, J., & Loe, H. (1964). PERIODONTAL DISEASE IN PREGNANCY. II. CORRELATION BETWEEN ORAL HYGIENE AND PERIODONTAL CONDTION. *Acta Odontologica Scandinavica, 22*(1), 121–135. DOI: 10.3109/00016356408993968 PMID: 14158464

Simpson, A.. (2025). Wastewater-based epidemiology: Methodological considerations for pathogen surveillance. *Current Opinion in Environmental Science & Health, 33*, 100432.

Simpson, D. D. (2011). A framework for implementing sustainable oral health promotion interventions. *Journal of Public Health Dentistry, 71*(s1, Suppl. 1), S84–S94. DOI: 10.1111/j.1752-7325.2011.00234.x PMID: 21499507

Simpson, T. C., Clarkson, J. E., Worthington, H. V., MacDonald, L., Weldon, J. C., Needleman, I., Iheozor-Ejiofor, Z., Wild, S. H., Qureshi, A., Walker, A., Patel, V. A., Boyers, D., & Twigg, J. (2022). Treatment of periodontitis for glycaemic control in people with diabetes mellitus. *Cochrane Database of Systematic Reviews, 4*(4), CD004714. Advance online publication. DOI: 10.1002/14651858.CD004714 PMID: 35420698

Singh, H., Fulton, J.IV, Mirzazada, S., Saragosa, M., Uleryk, E. M., & Nelson, M. L. A. (2023). Community-based culturally tailored education programs for Black communities with cardiovascular disease, diabetes, hypertension, and stroke: Systematic review findings. *Journal of Racial and Ethnic Health Disparities, 10*(6), 2986–3006. DOI: 10.1007/s40615-022-01474-5 PMID: 36508135

Singh, N., & Raza, K. (2022). Progress in deep learning-based dental and maxillofacial image analysis: A systematic review. *Expert Systems with Applications, 199*, 116968. DOI: 10.1016/j.eswa.2022.116968

Sivari, E., Senirkentli, G., Bostanci, E., Guzel, M., Açıcı, K., & Aşuroğlu, T. (2023). Deep Learning in Diagnosis of Dental Anomalies and Diseases: A Systematic Review. *Diagnostics (Basel)*, *13*(15), 2512. Advance online publication. DOI: 10.3390/diagnostics13152512 PMID: 37568875

Skillman, S. M., Doescher, M. P., Mouradian, W. E., & Brunson, D. K. (2010). The challenge to delivering oral health services in rural America. *Journal of Public Health Dentistry*, *70*(s1, Suppl 1), S49–S57. DOI: 10.1111/j.1752-7325.2010.00178.x PMID: 20806475

Sreedharan, J., Subbarayalu, A. V., Kamalasanan, A., Albalawi, I., Krishna, G. G., Alahmari, A. D., Alsalamah, J. A., Alkhathami, M. G., Alenezi, M., Alqahtani, A. S., Alahmari, M., Phillips, M. R., & MacDonald, J. (2024). Key Performance Indicators: A Framework for Allied Healthcare Educational Institutions. *ClinicoEconomics and Outcomes Research*, *16*, 173–185. DOI: 10.2147/CEOR.S446614 PMID: 38562567

Stankevic, E., Bjørnland, T., Kunzmann, A. T., Jansonius, N. M., & Magnusson, P. K. E. (2024). Genome-wide association study identifies host genetic variants influencing oral microbiota diversity and metabolic health. *Scientific Reports*, *14*(1), 14738. DOI: 10.1038/s41598-024-65538-8 PMID: 38926497

Steinsbekk, K. S., Kare Myskja, B., & Solberg, B. (2013). Broad consent versus dynamic consent in biobank research: Is passive participation an ethical problem? *European Journal of Human Genetics : EJHG*, *21*(9), 897–902. DOI: 10.1038/ejhg.2012.282 PMID: 23299918

Stephan, D., Bertsch, A., Burwinkel, M., Vinayahalingam, S., Al-Nawas, B., Kämmerer, P., & Thiem, D. G. E. (2024). AI in dental radiology—improving the efficiency of reporting with ChatGPT: Comparative study. *Journal of Medical Internet Research*, *26*, e60684. DOI: 10.2196/60684 PMID: 39714078

Strasser, S., Stauber, C., Shrivastava, R., Riley, P., & O'Quin, K. (2021). Collective insights of public-private partnership impacts and sustainability: A qualitative analysis. *PLoS One*, *16*(7), e0254495. DOI: 10.1371/journal.pone.0254495 PMID: 34283847

Stubbe, D. E. (2020). Practicing cultural competence and cultural humility in the care of diverse patients. *Focus - American Psychiatric Publishing*, *18*(1), 49–51. DOI: 10.1176/appi.focus.20190041 PMID: 32047398

Sun, X., Hu, C., & Gong, W. (2025). Follicular dendritic cell sarcoma of the stomach in a young male: A rare case report and literature review. *Medicine*, *104*(27), e43004. DOI: 10.1097/MD.0000000000043004 PMID: 40629639

Suzman, R., Beard, J. R., Boerma, T., & Chatterji, S. (2015). Health in an ageing world—What do we know? *Lancet*, *385*(9967), 484–486. DOI: 10.1016/S0140-6736(14)61597-X PMID: 25468156

Syed, S. T., Gerber, B. S., & Sharp, L. K. (2013). Traveling towards disease: Transportation barriers to health care access. *Journal of Community Health*, *38*(5), 976–993. DOI: 10.1007/s10900-013-9681-1 PMID: 23543372

Szabó, V., Szabó, B., Orhan, K., Veres, D., Manulis, D., Ezhov, M., & Sanders, A. (2024). Validation of artificial intelligence application for dental caries diagnosis on intraoral bitewing and periapical radiographs. *Journal of Dentistry*, *147*, 105105. DOI: 10.1016/j.jdent.2024.105105 PMID: 38821394

Tabatabaian, F., Vora, S. R., & Mirabbasi, S. (2023). Applications, functions, and accuracy of artificial intelligence in restorative dentistry: A literature review. *Journal of Esthetic and Restorative Dentistry : Official Publication of the American Academy of Esthetic Dentistry ... [et al.]*, *35*(6), 842–859. DOI: 10.1111/jerd.13079 PMID: 37522291

Taha, M. K., Martinon-Torres, F., Köllges, R., Bonanni, P., Safadi, M. A. P., Booy, R., Smith, V., Garcia, S., Bekkat-Berkani, R., & Abitbol, V. (2022). Equity in vaccination policies to overcome social deprivation as a risk factor for invasive meningococcal disease. *Expert Review of Vaccines*, *21*(5), 659–674. DOI: 10.1080/14760584.2022.2052048 PMID: 35271781

Tang, W. H. W., Kitai, T., & Hazen, S. L. (2017). Gut microbiota in cardiovascular health and disease. *Circulation Research*, *120*(7), 1183–1196. DOI: 10.1161/CIRCRESAHA.117.309715 PMID: 28360349

Taylor, G. W. (2001). Bidirectional interrelationships between diabetes and periodontal diseases: An epidemiologic perspective. *Annals of Periodontology*, *6*(1), 99–112. DOI: 10.1902/annals.2001.6.1.99 PMID: 11887478

Taylor, G. W., & Borgnakke, W. S. (2008). Periodontal disease: Associations with diabetes, glycemic control and complications. *Oral Diseases*, *14*(3), 191–203. DOI: 10.1111/j.1601-0825.2008.01442.x PMID: 18336370

Thacker, S. B. & Centers for Disease Control and Prevention. (2006). Epidemiology and public health at CDC. *MMWR Supplements*, *55*(2), 3–4. PMID: 17183233

Thaler, R. H., & Sunstein, C. R. (2008). *Nudge*. Yale University Press., DOI: 10.1016/j.soscij.2008.09.003

Thiébaut, R., & Thiessard, F. (2017). Public Health and Epidemiology Informatics. *Yearbook of Medical Informatics*, *26*(1), 248–251. DOI: 10.15265/IY-2017-036 PMID: 29063574

Thomson, K., Hillier-Brown, F., Todd, A., McNamara, C., Huijts, T., & Bambra, C. (2018). The effects of public health policies on health inequalities in high-income countries: An umbrella review. *BMC Public Health*, *18*(1), 869. DOI: 10.1186/s12889-018-5677-1 PMID: 30005611

Tiwari, T., Patel, J., & Nascimento, G. (2025). Big data and oral health disparities: A critical appraisal. *Journal of Dental Research*, *104*(2), 119–130. DOI: 10.1177/00220345241285847 PMID: 39629938

Tonetti, M. S., Jepsen, S., Jin, L., & Otomo-Corgel, J. (2017). Impact of the global burden of periodontal diseases on health, nutrition and wellbeing of mankind: A call for global action. *Journal of Clinical Periodontology*, *44*(5), 456–462. DOI: 10.1111/jcpe.12732 PMID: 28419559

Topol, E. J. (2019). High-performance medicine: The convergence of human and artificial intelligence. *Nature Medicine*, *25*(1), 44–56. DOI: 10.1038/s41591-018-0300-7 PMID: 30617339

Tracy, M., Cerdá, M., & Keyes, K. M. (2018). Agent-Based Modeling in Public Health: Current Applications and Future Directions. *Annual Review of Public Health*, *39*(1), 77–94. DOI: 10.1146/annurev-publhealth-040617-014317 PMID: 29328870

Tran, N. H., Zhang, X., Li, M., & Shan, B. (2021). Deep learning in cancer diagnosis, prognosis and treatment selection. *Genome Medicine*, *13*(1), 152. DOI: 10.1186/s13073-021-00968-x PMID: 34579788

Tu, C., Wang, G., Hu, Z., Wang, S., Yan, Q., & Liu, X. (2023). Burden of oral disorders, 1990–2019: Estimates from the global burden of disease study 2019. *Archives of Medical Science : AMS*, *19*(4), 930–940. DOI: 10.5114/aoms/165962 PMID: 37560733

Tyagi, P.. (2025). Artificial Intelligence Applications in Dentistry: A Systematic Review. *Cureus*. Advance online publication. DOI: 10.7759/cureus.85062

U.S. Food and Drug Administration. (2023). *Artificial intelligence and machine learning (AI/ML)-enabled medical devices*. https://www.fda.gov/medical-devices/software-medical-device-samd/artificial-intelligence-and-machine-learning-aiml-enabled-medical-devices

Uffelmann, E., Huang, Q. Q., Munung, N. S., de Vries, J., Okada, Y., Martin, A. R., Martin, H. C., Lappalainen, T., & Posthuma, D. (2021). Genome-wide association studies. *Nature Reviews. Methods Primers*, *1*(1), 59. DOI: 10.1038/s43586-021-00056-9

Unkel, S., Farrington, C. P., Garthwaite, P. H., Robertson, C., & Andrews, N. (2012). Statistical methods for the prospective detection of infectious disease outbreaks: A review. *Journal of the Royal Statistical Society. Series A, (Statistics in Society)*, *175*(1), 49–82. DOI: 10.1111/j.1467-985X.2011.00714.x

Uribe, S., Issa, J., Sohrabniya, F., Denny, A., Kim, N., Dayo, A., Chaurasia, A., Sofi-Mahmudi, A., Büttner, M., & Schwendicke, F. (2024). Publicly available dental image datasets for artificial intelligence. *Journal of Dental Research*, *103*(13), 1365–1374. DOI: 10.1177/00220345241272052 PMID: 39422586

van Nistelrooij, N.. (2025). A novel AI-powered radiographic analysis surpasses specialists in stage II–IV periodontitis detection: A multicenter diagnostic study. npj. *Digital Medicine*, *8*(1), 691. DOI: 10.1038/s41746-025-02077-0 PMID: 41254181

van Seventer, J. M., & Hochberg, N. S. (2017). Principles of Infectious Diseases: Transmission, Diagnosis, Prevention, and Control. *International Encyclopedia of Public Health*, 22–39. DOI: 10.1016/B978-0-12-803678-5.00516-6

VanderWeele, T. J. (2019). Principles of confounder selection. *European Journal of Epidemiology*, *34*(3), 211–219. DOI: 10.1007/s10654-019-00494-6 PMID: 30840181

Varela, A. R., Pratt, M., Powell, K., Lee, I.-M., Bauman, A., Heath, G., Martins, R. C., Kohl, H., & Hallal, P. C. (2017). Worldwide Surveillance, Policy, and Research on Physical Activity and Health: The Global Observatory for Physical Activity. *Journal of Physical Activity & Health*, *14*(9), 701–709. DOI: 10.1123/jpah.2016-0626 PMID: 28513338

Varoni, E. M., & Rimondini, L. (2022). Oral microbiome, oral health and systemic health: A multidirectional link. *Biomedicines*, *10*(1), 186. DOI: 10.3390/biomedicines10010186 PMID: 35052865

Varzakas, T., & Antoniadou, M. (2024). A holistic approach for ethics and sustainability in the food chain: The gateway to oral and systemic health. *Foods*, *13*(8), 1224. DOI: 10.3390/foods13081224 PMID: 38672896

Vashisht, R., Sharma, A., Kiran, T., Jolly, S. S., Brar, P. K., & Puri, J. V. (2024). Artificial intelligence in dentistry—A scoping review. *Journal of Oral and Maxillofacial Surgery, Medicine, and Pathology*, *36*(4), 579–592. DOI: 10.1016/j.ajoms.2024.04.009

Verhulst, M. J. L., Loos, B. G., Gerdes, V. E. A., & Teeuw, W. J. (2019). Evaluating all potential oral complications of diabetes mellitus. *Frontiers in Endocrinology, 10*, 56. DOI: 10.3389/fendo.2019.00056 PMID: 30962800

Vialas, V., Nogales-Cadenas, R., Nombela, C., Pascual-Montano, A., & Gil, C. (2009). Proteopathogen, a protein database for studying *Candida albicans*–host interaction. *Proteomics, 9*(20), 4664–4668. DOI: 10.1002/pmic.200900023 PMID: 19743419

Vidmar Šimic, M., Maver, A., Zimani, A. N., Hočevar, K., Peterlin, B., Kovanda, A., & Premru-Sršen, T. (2023). Oral microbiome and preterm birth. *Frontiers in Medicine, 10*, 1177990. DOI: 10.3389/fmed.2023.1177990 PMID: 37608830

Vieira, A. R. (2012). Genetics and dental caries: Prospects for the future. *Journal of Dental Research, 91*(Suppl.), S23–S28.

Viet, C. T., Asam, K. R., Yu, G., Dyer, E. C., Kochanny, S., Thomas, C. M., et al. (2024). Artificial intelligence-based epigenomic, transcriptomic, and histologic signatures of tobacco use in oral squamous cell carcinoma. npj Precision Oncology, 8, 130. https://doi.org/DOI: 10.1038/s41698-024-00605-x

Vilar-Compte, M., Burrola-Méndez, S., Lozano-Marrufo, A., Ferré-Eguiluz, I., Flores, D., Gaitán-Rossi, P., Teruel, G., & Pérez-Escamilla, R. (2021). Urban poverty and nutrition challenges associated with accessibility to a healthy diet: A global systematic literature review. *International Journal for Equity in Health, 20*(1), 40. DOI: 10.1186/s12939-020-01330-0 PMID: 33472636

Visentin, D., Gobin, I., & Maglica, Ž. (2023). Periodontal pathogens and their links to neuroinflammation and neurodegeneration. *Microorganisms, 11*(7), 1832. DOI: 10.3390/microorganisms11071832 PMID: 37513004

Visscher, C. M., Baad-Hansen, L., Durham, J., Goulet, J. P., Michelotti, A., Barraza, C. R., & Raphael, K. G. (2018). Benefits of implementing pain-related disability and psychological assessment in dental practice for patients with temporomandibular pain and other oral health conditions. *The Journal of the American Dental Association, 149*(6), 422–431. DOI: 10.1016/j.adaj.2017.12.031 PMID: 29653670

Vujicic, M., Buchmueller, T., & Klein, R. (2016). Dental Care Presents The Highest Level Of Financial Barriers, Compared To Other Types Of Health Care Services. *Health Affairs (Project Hope), 35*(12), 2176–2182. DOI: 10.1377/hlthaff.2016.0800 PMID: 27920304

Wallace, S., Nazroo, J., & Bécares, L. (2016). Cumulative effect of racial discrimination on the mental health of ethnic minorities in the United Kingdom. *American Journal of Public Health, 106*(7), 1294–1300. DOI: 10.2105/AJPH.2016.303121 PMID: 27077347

Wang, C. H., Chueh, L. H., Chen, S. C., Feng, Y. C., Hsiao, C. K., & Chiang, C. P. (2011). Impact of diabetes mellitus, hypertension, and coronary artery disease on tooth extraction after nonsurgical endodontic treatment. *Journal of Endodontics, 37*(1), 1–5. DOI: 10.1016/j.joen.2010.08.054 PMID: 21146066

Wang, C., Liu, W., Yao, L., Zhang, X., Zhang, X., Ye, C., Jiang, H., He, J., Zhu, Y., & Ai, D. (2017). Hydroxyeicosapentaenoic acids and epoxyeicosatetraenoic acids attenuate the early occurrence of nonalcoholic fatty liver disease. *British Journal of Pharmacology, 174*(14), 2358–2372. DOI: 10.1111/bph.13844 PMID: 28471490

Wang, H., Li, J., Lin, Y., Lin, C., Liu, C., Lin, T., Chan, C.-T., & Hsieh, C.-Y. (2025). Machine learning-based toothbrushing region recognition using smart toothbrush holder and wearable sensors. *Biosensors (Basel), 15*(12), 798. DOI: 10.3390/bios15120798 PMID: 41440279

Wang, Q., Nguyen, T.-T., Huang, J. Z., & Nguyen, T. T. (2018). An efficient random forests algorithm for high dimensional data classification. *Advances in Data Analysis and Classification, 12*(4), 953–972. DOI: 10.1007/s11634-018-0318-1

Wang, X., Wang, X., Lou, Y., Liu, J., Huo, S., Pang, X., Wang, W., Wu, C., Chen, Y., Chen, Y., Chen, A., Bi, F., Xing, W., Deng, Q., Jia, L., & Chen, J. (2022). Constructing tongue coating recognition model using deep transfer learning to assist syndrome diagnosis and its potential in noninvasive ethnopharmacological evaluation. *Journal of Ethnopharmacology, 285*, 114905. DOI: 10.1016/j.jep.2021.114905 PMID: 34896205

Washington, A. E., Coye, M. J., & Boulware, L. E. (2016). Academic Health Systems' Third Curve: Population Health Improvement. *Journal of the American Medical Association, 315*(5), 459–460. DOI: 10.1001/jama.2015.18550 PMID: 26836726

Watt, R. G. (2012). Social determinants of oral health inequalities: Implications for action. *Community Dentistry and Oral Epidemiology, 40*(s2, Suppl. 2), 44–48. DOI: 10.1111/j.1600-0528.2012.00719.x PMID: 22998304

Watt, R. G., Daly, B., Allison, P., Macpherson, L. M. D., Venturelli, R., Listl, S., Weyant, R. J., Mathur, M. R., Guarnizo-Herreño, C. C., Celeste, R. K., Peres, M. A., Kearns, C., & Benzian, H. (2019). Ending the neglect of global oral health: Time for radical action. *Lancet, 394*(10194), 261–272. DOI: 10.1016/S0140-6736(19)31133-X PMID: 31327370

Watt, R. G., & Sheiham, A. (2012). Integrating the common risk factor approach into a social determinants framework. *Community Dentistry and Oral Epidemiology*, *40*(4), 289–296. DOI: 10.1111/j.1600-0528.2012.00680.x PMID: 22429083

Weingart, J., Schlager, S., Metzger, M., Brandenburg, L., Hein, A., Schmelzeisen, R., Bamberg, F., Kim, S., Kellner, E., Reisert, M., & Russe, M. F. (2023). Automated detection of cephalometric landmarks using deep neural patchworks. *Dento Maxillo Facial Radiology*, *52*(6), 20230059. DOI: 10.1259/dmfr.20230059 PMID: 37427585

Wild, C. P. (2012). The exposome: From concept to utility. *International Journal of Epidemiology*, *41*(1), 24–32. DOI: 10.1093/ije/dyr236 PMID: 22296988

Wirtz, A.. (2023). Machine learning in dentistry: A scoping review. *Clinical Oral Investigations*, *27*(1), 45–63. PMID: 36459238

Wojtkowska, A., Zapolski, T., Wysokińska-Miszczuk, J., & Wysokiński, A. P. (2021). The inflammation link between periodontal disease and coronary atherosclerosis in patients with acute coronary syndromes: Case-control study. *BMC Oral Health*, *21*(1), 5. DOI: 10.1186/s12903-020-01356-4 PMID: 33407375

Wolf, T. G., Cagetti, M. G., Fisher, J.-M., Seeberger, G. K., & Campus, G. (2021). Non-communicable diseases and oral health: An overview. *Frontiers in Oral Health*, *2*, 725460. DOI: 10.3389/froh.2021.725460 PMID: 35048049

World Health Organisation. (2021). *Resolution WHA74.5: Oral health.* World Health Assembly.

World Health Organisation. (2022). *WHO global strategy on oral health.* World Health Organisation.

World Health Organization. (2022). *Global oral health status report: Towards universal health coverage for oral health by 2030.* https://www.who.int/publications/i/item/9789240061484

World Health Organization. (2022). *Global oral health status report: Towards universal health coverage for oral health by 2030.* World Health Organization. https://www.who.int/publications/i/item/9789240061484

World Health Organization. (2023). *Global oral health status report: Towards universal health coverage for oral health by 2030.* World Health Organization.

World Health Organization. (2023, November 29). *Comprehensive assessment of evidence on oral cancer prevention released.* https://www.who.int/news/item/29-11-2023-comprehensive-assessment-of-evidence-on-oral-cancer-prevention-released-29-november-2023

World Health Organization. (2025). *Bangkok declaration—No health without oral health: Towards universal health coverage for oral health by 2030*. https://www.who.int/publications/m/item/bangkok-declaration-no-health-without-oral-health

World Health Organization. Oral health. Geneva: World Health Organization (2025). Available at:https://www.who.int/news-room/fact-sheets/detail/oral-health(Accessed March 20, 2025).

Wu, W., Hu, L., Chen, Y., Cao, F., Ding, S., Wu, T., & Xu, J. (2022). Effectiveness of an online application of the health action process approach (HAPA) theory on oral hygiene intervention in young adults with fixed orthodontic appliances: A randomized controlled trial. *BMC Oral Health*, *22*(1), 192. DOI: 10.1186/s12903-022-02219-w PMID: 35590291

Wyper, G. M. A. (2024). The global burden of disease study and population health metrics. *Population Health Metrics*, *22*(1), 35. DOI: 10.1186/s12963-024-00357-7 PMID: 39673070

Xie, H., Qin, Z., Ling, Z., Ge, X., Zhang, H., Guo, S., Liu, L., Zheng, K., Jiang, H., & Xu, R. (2023). Oral pathogen aggravates atherosclerosis by inducing smooth muscle cell apoptosis and repressing macrophage efferocytosis. *International Journal of Oral Science*, *15*(1), 26. DOI: 10.1038/s41368-023-00232-5 PMID: 37380627

Xue, T., Chen, L., & Sun, Q. (2024). Deep learning method to automatically diagnose periodontal bone loss and periodontitis stage in dental panoramic radiograph. *Journal of Dentistry*, *150*, 105373. DOI: 10.1016/j.jdent.2024.105373 PMID: 39332519

Yactayo-Alburquerque, M. T., Alen-Méndez, M. L., Azañedo, D., Comandé, D., & Hernández-Vásquez, A. (2021). Impact of oral diseases on oral health-related quality of life: A systematic review of studies conducted in Latin America and the Caribbean. *PLoS One*, *16*(6), e0252578. DOI: 10.1371/journal.pone.0252578 PMID: 34077473

Yang, D. W., Wang, T. M., Zhang, J. B., Li, X. Z., He, Y. Q., Xiao, R., Xue, W. Q., Zheng, X. H., Zhang, P. F., Zhang, S. D., Hu, Y.-Z., Shen, G.-P., Chen, M., Sun, Y., & Jia, W.-H. (2020). Genome-wide association study identifies genetic susceptibility loci and pathways of radiation-induced acute oral mucositis. *Journal of Translational Medicine*, *18*(1), 224. DOI: 10.1186/s12967-020-02390-0 PMID: 32503578

Yang, G., Feng, D., Li, F., Luo, B., Zhu, J., Yang, Q., Zheng, L., Dong, Q., Chen, M., Xu, Z., Li, L., Chen, P., & Sun, J. (2021). A randomized controlled phase II trial of maxillofacial and oral massage in attenuating severe radiotherapy-induced oral mucositis and lipid metabolite changes in nasopharyngeal carcinoma. *Radiotherapy and Oncology : Journal of the European Society for Therapeutic Radiology and Oncology*, *163*, 76–82. DOI: 10.1016/j.radonc.2021.07.024 PMID: 34343545

Yan, Y., Mao, M., Li, Y. Q., Chen, Y. J., Yu, H. D., Xie, W. Z., Huang, Q., Leng, W. D., & Xiong, J. (2022). Periodontitis Is Associated With Heart Failure: A Population-Based Study (NHANES III). *Frontiers in Physiology*, *13*, 854606. DOI: 10.3389/fphys.2022.854606 PMID: 35514329

Yarlagadda, S. K., Samavati, N., Ghorbanifarajzadeh, M., Levinta, V., Sojoudi, A., Inam, W., & Dolan, T. A. (2025). Development and validation of an AI-enabled oral score using large-scale dental data. *Scientific Reports*, *15*(1), 20398. DOI: 10.1038/s41598-025-07484-7 PMID: 40593131

Yaya, S., & Ghose, B. (2019). Global Inequality in Maternal Health Care Service Utilization: Implications for Sustainable Development Goals. *Health Equity*, *3*(1), 145–154. DOI: 10.1089/heq.2018.0082 PMID: 31289773

Yekani, M., Dastgir, M., Fattahi, S., Shahi, S., Maleki Dizaj, S., & Memar, M. Y. (2025). Microbiological and molecular aspects of periodontitis pathogenesis: An infection-induced inflammatory condition. *Frontiers in Cellular and Infection Microbiology*, *15*, 1533658. DOI: 10.3389/fcimb.2025.1533658 PMID: 40406516

Yeslam, H. E., Freifrau von Maltzahn, N., & Nassar, H. M. (2024). Revolutionizing CAD/CAM-based restorative dental processes and materials with artificial intelligence: A concise narrative review. *PeerJ*, *12*, e17793. DOI: 10.7717/peerj.17793 PMID: 39040936

Yuan, M., Lin, H., Wu, H., Yu, M., Tu, J., & Lü, Y. (2021). Community engagement in public health: A bibliometric mapping of global research. *Archives of Public Health = Archives Belges de Santé Publique*, *79*(1), 6. DOI: 10.1186/s13690-021-00525-3 PMID: 33436063

Yu, L., & Zhai, X. (2024). Use of artificial intelligence to address health disparities in low- and middle-income countries: A thematic analysis of ethical issues. *Public Health*, *234*, 77–83. DOI: 10.1016/j.puhe.2024.05.029 PMID: 38964129

Yu, S., Huang, S., Song, S., Lin, J., & Liu, F. (2024). Impact of oral health literacy on oral health behaviors and outcomes among the older adults: A scoping review. *BMC Geriatrics*, *24*(1), 858. DOI: 10.1186/s12877-024-05469-1 PMID: 39438807

Zaas, A. K., Aziz, H., Lucas, J., Perfect, J. R., & Ginsburg, G. S. (2010). Blood gene expression signatures predict invasive candidiasis. *Science Translational Medicine*, *2*(21), 21ra17. DOI: 10.1126/scitranslmed.3000715 PMID: 20374997

Zavala-Medina, L. C., Salas-Leiva, J. S., Villegas-Mercado, C. E., Arreguín-Cano, J. A., Soto-Barreras, U., Santana-Delgado, S. A., Larrinua-Pacheco, A. D., García-Vega, M. F., & Bermúdez, M. (2026). Oral Dysbiosis and Neuroinflammation: Implications for Alzheimer's, Parkinson's and Mood Disorders. *Microorganisms*, *14*(1), 143. DOI: 10.3390/microorganisms14010143 PMID: 41597661

Zhang, A., Sun, H., & Wang, X. (2012). Metabolomics in biomarker discovery. *Mass Spectrometry Reviews*, *31*(2), 270–298.

Zhang, Q., Zhang, R., Xiong, Y., Sui, Y., Tong, C., & Lin, F. H. (2025). Generative AI Mental Health Chatbots as Therapeutic Tools: Systematic Review and Meta-Analysis of Their Role in Reducing Mental Health Issues. *Journal of Medical Internet Research*, *27*, e78238. DOI: 10.2196/78238 PMID: 41401240

Zhang, X., Wang, X., Wu, J., Wang, M., Hu, B., Qu, H., Zhang, J., & Li, Q. (2024). The global burden of periodontal diseases in 204 countries and territories from 1990 to 2019. *Oral Diseases*, *30*(2), 754–768. DOI: 10.1111/odi.14436 PMID: 36367304

Zhang, Z., Dou, Z., Zhang, X., Wang, D., Abudoureheman, K., Yan, Y., Kang, F., Zhang, W., Meng, W., Zhang, K., Li, Z., Zhang, J., Liu, B., & Zhang, B. (2025). Development and validation of a novel public prediction platform for deciduous caries in preschool children: An observational study from Northwest China. *BMC Pediatrics*, *25*(1), 600. DOI: 10.1186/s12887-025-05763-w PMID: 40764955

Zhao, X., Liu, L., Zhao, P., Jiang, W., & Nahata, M. (2024). The Global Burden and Trends of Mental Disorders and Substance Use Disorders Among Adolescents and Young Adults: Findings from the Global Burden of Disease Study 1990–2021. *Available at SSRN* 4957498. DOI: 10.2139/ssrn.4957498

Zhou, B., Yang, G., Shi, Z., & Ma, S. (2024). Natural Language Processing for Smart Healthcare. *IEEE Reviews in Biomedical Engineering*, *17*, 4–18. DOI: 10.1109/RBME.2022.3210270 PMID: 36170385

Zhou, T., Xu, W., Wang, Q., Jiang, C., Li, H., Chao, Y., Sun, Y., & A, L. (2023). The effect of the "oral–gut" axis on periodontitis in inflammatory bowel disease: A review of microbe and immune mechanism associations. *Frontiers in Cellular and Infection Microbiology*, *13*, 1132420. DOI: 10.3389/fcimb.2023.1132420 PMID: 36923589

Zhuang, T., & Liu, B. (2022). Sustaining Higher Education Quality by Building an Educational Innovation Ecosystem in China—Policies, Implementations and Effects. *Sustainability (Basel)*, *14*(13), 7568. DOI: 10.3390/su14137568

Zhu, J. (2021). Artificial intelligence in the diagnosis of dental diseases on panoramic radiographs: A preliminary study. *BMC Oral Health, 21*, 158. DOI: 10.1186/s12903-021-01592-6 PMID: 37270488

Zhu, N., Bian, J., Dong, Z., & Zhu, N. (2025). An empirical study on the psychological impact of medical AI on patients undergoing dental surgery. *Scientific Reports, 16*(1), 401. DOI: 10.1038/s41598-025-29754-0 PMID: 41339456

Zhu, S., Gilbert, M., Chetty, I., & Siddiqui, F. (2022). The 2021 landscape of FDA-approved artificial intelligence/machine learning-enabled medical devices: An analysis of the characteristics and intended use. *International Journal of Medical Informatics, 165*, 104828. DOI: 10.1016/j.ijmedinf.2022.104828 PMID: 35780651

Zimmerman, B., Tsoi, S., Khosrowpour, B., & Ghazali, M. (2022). The state of dental electronic health records and opportunities for FHIR integration. *Journal of the American Medical Informatics Association : JAMIA, 29*(4), 703–710. DOI: 10.1093/jamia/ocab282

Zolfaghari, M., Shirmohammadi, M., Shahhosseini, H., Mokhtaran, M., & Mohebbi, S. (2021). Development and evaluation of a gamified smart phone mobile health application for oral health promotion in early childhood: A randomized controlled trial. *BMC Oral Health, 21*(1), 18. DOI: 10.1186/s12903-020-01374-2 PMID: 33413304

Zuckerman, M. K., Harper, K. N., Barrett, R., & Armelagos, G. J. (2014). The evolution of disease: Anthropological perspectives on epidemiologic transitions. *Global Health Action, 7*(1), 23303. DOI: 10.3402/gha.v7.23303 PMID: 24848652

Zwarenstein, M., Treweek, S., Gagnier, J. J., Altman, D. G., Tunis, S., Haynes, B., Oxman, A. D., & Moher, D.CONSORT group. (2008). Improving the reporting of pragmatic trials: An extension of the CONSORT statement. *BMJ (Clinical Research Ed.), 337*(nov11 2), a2390. DOI: 10.1136/bmj.a2390 PMID: 19001484

About the Contributors

Muhammad Farooq Umer is a public health specialist and epidemiologist with over 18 years of progressive experience spanning clinical dentistry, field public health, international research, and higher education leadership. Registered as Consultant in Public Health with the Saudi Commission for Health Specialties, holds a PhD in Epidemiology and Health Statistics, and is a Senior Fellow of the Higher Education Academy (SFHEA) and Fellow of the Royal Society of Public Health (FRSPH). Currently serving as Assistant Professor of Dental Public Health at the College of Dentistry, King Faisal University, Al-Ahsa, Saudi Arabia, combining an active research programme with recognised excellence in teaching, curriculum leadership, and postgraduate supervision. Academic Editor for PLOS ONE and Approved PhD supervisor under the Higher Education Commission of Pakistan, Lincoln University College Malaysia, and Shaheed Zulfiqar Ali Bhutto Medical University Pakistan.

***

Muhammad Adeel Ahmed is an Associate Professor of Restorative Dentistry at King Faisal University, Saudi Arabia. He holds multiple qualifications including PhD, FCPS, and CHPE, reflecting his strong academic and clinical expertise. His research interests focus on restorative dentistry, endodontics, and dental materials, with a notable publication record. Dr. Ahmed has contributed to high-impact studies in areas such as dental anxiety, COVID-19 practice adaptations, and esthetic dentistry. Alongside his research, he is actively engaged in teaching, academic leadership, and mentoring dental students and professionals.

Syed Fauzan Ali serves as Manager Innovation and Commercialization and Assistant Dean of the Faculty of Health Management Sciences at Baqai Medical University. With extensive corporate and academic expertise, he drives strategic growth, fosters industry-academia partnerships, and mentors professionals. An active researcher and APA affiliate, he excels in leadership, innovation, and multidisciplinary collaboration.

Muhammad Arshed, MBBS, MPH, PhD (Public Health) is an Assistant Professor in the Department of Community Medicine and Director of the Master of Public Health (MPH) Program at Baqai Medical University, Karachi, Pakistan. He earned his PhD in Public Health from Universiti Putra Malaysia. His research focuses on epidemiology, implementation science, digital health, chronic disease prevention, medication adherence, oral health, and health systems research. He has led several randomized controlled trials and implementation studies evaluating scalable, theory-informed interventions in low- and middle-income countries. Dr. Arshed has published extensively in international peer-reviewed journals and serves as a reviewer for several leading scientific journals. He supervises postgraduate research and is actively involved in developing evidence-based interventions and implementation frameworks that translate research into policy and practice. His current work emphasizes behavioral interventions, implementation effectiveness, health equity, and economic evaluation to strengthen healthcare systems and improve population health.

Waseela Ashraf (PhD Epidemiology, MSc Data Science and Machine Learning) is an emerging interdisciplinary researcher specializing in the integration of epidemiology with advanced data science techniques. Her work focuses on leveraging machine learning, big data analytics, and statistical modeling to address complex public health challenges. She has expertise in predictive modeling, disease surveillance, and data-driven decision-making for health systems. Dr. Ashraf is actively engaged in research that bridges traditional epidemiological methods with modern computational approaches, contributing to innovative solutions for population health improvement, digital health, and precision public health.

Muralidhar L B is a professionally qualified dental surgeon. He holds Ph.D. from Canara Bank School of Management Studies, Bangalore University after his MBA from Christ University. He has 18 years of total teaching experience spanning across dental education, healthcare management and general management and 4 years of corporate experience. He has worked as research associate in Institute for Social and Economic Change, Bangalore in a project entitled as "Management By and For Common Man: An Exploration of the Concept and Direction for Future"post Ph.D. He had secured 28th rank in S.S.L.C (10th Standard) examination for Karnataka State in 1993. His 31 patents have been published and 2 design patents have been granted. He has 41 research publications to his credit out of which 36 are Scopus-indexed and 5 are ABDC indexed. He has co-authored 13 books. He is currently working as Assistant Professor (Grade-3) in Department of Business Management Studies, School of Commerce, Jain Deemed to be University, Bangalore.

Awais Farid, (MBBS, MPH, PhD) is a physician, public health researcher, and health systems leader currently serving as Director of Health and Wellbeing. He formerly held the position of Associate Professor at James Cook University, Australia. He earned his PhD from the Hong Kong University of Science and Technology (HKUST) and has extensive experience as a clinical research scientist, leading multidisciplinary research across public health, implementation science, infectious disease control, and healthcare innovation. Dr. Farid has collaborated with international academic institutions, healthcare organizations, and government agencies, contributing to research, policy, and evidence-based practice. His scholarly interests include psychodental health, health equity, implementation science, infection prevention, and digital health technologies. He has published widely in peer-reviewed journals and contributed to several international book chapters.

Mohamad Syahrizal Halim is a dental academic at the School of Dental Sciences, Universiti Sains Malaysia. He specializes in conservative dentistry, endodontics, aesthetic dentistry, and dental implantology. Dr. Halim has a strong research portfolio, with impactful publications in artificial intelligence applications, teledentistry, and clinical endodontics. His work includes systematic reviews and clinical studies contributing to modern digital and evidence-based dentistry. In addition to research, he is actively involved in teaching, supervision, and advancing dental education at both undergraduate and postgraduate levels.

Rizwan Jouhar is a dental academic and researcher affiliated with the College of Dentistry at King Faisal University, Saudi Arabia. He specializes in restorative dentistry and endodontics, with a strong focus on clinical innovation and biomaterials research. Dr. Jouhar has an extensive publication record with significant citation impact, contributing to global dental research literature. His work spans topics such as COVID-19-related dental practices, tooth shade selection, and advanced restorative techniques. In addition to research, he is actively involved in teaching, curriculum development, and mentoring dental students at undergraduate and postgraduate levels.

Slesha is a dedicated dental professional with a strong commitment to advancing oral health through clinical excellence, research, innovation, and healthcare management. With a patient-centric approach at the core of her practice, she focuses on delivering quality care while promoting preventive and community-oriented oral healthcare. She has contributed to the scientific community through multiple research articles, scholarly publications, and patents, reflecting her passion for innovation and evidence-based practice. Her professional interests span dentistry, public health, healthcare management, healthcare innovation, and interdisciplinary research. Driven by a commitment to continuous learning and professional growth, Dr. Slesha strives to integrate clinical expertise, research, and healthcare management principles to enhance patient outcomes, strengthen healthcare systems, and contribute meaningfully to the advancement of healthcare delivery.

Rajashree K. C is a Biomedical Engineer with a Master's in Business Administration from Saveetha University, specializing in Hospital Management and Marketing, and holds a Ph.D. in Healthcare Management. An energetic and enthusiastic professor, she excels in academics and as a multitasker, organizing seminars, workshops, cultural programs, and other extra-curricular activities. She serves as the Coordinator of NSS Unit of Saveetha School of Management, leading them to achieve multiple accolades including the Best Club award. A prominent researcher with publications in Web of Science, Scopus, and UGC-listed journals, she actively enhances her expertise through conferences, workshops, MOOCs, and certifications, including Quality Coordination in Hospitals. Awarded the "Young Academician Award" and "Young Teacher Award," she is passionate about innovation, student skill development, and inspiring young minds through exemplary teaching and mentorship.

Amany Osama Kassem is a Lecturer in Dental Public Health at Riyadh Elm University, Saudi Arabia. She holds a Master's degree in Dental Public Health from King Faisal University. Her research interests include oral epidemiology, preventive dentistry, and the application of public health approaches in oral healthcare. She has contributed to research on oral hygiene practices and the role of healthcare providers in improving oral health outcomes.

Abdul Kabeer Kazi (PhD) is the Dean of the Baqai Institute of Health Sciences, Karachi, and a distinguished public health academic with extensive research and leadership experience. He has made significant contributions to health systems strengthening, epidemiology, and community-based research, with a strong focus on improving population health outcomes in low- and middle-income settings. With a vast academic career, he has supervised numerous postgraduate students and contributed to impactful publications. His leadership at Baqai has fostered academic excellence, research innovation, and capacity building, positioning the institute as a leading center for public health education and research in Pakistan.

Mehwish Kiran is a medical doctor (MBBS) currently pursuing her Master's in Public Health (MPH). She is an active public health researcher with a growing portfolio, including around five peer-reviewed publications in prestigious Q1 journals. Passionate about improving health outcomes, she is involved in various health projects addressing critical public health issues. Dr. Kiran is committed to advancing evidence-based solutions in health systems and community well-being.

Pardeep Kumar Assistant Professor, Department of Mathematics, Lovely Professional University, Phagwara, Punjab, India Dr. Pardeep Kumar holds a Ph.D. in Mathematics from Lovely Professional University (2021). His research expertise lies in Stochastic Processes, with a specialized focus on Markov Models, Engineering System Reliability, and Reliability Theory. He actively contributes to the modeling and reliability analysis of IoT-enabled and sensor-integrated systems for next-generation engineering applications. Dr. Kumar has a profound command of Stochastic Modelling, Reliability Testing, and advanced analytical methods for complex system behavior under uncertainty. His work emphasises practical implementations in smart technologies and cyber-physical systems. He has an exceptional academic track record, having qualified the prestigious CSIR-UGC NET twice, securing All India Ranks (AIR) of 15 and 32, respectively. To date, Dr. Kumar has published 26 high-quality research papers in reputed national and international journals, reflecting his continued contribution to the advancement of mathematical reliability and its engineering applications.

Sanjeev Kumar Is a Professor in Lovely Professional University Punjab India. He received Undergraduate in Hotel Management from Osmania University, Postgraduate in Tourism Management from Madurai Kamaraj University. He completed Doctor of Philosophy in Hospitality Management in 2019 from Amity University Jaipur India. His research areas lies in food Service Industry, his research focuses on Alcoholic beverages, Event management and Sustainable Management Practices, Metaverse, AI Machine Learning and Artificial Intelligence. He published more than 80 research papers, articles and chapters in Scopus Indexed, UGC Approved and peer reviewed Journals and books. Dr. Sanjeev Kumar participated and acted as resource person in various National and International conferences, seminars, session chair, research workshops and industry talks and his work has been widely cited. Dr. Sanjeev also edited more than 20 books with various International Publishers such as IGI Global, Cambridge Scholars, Emerald, CABI, Bentham Science, Taylor & Francis. Dr Sanjeev is an active researcher and has published numerous research articles in prestigious National and International journals and books.

Aidalina Mahmud (MBChB, MPH, PhD) is an Associate Professor in the Department of Community Health at the Faculty of Medicine and Health Sciences,

Universiti Putra Malaysia (UPM). With over 15 years of experience in academia and research, she has established herself as a prominent scholar in the field of public health. Dr. Mahmud has an extensive publication record, with more than 60 peer-reviewed articles contributing to the advancement of population health, health systems, and evidence-based policy. Her research expertise spans mixed-methods research, randomized controlled trials (RCTs), and the development and application of surveillance models and frameworks for public health improvement. Her work focuses on strengthening health systems through innovative research designs, integrating quantitative and qualitative approaches to generate robust, policy-relevant evidence. She has been actively involved in designing and evaluating public health interventions, particularly those aimed at improving disease surveillance, health service delivery, and community health outcomes. In addition to her research contributions, Dr. Mahmud is deeply engaged in academic leadership, teaching, and mentorship, guiding undergraduate and postgraduate students in public health research. Her commitment to capacity building and methodological rigor has positioned her as a respected expert in advancing public health development at both national and international levels.

Sakhaudiin Ahmed Mohamud is a medical doctor, public health consultant and director of research at Wellshare International in United States.

Fayez Hussain Niazi is a dental academic affiliated with Dar Al Uloom University, Saudi Arabia. His research interests span general dentistry, oral health, and preventive dental care. Dr. Niazi has contributed to impactful studies on maternal oral health, miswak use, and root canal morphology. His work also explores interdisciplinary areas such as salivary biomarkers and systemic health links. In addition to research, he is involved in teaching and promoting evidence-based dental practices.

Praveen KumarP holds an MCom, MBA, and PhD in Finance from Pondicherry University. He secured the University 1st Rank in his Under Graduation. His teaching interests include Financial Accounting, Financial Management, Mergers & Acquisitions, Security Analysis & Portfolio Management, and other finance-related courses. His research interests extend to interdisciplinary areas.

P. Saranraj holds a Ph.D. in Microbiology from Annamalai University, Chidambaram, India, and is NET (ASRB–ICAR) qualified in Microbiology. He is currently serving as Assistant Professor and Head, Department of Microbiology, at Sacred Heart College (Autonomous), Tirupattur, Tamil Nadu, India. In addition, he is the Proprietor and Managing Director of JPS Scientific Publications, contributing actively to academic publishing and research dissemination. Dr. Saranraj has over

15 years of research experience and 10 years of teaching experience in the fields of Environmental Microbiology, Agricultural Microbiology, Industrial Microbiology, Bioremediation, Microbial Biotechnology, and Sustainable Ecosystem Management. His research work has focused on Microbial degradation of pollutants, Effluent treatment, Soil health improvement, Plant–microbe interactions, and Applied environmental sustainability. He has an extensive publication record, with more than 240 international research articles, over 90 books (international and national), and 70+ book chapters published with reputed academic publishers.

S. Kanshiya, PG and Research Department of Microbiology, Sacred Heart College (Autonomous), Tirupattur, Tamil Nadu, India

T. Elavarasi, PG and Research Department of Microbiology, Sacred Heart College (Autonomous), Tirupattur, Tamil Nadu, India

Fahim Vohra is a Professor of Prosthodontics with extensive academic and clinical experience in dental sciences. He holds multiple prestigious qualifications, including PhD and memberships from the Royal Colleges in Edinburgh and Glasgow. His research interests include prosthodontics, implant dentistry, restorative dentistry, and dental education. Dr. Vohra has a highly impactful publication record with significant citations, particularly in COVID-19-related healthcare research and dental materials. Alongside his research, he plays a key role in academic leadership, teaching, and advancing dental education at an international level.

Shumaila Zofeen is affiliated with the School of Public Health at Xi'an Jiaotong University, China. She holds a Bachelor of Dental Surgery (BDS), a Certificate in Health Professions Education (CHPE), and a Master's degree in Epidemiology and Health Statistics. Her research interests include epidemiology, public health, and the application of statistical methods in health research.

Index

A

B

C

D

E

G

H

I

M

R

S

www.ingramcontent.com/pod-product-compliance
Lightning Source LLC
LaVergne TN
LVHW061526290926
849162LV00004B/676
* 9 7 9 8 3 3 7 3 8 4 0 2 3 *